Guidelines for Perinatal Care

Fourth Edition

American Academy of Pediatrics

The American College of Obstetricians and Gynecologists

Supported in part by

March of Dimes
BIRTH DEFECTS FOUNDATION

Guidelines for Perinatal Care was developed through the cooperative efforts of the American Academy of Pediatrics (AAP) Committee on Fetus and Newborn and the American College of Obstetricians and Gynecologists (ACOG) Committee on Obstetric Practice. The guidelines should not be viewed as a body of rigid rules. They are general and intended to be adapted to many different situations, taking into account the needs and resources particular to the locality, the institution, or type of practice. Variations and innovations that improve the quality of patient care are to be encouraged rather than restricted. The purpose of these guidelines will be well served if they provide a firm basis on which local norms may be built.

Library of Congress Cataloging-in-Publication Data

American Academy of Pediatrics.
    Guidelines for perinatal care / American Academy of Pediatrics [and] American College of Obstetricians and Gynecologists. — 4th ed.
      p.   cm.
    "Developed through the cooperative efforts of the American Academy of Pediatrics (AAP) Committee on Fetus and Newborn and the American College of Obstetricians and Gynecologists (ACOG) Committee on Obstetric Practice"— T.p. verso.
    Rev. ed. of: Guidelines for perinatal care. 3rd ed. c1992.
    Includes bibliographical references and index.
    ISBN 0-915473-35-6: $60.00
    1. Perinatology—Standards. I. American College of Obstetricians and Gynecologists. II. American Academy of Pediatrics. Committee on Fetus and Newborn. III. American College of Obstetricians and Gynecologists. Committee on Obstetric Practice. IV. Guidelines for perinatal care. V. Title. VI. Title: Perinatal care.
    [DNLM: 1. Perinatology—standards. WQ 210 A512g 1997]
    RG600.A45 1997
    618.3'2—DC21
    DNLM/DLC
    for Library of Congress   97-19319
                                                                CIP

ISBN 0-915473-35-6

Single copy price is $60 for nonmembers and $50 for ACOG/AAP members. Quantity prices available on request. Address all orders to AAP; inquiries regarding content may be directed to the respective organizations:

American Academy of Pediatrics
141 Northwest Point Boulevard
PO Box 927
Elk Grove Village, IL 60009-0927

American College of Obstetricians and Gynecologists
409 12th Street, SW
PO Box 96920
Washington, DC 20090-6920

Editorial Committee

Editors
John C. Hauth, MD, FACOG
Gerald B. Merenstein, MD, FAAP

Associate Editors
Sharon L. Dooley, MD, MPH, FACOG
Michael T. Mennuti, MD, FACOG
William Oh, MD, FAAP

Staff
ACOG
Stanley Zinberg, MD, MS, FACOG
Debra A. Hawks, MPH
Shirley A. Shelton
Rebecca D. Rinehart

AAP
Susan M. Tellez

ACOG Committee on Obstetric Practice

Members, 1996–1997
Larry C. Gilstrap III, MD (Chair)
David B. Cotton, MD
Michael F. Greene, MD
Gay P. Hall, CNM
Peter S. Heyl, MD
Iffath A. Hoskins, MD
Edward C. Maeder, Jr, MD
Sharon T. Phelan, MD

Liason Representatives
Joy L. Hawkins, MD
William Oh, MD

Members, 1995–1996
Michael T. Mennuti, MD (Chair)
Larry C. Gilstrap III, MD
Gay P. Hall, CNM
Peter S. Heyl, MD
Iffath A. Hoskins, MD
Edward C. Maeder, Jr, MD
James N. Martin, Jr, MD
Sharon T. Phelan, MD

Liason Representatives
Joy L. Hawkins, MD
William Oh, MD

Members, 1994–1995
Michael T. Mennuti, MD (Chair)
Vivian M. Dickerson, MD
Larry C. Gilstrap III, MD
Gay P. Hall, CNM
Peter S. Heyl, MD
Iffath A. Hoskins, MD
James N. Martin, Jr, MD
Sharon T. Phelan, MD

Liason Representatives
David H. Chestnut, MD
William Oh, MD

AAP Committee on Fetus and Newborn

Contents

Chapter 4
Antepartum Care *(continued)*

Chapter 5
Intrapartum Care   93

Chapter 6
Obstetric Complications   127

Chapter 6
Obstetric Complications *(continued)*

Chapter 7
Postpartum and Follow-Up Care   147

Preface

The fourth edition of *Guidelines for Perinatal Care* provides updated and expanded information from the preexisting edition as well as incorporates the philosophy of the March of Dimes Birth Defects Foundation *Toward Improving the Outcome of Pregnancy: The 90s and Beyond* (TIOP II). The American College of Obstetricians and Gynecologists (ACOG) and the American Academy of Pediatrics (AAP) led a call for action to develop TIOP II to respond to a changing environment and to make further recommendations for the regionalization of perinatal care in the 1990s and beyond. To update the vision for delivery of perinatal services, TIOP II focused on four key areas: (1) care before and during pregnancy; (2) care during birth and beyond; (3) data documentation and evaluation; and (4) financing.

Guidelines for Perinatal Care, Fourth Edition, embraces these concepts by encouraging all health care providers to use reproductive health screening to reduce risks, by outlining the capabilities and accountability of perinatal regional programs, and by emphasizing preconception care and ongoing antepartum risk assessment as standard components of care. *Guidelines* describes the roles of regions, institutions, and individuals in providing perinatal care. It defines levels of care in terms of facilities, equipment, and personnel, from both an obstetric and a pediatric standpoint. The integral parts of a regional program are delineated, along with what is expected of all members of such a program in an attempt to clarify and evaluate what constitutes quality health care.

Guidelines for Perinatal Care represents a cross-section of different disciplines within the perinatal community. It is designed for use by all personnel who are involved in the care of pregnant women, their fetuses, and their neonates in community programs, hospitals, and medical centers. An intermingling of information of all kinds in varying degrees of detail is provided to address their collective needs. The result is a unique resource that complements the educational documents listed in Appendix G, which provide more specific information. Readers are encouraged to refer to the appendix for related documents to supplement those listed at the end of each chapter. The fourth edition of the *Guidelines* has been reorganized to include a new chapter on obstetric complications. Antepartum care and intrapartum care as well as organization of perinatal services have been separated into respective chapters that focus on these important areas. New information has been added on substance use and domestic violence to encourage provider awareness and screening to address these problems of increasing concerns during pregnancy. The recommendations for prevention of early-onset group B streptococcus in the newborn, additional prenatal screening tests, prenatal folic acid intake, postpartum length of stay, prevention of respiratory syncytial virus in high-risk infants, and prenatal human immunodeficiency virus counseling and testing have been updated from the third edition. The new guidelines on isolation precautions by the Centers for Disease Control and Prevention have been incorporated. Revised recommendations combine the major features of universal precautions (now termed standard precautions) with transmission-based precautions for infection control in acute-care hospitals. Information on adolescent pregnancy and psychosocial services has been incorporated from ACOG's *Standards for Obstetric–Gynecologic Services*, which has been replaced by *Guidelines for Perinatal Care* and its companion volume, ACOG's *Guidelines for Women's Health Care*. Both AAP and ACOG will continue to update information presented here through policy statements and recommendations that both organizations issue periodically, particularly with regard to rapidly evolving technologies and areas of practice such as genetics (including cystic fibrosis) and treatment of human immunodeficiency virus.

The most current scientific information, professional opinions, and clinical practices have been assembled and received in the formulation of the information in this manual, which is intended to offer guidelines, not strict operating rules. Local circumstances must dictate the way in which these guidelines are best interpreted to meet the needs of a particular hospital, community, or system. For instance, the term *readily available*, used to designate acceptable levels of care, should be defined by each institution within the context of its resources and geographic location. Emphasis has been placed on identifying those areas to be covered by specific, locally defined protocols rather than on promoting rigid recommendations. The content of this newest edition of *Guidelines* has undergone careful review to ensure accuracy and consistency with the policies of both groups. The guidelines are not meant to be exhaustive, nor do they always agree with those of other organizations; however, they reflect the latest recommendations of AAP and ACOG in areas that are subject to constant updating. The text was written, revised, and reviewed by members of the AAP Committee on Fetus and Newborn and the ACOG Committee on Obstetrics, and consultants in a variety of specialized areas have contributed to the content. The pioneering efforts of those who developed the previous editions must also be acknowledged. To each and every one of them our sincere appreciation is extended.

Editorial Committee

Introduction

The 20th century has brought an unprecedented rate of change in approaches to improving maternal and infant health in the United States, resulting in a 95–99% reduction in both maternal and infant mortality since 1900. In 1913, the U.S. Children's Bureau began to study factors influencing infant mortality based on each topic's "fundamental social importance." The results of these early studies indicated that many pregnant women did not receive appropriate prenatal, birth, and postpartum services. Expanded public health services, new knowledge of the causes of maternal mortality, and increased use of hospital-based labor and delivery services led to improvements in pregnancy outcome during the first half of the century.

In the 1960s and 1970s, there was a focus on new technology and the delivery of inpatient care. A regional perinatal care structure emerged, reflecting increased interest in addressing the management of preterm birth and low-birth-weight babies. With the development of neonatal intensive care units, new professional roles were created. Out of local models, a national framework for the organization of perinatal care evolved. These interwoven trends were part of a broader effort to maximize the efficiency and cost-effectiveness of several new types of "intensive care" medicine. For maternal and infant health, they culminated in the concept of "regionalized perinatal care."

In the early 1970s, the March of Dimes Birth Defects Foundation assembled a multidisciplinary group of professionals representing all aspects of perinatal care. The group, called the Committee on Perinatal Health, developed the 1976 publication *Toward Improving the Outcome of Pregnancy*, in which a model system for regionalized perinatal care was proposed and three levels of inpatient hospital care defined. That approach, which focused primarily on inpatient levels of emergency neonatal care, has served newborns well for two decades. It fostered a continuation of improved perinatal outcome and survival for high-risk infants (Fig. I–1 and I–2), although the quality of long-term survival of these infants has not been significantly altered. Consistent with the goals of regional coordination, improved outcomes have been associated with risk identification, care in a setting appropriate for the level of risk, and transport when necessary. Specifically, premature (born at <37 weeks) and low-birth-weight (weighing <2,500 g at birth) infants born in subspecialty hospitals with neonatal care have better survival rates, even after controlling for interhospital differences in birth-weight distribution, race, gestational age, and multiple births. The greatest impact has been in reducing the mortality of very low-birth-weight neonates (weighing <1,500 g at birth).

Although the reported incidence of low birth weight and very low birth weight in the United States is higher than in at least a dozen other industrialized nations, the birth-weight-specific survival rates among infants in this country are among the best in the world. This phenomenon has been attributed to the technologically advanced care provided to newborns through regionalized inpatient services.

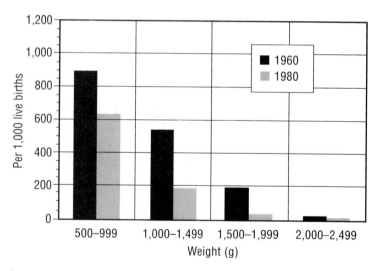

Fig. I–1. Neonatal mortality risk for low-birth-weight infants in the United States, 1960 and 1980. (Modified from March of Dimes Birth Defects Foundation, Committee on Perinatal Health. Toward improving the outcome of pregnancy: the 90s and beyond. White Plains, New York: March of Dimes Birth Defects Foundation, 1993.)

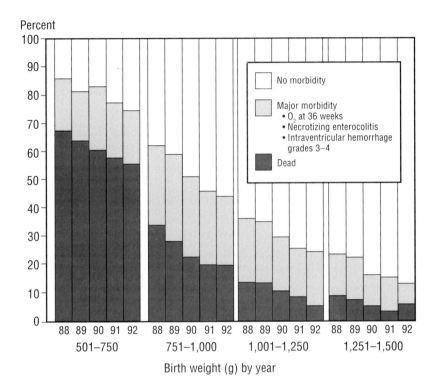

Fig. I–2. Birth weight, by year, 1988–1992. (Fanaroff AA, Wright LL, Stevenson DK, Shankaran S, Donovan EF, Ehrenkranz RA, et al. Very-low-birth-weight outcomes of the National Institute of Child Health and Human Development Neonatal Research Network, May 1991 through December 1992. Am J Obstet Gynecol 1995;173:1423–1431.)

In sharp contrast with the dramatic improvement in health care utilization and infant survival of the 1970s, progress slowed during the 1980s. The overall national rate of decline in infant mortality slowed from 4.7% per year during the 1970s to 2.8% per year from 1980 to 1988. Although gestational age-specific survival continues to improve, the incidence of low birth weight and the number of women receiving early prenatal care showed no improvement between 1979 and 1989. During the late 1980s and early 1990s, adolescent childbearing increased, and one third of births were to unmarried women.

In the 1990s, it became apparent that there was a need to refine and augment the levels of care designated in a regionalized system of care.

At the request of the American Academy of Pediatrics and the American College of Obstetricians and Gynecologists, a new Committee on Perinatal Health was assembled by the March of Dimes Birth Defects Foundation to respond to a changing environment and to make further recommendations for the regional coordination of perinatal care in the 1990s and beyond. Charged with updating the vision of content and organization developed by the original Committee on Perinatal Health, the group focused on what it considered to be four key areas: (1) care before and during pregnancy, (2) care during birth and beyond, (3) data documentation and evaluation, and (4) financing. The recommendations broadened the concept of regionalized services to address perinatal care from before conception through infancy, proposing practical strategies for implementation on a national basis. These recommendations are presented in *Toward Improving the Outcome of Pregnancy: The 90s and Beyond*, published in 1993, and some aspects of these recommendations have been incorporated into this edition of *Guidelines for Perinatal Care*. A guide to the functional organization of individual regional programs is described in *Toward Improving the Outcome of Pregnancy: The 90s and Beyond*, and it can be modified according to local needs and resources.

At the end of the 20th century, the technologic revolution of communication and information systems is being harnessed to improve not only the ability to provide comprehensive and state-of-the-art health care, but also to assess the outcomes of such efforts. Only with such reassessment and quality management can our health care systems continue to evolve so that they can be comprehensive, current, fiscally efficient, and responsible, yet sensitive to the particular needs of individual mothers and babies. It is encouraging to note that there is increasing use of single and multicenter trials to assess the efficacy and safety of therapeutic interventions in both maternal–fetal medicine and neonatology. Examples include evaluation of the safety of prenatal diagnostic techniques, antibiotics for preterm premature rupture of membranes, and surfactant therapy for newborn respiratory distress syndrome. Utilization of well-designed randomized clinical trials will improve the ability to provide the most appropriate care to mothers and their newborns.

Chapter 1

Organization of Perinatal Health Care

A regionally coordinated system focusing on levels of hospital-based perinatal care has been shown to be effective and to result in improved outcomes for both mothers and newborns. Such a system can be extended to encompass preconception evaluation and early pregnancy risk assessment in both an ambulatory and a hospital-based setting. The recommendations regarding regional perinatal care services in *Toward Improving the Outcome of Pregnancy: The 90s and Beyond,* from the Committee on Perinatal Health of the March of Dimes Birth Defects Foundation, have been incorporated in this chapter. These recommendations emphasize early recognition and triage of potential prenatal problems before or early in pregnancy. The functional capabilities of providers are defined on the basis of the level of care provided to address both inpatient maternal and neonatal needs.

At all levels of care, the health care system should foster an atmosphere of family-centered care. Women and their families should be encouraged to take an active role in their pregnancy care and to participate in the development and evaluation of perinatal care systems. Efforts should be undertaken to ensure access to care at all levels on a regional basis.

Clinical Components of Regionalized Perinatal Services

Ambulatory Prenatal Care

The overall goals for regional coordination of ambulatory prenatal care are to ensure appropriate care for all women, to better utilize available resources, and to improve the outcome of pregnancy. Prenatal care can be delivered more effectively and efficiently by defining the capabilities and expertise (basic, specialty, and subspecialty) of providers and ensuring that pregnant women receive risk-appropriate care (Table 1–1). Developments in maternal–fetal risk assessment and diagnosis, as well as interventions to change behavior, make early and continuous prenatal care more effective in improving pregnancy outcome.

The content and timing of prenatal care should vary according to the risk status of the mother and the fetus. Use of a standardized prenatal record (Appendix A) by public and private providers within a perinatal region helps to document risk assessment and intervention activities and facilitates communication in providing continuity of care.

Prenatal care may call upon the services of many kinds of providers, including the early involvement of pediatricians. The frequency and content of prenatal care should be risk responsive and should take into account the need for intervention.

Early and ongoing risk assessment should be an integral component of perinatal care. All providers of prenatal care should be able to identify a full range of medical and psychosocial risks and to refer patients for appropriate care throughout pregnancy. Early prenatal risk assessment facilitates development of a specific plan of care and referral and consultation among providers of basic, specialty, and subspecialty levels of prenatal care on the basis of the individual patient's circumstances and the expertise of the individual provider (Appendixes B and C).

The primary goals of early and ongoing risk assessment are to prevent or treat conditions associated with morbidity and mortality and to improve linkages to inpatient care through more effective

Table 1–1. Ambulatory Prenatal Care Provider Capabilities and Expertise

Level of Prenatal Care	Capabilities	Provider Types
Basic	Risk-oriented prenatal care record, physical examination and interpretation of findings, routine laboratory assessment, assessment of gestational age and normal progress of pregnancy, ongoing risk identification, mechanisms for consultation and referral, psychosocial support, childbirth education, and care coordination (including referral for ancillary services such as transportation, food, and housing assistance)	Obstetricians, family physicians, certified nurse–midwives, and other advanced-practice nurses with experience, training, and demonstrated competence
Specialty	Basic care plus fetal diagnostic testing (eg, biophysical tests, amniotic fluid analysis, basic ultrasound); expertise in management of medical and obstetric complications	Obstetricians
Subspecialty	Basic and specialty care plus advanced fetal diagnoses (eg, targeted ultrasound, fetal echocardiology); advanced fetal therapy (eg, intrauterine fetal transfusion and treatment of cardiac arrhythmias); medical, surgical, neonatal, and genetic consultation; and management of severe maternal complications	Maternal–fetal medicine specialists and reproductive geneticists with experience, training, and demonstrated competence

Modified from March of Dimes Birth Defects Foundation, Committee on Perinatal Health. Toward improving the outcome of pregnancy: the 90s and beyond. White Plains, New York: March of Dimes Birth Defects Foundation, 1993.

mechanisms for referral and consultation. Overall, early systematic risk assessment will accomplish the following:

- Better match of care to patients' needs
- More efficient use of resources
- Expeditious and appropriate transfers and referrals
- Reduced need for emergency transfer and referral

In-Hospital Perinatal Care

In 1976, the March of Dimes designated three levels of perinatal care—levels I, II, and III. Since then, financial and marketing pressures have encouraged some hospitals to raise their level designation for perinatal care services, primarily with regard to patient care activities. This tendency contrasts with the classic concept of regional coordination, in which tertiary or subspecialty care centers have the capability to provide complex patient care and to assume regional responsibilities for transport, outreach education, research, and quality control. Attempts to share responsibilities among hospitals have not been uniformly successful and have resulted in different levels of care for different services at a single hospital. The imbalance in the provision of services that have been traditionally delivered by a regional perinatal center (including patient care, research, and regional education programs) has resulted from a growing market of competitive health care and prepaid health plans. Another complicating factor is the uneven distribution of subspecialists in neonatal and maternal–fetal medicine throughout the United States. Rather than a numerical designation (ie, levels I, II, III), a functional descriptive designation of basic, specialty, and subspecialty is used.

Following are the responsibilities of in-hospital perinatal services, designated by basic, specialty, and subspecialty levels of care. The level of care is based on the individual needs of the mother and baby. Although they may require different levels of care, an effort should be made to keep them together to maintain the mother–infant dyad.

1. Basic care
   - Surveillance and care of all patients admitted to the obstetric service, with an established triage system for identifying high-risk patients who should be transferred to a facility that provides specialty or subspecialty care
   - Proper detection and supportive care of unanticipated maternal–fetal problems that occur during labor and delivery
   - Capability to begin an emergency cesarean delivery within 30 minutes of the decision to do so (see "Cesarean Delivery" in Chapter 5)
   - Availability of blood and fresh-frozen plasma for transfusion

- Availability of anesthesia, radiology, ultrasound, and laboratory services on a 24-hour basis
- Care of postpartum conditions
- Evaluation of the condition of healthy neonates and continuing care of these neonates until their discharge
- Resuscitation and stabilization of all neonates born in hospital
- Stabilization of small or ill neonates before transfer to a specialty or subspecialty care facility
- Consultation and transfer arrangements
- Nursery care
- Parent–sibling–neonate visitation
- Data collection and retrieval

Some basic care facilities may provide continuing care for neonates who have relatively minor problems that do not require advanced laboratory, radiologic, or pediatric consultation. Many basic care facilities provide care for convalescing babies who have been returned from specialty and subspecialty facilities.

2. Specialty care
   - Performance of basic care services as described above
   - Care of high-risk mothers and fetuses, both admitted and transferred from other facilities
   - Stabilization of ill newborns prior to transfer
   - Care of preterm infants with a birth weight of 1,500 g or more

Some specialty hospitals also have neonatal intensive care facilities. The needed subspecialty expertise is almost always neonatal medicine and not maternal–fetal medicine. Specialty care should be reserved for stable or moderately ill newborns who have problems that are expected to resolve rapidly. These situations usually occur as a result of preterm labor or preterm premature rupture of membranes at 32 weeks of gestation or later. Preterm labor and impending delivery at less than 32 weeks of gestation warrant maternal transfer to a subspecialty center. Other examples warranting maternal transfer might include intrauterine growth restriction with oligohydramnios, severe preeclampsia, placenta previa, or chorioamnionitis. Infants with birth weights of less than 1,500 g and born at less than 32 weeks of gestation should usually be transferred to a subspecialty center. Mothers with complex medical or surgical problems requiring early intervention should be transferred to a subspecialty center.

3. Subspecialty care
   - Provision of comprehensive perinatal care services for both admitted and transferred mothers and neonates of all risk categories, including basic and specialty care services as described above
   - Research and educational support
   - Analysis and evaluation of regional data, including those on complications
   - Initial evaluation of new high-risk technologies

The services needed at a subspecialty facility vary markedly from those at a specialty facility. At less than 32 weeks of gestation, subspecialty care usually requires expertise in neonatal and maternal–fetal medicine. Fetuses that may require immediate complex care should be delivered at a subspecialty care center. These fetuses include—but are not limited to—those with severe immune or nonimmune hydrops fetalis or fetal anomalies such as congenital heart disease, open neural tube defects, abdominal wall defects, or diaphragmatic hernias requiring pediatric specialty surgical capabilities to manage these conditions.

When subspecialty maternal care is needed, care of the neonate by basic or specialty neonatal services may be adequate. Instances in which maternal intensive care may be needed include—but are not limited to—severe maternal cardiac, endocrine, or pulmonary disease; severe pregnancy-associated hypertensive conditions; severe hemoglobinopathies; and active collagen vascular disease.

Maternal and Infant Postdischarge Care

Primary or basic perinatal care includes ambulatory care of mother and baby after discharge. Decreasing lengths of hospital stays have increased the importance of organization and coordination of care as well as the need for evaluation and monitoring of outcomes. Infant follow-up and early intervention services are important components of perinatal care, as is collection of data on long-term outcomes, which are essential to evaluate new interventions and technologies.

Comprehensive Care

The integration of clinical activities, on basic through subspecialty levels, in one geographic location provides comprehensive and immediate care for the population. When people needing reproductive health care are dispersed over a wide area, a carefully structured, well-organized system of services becomes necessary. Networks and other forms of vertically integrated systems can be structured to ensure that they provide all necessary services. These services include public and professional education, research, and outcome evaluations. The broad goals of a program should include reduction of perinatal mortality and morbidity and efficient use of resources.

Manpower: The Distribution and Supply of Perinatal Care Providers

The distribution and supply of physicians providing perinatal services has been changing. Although the number of physicians has increased substantially over the past 20 years, the percentage of all physicians who provide obstetric care has declined. Published data indicate that there appears to be a sufficient number of physician specialists in neonatal care at present. However, providers of perinatal care are unevenly distributed among geographic areas and types of facilities. A team approach to perinatal care is essential to improving the outcome of pregnancy. Certified nurse–midwives, physicians' assistants, advanced-practice nurses, perinatal social workers, and other professionals are also important providers of perinatal services.

Strategies should be aimed at increasing recruitment and retention of perinatal care providers, particularly in rural and urban medically underserved areas. More than 2,000 areas are designated as federal health professional shortage areas, and most of the people in need of services in these areas are women of childbearing age and young children. Rural communities are particularly likely to be medically underserved. The poorest urban areas often are underserved because of insufficient funding to support perinatal services. Supports and incentives should be developed to encourage qualified professionals to provide perinatal care in these underserved areas.

Examples of regional programs that have been successfully used to increase access to care include liability cost relief, locum tenens programs (with physicians to serve as backup or relief), satellite practice models, financial incentives to establish or maintain a practice, innovative approaches to continuing education, and programs to provide technical support. The National Health Service Corps and state scholarship and loan repayment programs for the education of health professionals, which include a special requirement for service in underserved areas, provide another important incentive. Such programs should give priority to perinatal providers and should be strengthened and adequately funded.

The Social Context for Perinatal Care

In recent years, a number of national reports have documented gaps in the organization and delivery of care. Strategies have been proposed for filling these gaps:

- Improving access to services
- Identifying risks early and providing linkages to appropriate care of women, children, and families
- Ensuring continuity and comprehensiveness of and compliance with care

A health care system that is responsive to the needs of women will help them to reduce their risk behaviors and gain access to appropriate health services. Structural and cultural barriers to appropriate health care should be eliminated. All counseling should be sensitive to cultural diversity, and a skilled translator should be sought for women and their families whose primary language is not that of the care providers.

Reproductive Awareness

Patient awareness of reproductive risks, health-enhancing behaviors, and family planning options are essential to improving the outcome of pregnancy. Reproductive awareness must be better integrated into the health care system and society at large. That less than half of pregnancies in the United States are planned suggests the need for a new approach to reproductive awareness. Because unintended pregnancies and reproductive health hazards—including the use of alcohol, tobacco, and other drugs—occur across all socioeconomic groups, the target group for reproductive awareness must include all women of childbearing age.

Every encounter with the health care system should be viewed as an opportunity to reinforce reproductive awareness in women of childbearing age. New reproductive awareness messages, and strategies to deliver them, should also be developed for men. Marketing techniques may be effective in changing attitudes and behaviors among both women and men. To implement this new strategy, health providers should ask one basic question when providing care for women: Is the patient in her reproductive years? If the answer is yes, a dialogue about reproductive awareness should take place. Reproductive health screening should be used by all health care professionals serving women in their reproductive years. A sample form that may be useful in facilitating appropriate selective reproductive health screening is shown in Table 1–2.

Family-Centered Care

The health care system should be oriented toward providing family-centered care, the underlying assumption of which is that the family is the primary source of support for anyone receiving health care services. Family-centered health care professionals engage parents as caregivers and partners and seek to ensure that every encounter builds on the family's strengths, preserves their dignity, and enhances their confidence and competence. These health care professionals strive to understand each family's priorities and needs, incorporating the family's perspectives into an individualized plan of care for each infant.

Table 1-2. Health Screening for Women of Reproductive Age

Selective Reproductive Health Screening (Menarche to Menopause)	Done	Referred
Reproductive awareness		
Pregnancy prevention counseling	☐	☐
Preconception and nutrition counseling	☐	☐
Medical diseases (counsel regarding effects on future pregnancies)		
Diabetes mellitus	☐	☐
Hypertension	☐	☐
Epilepsy	☐	☐
Other chronic illness	☐	☐
Infectious diseases (counsel, test, or refer)		
Sexually transmissible infections, including human immunodeficiency virus	☐	☐
Hepatitis B (immunize if at high risk)	☐	☐
Rubella (test; if nonimmune, immunize)	☐	☐
Teratogens/genetics (counsel regarding effects on future pregnancies)		
Hemoglobinopathy	☐	☐
Medication and vitamin use (eg, isotretinoin/vitamin A [retinoic acid])	☐	☐
Self or prior child with congenital defect	☐	☐
Family history of genetic disease	☐	☐
Environmental exposure at home or in workplace	☐	☐
Behavior (counsel regarding effects on future pregnancies)		
Alcohol use	☐	☐
Tobacco use	☐	☐
Use of illicit substances (eg, cocaine, crack)	☐	☐
Social support		
Safety (eg, domestic violence)	☐	☐
Personal resources (eg, transportation, housing)	☐	☐

Modified from March of Dimes Birth Defects Foundation, Committee on Perinatal Health. Toward improving the outcome of pregnancy: the 90s and beyond. White Plains, New York: March of Dimes Birth Defects Foundation, 1993.

Such an approach offers families real choices and respects the decisions they make for themselves and their children.

In family-centered perinatal services, women and their families are involved in all aspects of planning, delivering, and evaluating health care services. This approach creates a climate in which decisions at all levels throughout the perinatal program and hospital are based not only on the expertise and assumptions of health care professionals, but also on the needs, values, and strengths of the newborns and their families. Focus groups and surveys can provide information about personal and system barriers to the use of appropriate care.

Hospital and program leaders should communicate the concepts of family-centered care consistently and clearly to staff, students, families, and communities through vision, mission, and philosophy statements. This includes respecting the choices, values, and cultural backgrounds of expectant and new mothers and other family members; communicating honestly and openly; realizing opportunities for mutual support and information sharing; and collaborating in the development and evaluation of services.

Family-centered practices can help expectant and new parents become nurturing caregivers. Efforts should be made throughout the newborn period to minimize separation of infants and families. Staff interactions and unit policies should consistently reinforce the importance of mothers, fathers, and other family members to the health and well-being of their infants. Families' strengths and capabilities should be built upon in order to further their competence and confidence in their caregiving abilities. A patient's sense of personal responsibility and identity is important for the optimum outcome of pregnancy and family life.

Data Collection and Documentation

To improve patient outcomes, an organization must be able to track patients and have some indicators or measures of success. Significant progress has been made in methods for gathering vital statistics (eg, matched birth and death certificates) and in collecting data (eg, prenatal records). The concept of key indicators has been used to signal inadequate access to perinatal care and to predict or measure poor pregnancy outcome. For example, rates of unintended pregnancy, prenatal care utilization, and infant mortality are used to measure access and outcome at three different points along the continuum of perinatal health. These indicators serve as a baseline against which future progress may be measured. However, perinatal medicine has yet to benefit fully from information systems. Better data management is required to derive a benefit from evaluative clinical sciences.

Accountability

Accountability for actions is a fundamental principle of perinatal care, as well as a valuable attribute of professional practice that benefits all patients. However, accountability is often solely associated with individual patient care. The principle of accountability must also include perinatal program efforts such as planning and education so that the patient population can be assured of access to quality care.

Women should participate in the development and evaluation of perinatal care systems. Focus groups or surveys are two methods used to collect the views of women. These methods can provide information about both personal and systems barriers to the use of appropriate care.

Bibliography

Brown S, ed, Institute of Medicine. Including children and pregnant women in health care reform. Washington, DC: National Academy Press, 1992

Committee on Perinatal Health. Toward improving the outcome of pregnancy: recommendations for the regional development of maternal and perinatal health services. White Plains, New York: National March of Dimes Birth Defects Foundation, 1976

Committee on Perinatal Health. Toward improving the outcome of pregnancy: the 90s and beyond. White Plains, New York: March of Dimes Birth Defects Foundation, 1993

Congressional Budget Office. Factors contributing to the infant mortality ranking of the United States. Washington, DC: Congressional Budget Office, 1992

Makuc DM, Haglund B, Ingram DD, Kleinman JC, Feldman JJ. Health service areas for the United States. Vital and Health Statistics. Series 2. Data evaluation and methods research; vol. 112. Hyattsville, Maryland: National Center for Health Statistics, 1991

Public Health Service. Caring for our future: the content of prenatal care. Washington, DC: Department of Health and Human Services, 1989

Chapter 2

Inpatient Perinatal Care Services

This chapter outlines recommendations regarding medical expertise, nursing ratios, staffing guidelines, support services, perinatal outreach education, and physical facilities required for providing hospital-based perinatal care. These components have been defined for facilities providing basic, specialty, and subspecialty care.

Personnel

Factors critical to planning and evaluating the quality and level of personnel required to meet patients' needs in perinatal settings include the mission, geographic location, and design of the facility; patient population; scope of practice; qualifications of staff; and obligations for education or research. Perinatal care programs at basic, specialty, and subspecialty hospitals should be coordinated jointly by medical and nursing directors for obstetric and pediatric services.

Medical Providers

Individuals are granted privileges to practice by an institution's governing body by virtue of their qualifications. A hospital is responsible for granting privileges and verifying the applicant's credentials from the primary source. The credentials required and the privileges extended vary according to the level of care provided.

Basic Care Facility

The perinatal care program at a hospital providing basic care should be coordinated jointly by the chiefs of the obstetric, pediatrics, nursing, and midwifery services. This administrative approach requires close coordination and unified policy statements. The coordinators of perinatal care at a basic care hospital are responsible for developing policy, maintaining standards of care, and collaborating and consulting with professional staff of hospitals providing specialty and subspecialty care in the region. In hospitals that do not separate these services, one person may be given the responsibility for coordinating perinatal care.

A qualified physician or certified nurse–midwife should attend all deliveries. Collaborative practice involving a multidisciplinary team is encouraged. This team may consist of obstetrician–gynecologists and certified nurse–midwives as well as other health care professionals who function within the context of their educational preparation and scope of practice. For example, certified nurse–midwives are educated in the disciplines of nursing and midwifery and possess evidence of certification meeting the requirements of the American College of Nurse–Midwives. Certified nurse–midwives may provide care for low-risk women in the antepartum, intrapartum, and postpartum periods; manage normal newborns; and provide primary gynecologic services in accordance with state law or regulations. Obstetrician–gynecologists' training, credentials, and responsibilities place them in the role of team leaders, but various other providers are needed for unique contributions that are valuable and important to the quality of patient outcomes. Practice agreements and protocols should be established for communication between other practitioners providing obstetric care (eg, a nurse–midwife or family physician) and obstetricians who have agreed to provide specialty coverage. The obstetrician should be informed of the patient's condition and progress as appropriate for the situation.

Hospitals should ensure the availability of skilled personnel for perinatal emergencies. Anesthesia personnel with credentials to administer obstetric anesthesia should be available on a 24-hour basis. At least one person capable of initiating neonatal resuscitation should be present at every delivery. This resuscitation should be performed according to the American Heart Association/American Academy of Pediatrics Neonatal Resuscitation Program or an equivalent formal program. When required, one or two additional persons should be available to provide neonatal resuscitation (see Chapter 5).

Specialty Care Facility

A board-certified obstetrician with special interest, experience, and, in some situations, certification of special competence in maternal–fetal medicine should be chief of the obstetric service at a specialty care hospital. A board-certified pediatrician with special interest, experience, and, in some situations, subspecialty certification in neonatal–perinatal medicine should be chief of the neonatal care service. These physicians should coordinate the hospital's perinatal care services and, in conjunction with other medical, anesthesia, nursing, respiratory therapy, and hospital administration staff, develop policies concerning staffing, procedures, equipment, and supplies.

Care of high-risk neonates should be provided by appropriately qualified physicians. A general pediatrician should have the expertise to assume responsibility for acute, though less critical, care of infants; understand the need for proper continuity of care and be capable of providing it; and share responsibility with the neonatologist for the development and delivery of effective services for newborns at risk in the hospital and community. In collaboration with a physician, care may be provided by qualified advanced-practice nurses (APNs) who have formal education and training as well as supervised clinical experience in the care of newborns.

The director of obstetric anesthesia services should be board certified in anesthesia and should have training and experience in obstetric anesthesia. Anesthesia personnel who have credentials to administer obstetric anesthesia should be readily available. Policies regarding the provision of obstetric anesthesia, including the necessary qualifications of personnel who are to administer anesthesia and their availability for both routine and emergency deliveries, should be developed.

The hospital staff should also include a radiologist and a clinical pathologist who are available 24 hours a day. Specialized medical and surgical consultation should be readily available.

Subspecialty Care Facility

Ideally, the director of the maternal–fetal medicine service at a hospital providing subspecialty care should be a full-time, board-certified obstetrician with subspecialty certification in maternal–fetal medicine. The director of the regional newborn intensive care unit should be a full-time, board-certified pediatrician with subspecialty certification in neonatal–perinatal medicine. As codirectors of the perinatal service, these physicians are responsible for maintaining standards of care; developing the operating budget; evaluating and purchasing equipment; planning, developing, and coordinating in-hospital and outreach educational programs; and participating in the evaluation of perinatal care in the region. They should devote their time to patient care services, research, and teaching and should coordinate the services provided at their hospital with those provided at basic- and specialty-care hospitals in the region.

Other maternal–fetal medicine specialists and neonatologists who practice in the subspecialty care facility should have qualifications similar to those of the chief of their service. A maternal–fetal medicine specialist and a neonatologist should be readily available for consultation 24 hours a day. Personnel qualified to manage obstetric or neonatal emergencies should be in-house.

Obstetric and neonatal diagnostic imaging, provided by obstetricians or radiologists with special interest and competence in maternal and neonatal disease and its complications, should be available 24 hours a day. Pediatric subspecialists in cardiology, neurology, hematology, and genetics should be available for consultation. Consultant services in pediatric nephrology, metabolism, endocrinology, gastroenterology–nutrition, infectious diseases, pulmonology, immunology, and pharmacology are also needed. In addition, pediatric surgeons and pediatric surgical subspecialists (eg, cardiovascular surgeons; neurosurgeons; and orthopedic, ophthalmologic, urologic, and otolaryngologic surgeons) should be available for consultation and care. Pathologists with special competence in placental, fetal, and neonatal disease should also be members of the subspecialty hospital staff.

A board-certified anesthesiologist with special training or experience in maternal–fetal anesthesia should be in charge of obstetric anesthesia services at a subspecialty care hospital. Personnel with credentials in the administration of obstetric anesthesia should be available in the hospital. Personnel with credentials in the administration of neonatal and pediatric anesthesia should be available as needed.

Nurse Providers

Delivery of safe and effective perinatal nursing care requires appropriately qualified registered nurses in adequate numbers to meet the needs of each patient in accordance with the care setting. The number of staff and level of skill required are influenced by the scope of nursing practice and the degree of nursing responsibilities within an institution. Nursing responsibilities in individual hospitals vary according to the level of care provided by the facility, practice procedures, number of professional registered nurses and ancillary staff, and professional nursing activities in continuing education and research. Intrapartum care requires the same labor intensiveness and expertise as any other intensive care unit, and, accordingly, intrapartum units should have the same adequately trained personnel and fiscal support.

Changing trends in medical management and technologic advances influence and may increase the nursing workload. Each hospital should determine the scope of nursing practice for each nursing unit and specialty department. The scope of practice should be based on national nursing standards and guidelines for the specialty area of practice and should be in accordance with state law or regulations. A multidisciplinary committee comprising representatives from hospital, medical, and nursing administration should follow published professional standards and guidelines, consult state nurse practice acts and any accompanying regulations, identify the types and numbers of procedures performed on each unit, delineate direct and indirect nursing care activities performed, and identify activities that are to be performed by nonnursing personnel.

Trends in neonatal care have resulted in an increased use of APNs. An advanced-practice neonatal nurse (APNN) must have completed an educational program of study and supervised practice beyond the level of basic nursing. Included in this category are the following nursing professionals (note that the term *neonatal nurse clinician* is imprecise and should no longer be used):

• A *neonatal clinical nurse specialist* is a registered nurse with a master's degree who, through study and supervised practice at the graduate level, has become expert in the theory and practice of neonatal nursing.

• A *neonatal nurse practitioner* (NNP) is a registered nurse with clinical expertise in neonatal nursing who has received a formal education with supervised clinical experience in the care of newborns. These nurses manage a caseload of neonatal patients with consultation, collaboration, and medical supervision. Using their acquired knowledge of pathophysiology, pharmacology, and physiology, NNPs exercise independent judgment in the assessment and diagnosis of infants and in the performance of certain delegated procedures. Additionally, NNPs are involved in education, consultation, and research at various levels.

The spectrum of duties performed by an APNN will vary according to the institution and may be determined by state laws or regulations. Each of these duties requires advanced education. Nationally recognized certification examinations exist for each category of an APNN. The following guidelines are recommended:

1. Medical care provided by an APNN in a newborn intensive care unit should be supervised by a neonatologist. In basic and specialty nursery units, a board-certified pediatrician with special interest and experience in neonatal medicine should provide supervision.

2. Collaboration and consultation with other health professionals is an important aspect of the APNN's role.

3. Certification by a nationally recognized organization is recommended.

4. An APNN is responsible for maintaining clinical expertise and knowledge of current therapy by participating in continuing education and scholarly activities.

Recommended nurse/patient ratios for perinatal services are shown in Table 2–1. Additional personnel are necessary for indirect patient care activities. Close evaluation of all factors involved in a

Table 2–1. Recommended Nurse/Patient Ratios for Perinatal Care Services

Nurse/Patient Ratio	Care Provided
Intrapartum	
1:2	Patients in labor
1:1	Patients in second stage of labor
1:1	Patients with medical or obstetric complications
1:2	Oxytocin induction or augmentation of labor
1:1	Coverage for initiating epidural anesthesia
1:1	Circulation for cesarean delivery
Antepartum/ postpartum	
1:6	Antepartum/postpartum patients without complications
1:2	Patients in postoperative recovery
1:3	Antepartum/postpartum patients with complications but in stable condition
1:4	Recently born infants and those requiring close observation
Newborns	
1:6–8*	Newborns requiring only routine care
1:3–4	Normal mother–newborn couplet care
1:3–4	Newborns requiring continuing care
1:2–3	Newborns requiring intermediate care
1:1–2	Newborns requiring intensive care
1:1	Newborns requiring multisystem support
1:1 or greater	Unstable newborns requiring complex critical care

* This ratio reflects traditional newborn nursery care. If couplet care or rooming-in is used, a professional nurse who is responsible for the mother should coordinate and administer neonatal care. If direct assignment of the nurse is also made to the nursery to cover the newborn's care, there may be double assigning (one nurse for the mother–neonate couplet and one for just the neonate if returned to the nursery). A nurse should be available at all times, but only one may be necessary, as most neonates will not be physically present in the nursery. Direct care of neonates in the nursery may be provided by ancillary personnel under the nurse's direct supervision. Adequate staff are needed to respond to acute and emergency situations.

specific case is essential in establishing an acceptable nurse/patient ratio. Variables such as birth weight, gestational age, and diagnosis of patients; patient turnover; acuity of patients' conditions; patient or parent education needs; bereavement care; mixture of skills of the staff; environment; types of delivery; and use of anesthesia must be taken into account in determining appropriate nurse/patient ratios. The efficiency of nursing care can be enhanced by a team approach.

Basic Care Facility

Perinatal nursing care at a basic care facility should be under the direction of a registered nurse. This person's responsibilities include directing perinatal nursing services, guiding the development and implementation of perinatal policies and procedures, collaborating with medical staff, and consulting with hospitals that provide specialty and subspecialty care in the region.

For antepartum care, it is recommended that a registered nurse be on duty whose responsibilities include the organization and supervision of antepartum, intrapartum, and neonatal nursing services. The presence of one or more registered nurses or licensed practical nurses with demonstrated knowledge and clinical competence in the nursing care of mothers, fetuses, and newborns during labor, delivery, and the postpartum and neonatal periods is suggested. Ancillary personnel, supervised by a registered nurse, may provide support to the mother and attend to her personal comfort.

Intrapartum care should be under the direct supervision of a registered nurse. Responsibilities of this individual include initial evaluation and admission of patients in labor; continuing assessment and evaluation of patients in labor, including checking the status of the fetus, recording vital signs, observing the fetal heart rate, performing obstetric examinations, observing uterine contractions, and supporting the patient; determining the presence or absence of complications; supervising the performance of nurses with less training and experience and of ancillary personnel; and staffing of the delivery room at the time of delivery. This registered nurse should also be capable of monitoring the fetal heart rate. A licensed practical nurse or nurse assistant, supervised by a registered nurse, may provide support to the mother and attend to her personal comfort.

Postpartum care of the mother and infant should be supervised by a registered nurse whose responsibilities include initial and ongoing assessment, infant care education, preparation for discharge, and follow-up for mother and newborn. This nurse should have training and experience in the recognition of normal and abnormal physical and emotional characteristics of the mother and newborn. A licensed practical nurse or nurse assistant, supervised by a registered nurse, may provide support to the mother and attend to her personal comfort.

Specialty Care Facility

Specialty care hospitals should have a director of perinatal/neonatal nursing services who has overall responsibility for inpatient activities in the respective obstetric and neonatal areas. This registered nurse should be an APN with specialized education in obstetric or neonatal care.

In addition to fulfilling nursing responsibilities in basic care hospitals, nursing staff in the labor, delivery, and recovery areas should be able to identify and respond to the obstetric and medical complications of pregnancy, labor, and delivery. A registered nurse with advanced training and experience in routine and high-risk obstetric care should be assigned to the labor and delivery area at all times. In the postpartum period, a registered nurse is responsible for providing support for mothers and families with infants who require intensive care and for facilitating visitation and communication with the neonatal intensive care unit (NICU).

Direct patient care should be provided by a registered nurse who has education or experience in neonatal nursing and experience in the care of ill newborns. All nurses caring for ill newborns must possess demonstrated knowledge in the observation and treatment of newborns, including cardiorespiratory monitoring. Furthermore, the registered nursing staff of an intermediate-care nursery in a specialty care hospital should be able to monitor and maintain the stability of cardiopulmonary, neurologic, metabolic, and thermal functions; assist with special procedures, such as lumbar puncture, endotracheal intubation, and umbilical vessel catheterization; and perform emergency resuscitation. They should be specially trained and able to initiate, modify, or stop treatment when appropriate, according to established protocols, even when a physician or APN is not present. In units where neonates receive mechanical ventilation, medical, nursing, or respiratory therapy staff who have demonstrated ability to intubate the trachea, manage mechanical ventilation, and decompress a pneumothorax should be continually available (see Table 2–1). The nursing staff should be formally trained in neonatal resuscitation. These activities may be performed by APNNs. The unit's medical director should supervise the delegated medical functions, processes, and procedures performed by APNNs.

Subspecialty Care Facility

The director of perinatal/neonatal nursing services should have overall responsibility for inpatient activities in the maternity–newborn care units. This nurse should have experience and training in obstetric or neonatal nursing or both, as well as in the care of patients at high risk. Preferably, this individual has an advanced degree.

For antepartum care, a registered nurse should be responsible for the direction and supervision of nursing care. All nurses working with high-risk antepartum patients should have evidence of continuing education in maternal–fetal nursing. An APN who has been educated and prepared at the master's level should be on staff to coordinate education.

For intrapartum care, a registered nurse should be in attendance within the labor and delivery unit at all times. This nurse should be skilled in the recognition and nursing management of complications of labor and delivery.

For postpartum care, a registered nurse should be in attendance at all times. This nurse should be skilled in the recognition and nursing management of complications of mothers and newborns.

Registered nurses in the NICU should have specialty certification or advanced training and experience in the nursing management of high-risk neonates and their families. They should also be experienced in caring for unstable neonates with multiorgan system problems and in specialized care technology. An APN should be available to the staff for consultation and support on nursing care issues. Additional nurses with special training are required to fulfill regional center responsibilities such as outreach and transport (see Chapter 3).

The obsetric and neonatal areas may be staffed by a mix of professional and technical personnel. Assessment and monitoring activities should remain the responsibility of a registered nurse or an APN in obstetric–neonatal nursing, even when personnel with a mixture of skills are used.

Support Providers

All Facilities

Personnel who are capable of determining blood type, cross-matching blood, and performing antibody testing should be available on a 24-hour basis. The hospital's infection control personnel should be responsible for surveillance of infections in mothers and neonates, as well as for the development of an appropriate environmental control program (see Chapter 10). A radiologic technician should be readily available 24 hours a day to perform portable X-rays. Availability of a postpartum-care provider with expertise in lactation is strongly encouraged. The need for other support personnel depends on the intensity and level of sophistication of the other support services provided. An organized plan of action that includes personnel and equipment should be established for identification and immediate resuscitation (see the section "Neonatal Resuscitation" in Chapter 5).

Specialty and Subspecialty Care Facilities

The following support personnel should be available to the perinatal care service of specialty and subspecialty care hospitals:

- At least one full-time, master's degree–level, medical social worker (for every 30 beds) who has experience with the socioeconomic and psychosocial problems of high-risk mothers and fetuses, ill neonates, and their families. Additional medical social workers are required when there is a high volume of medical or psychosocial activity.

- At least one occupational or physical therapist with neonatal expertise

- At least one registered dietitian/nutritionist who has special training in perinatal nutrition and can plan diets that meet the special needs of high-risk mothers and neonates

• Qualified personnel for support services such as laboratory studies, radiologic studies, and ultrasound examinations (these personnel should be available 24 hours a day)
• Respiratory therapists or nurses with special training who can supervise the assisted ventilation of neonates with cardiopulmonary disease

The hospital's engineering department should include air-conditioning, electrical, and mechanical engineers and biomedical technicians who are responsible for the safety and reliability of the equipment in all perinatal care areas.

Education

In-Service and Continuing Education

The medical and nursing staff of any hospital providing perinatal care at any level should be knowledgeable about current maternal and neonatal care through joint in-service sessions. These sessions should cover the diagnosis and management of perinatal emergencies, as well as the management of routine problems. The staff of each unit should also have a monthly multidisciplinary conference at which the patient care problems that arose during the previous month are presented and discussed.

The staff of regional centers should be capable of assisting with the in-service programs of other hospitals in their region on a regular basis. Such assistance should include periodic visits to those hospitals, as well as periodic review of the quality of patient care provided by those hospitals. Regional center staff should be accessible for consultation at all times. The medical and nursing staff of hospitals providing specialty and subspecialty care should participate in formal courses or conferences sponsored by a regional perinatal center. Regularly scheduled regional conferences should include subjects such as the following:

• Review of the major perinatal illnesses and their treatment and nursing care

- Review of perinatal statistics, the pathology related to all deaths, and significant surgical specimens
- Review of current X-ray films and ultrasound material
- Administrative staff review of procedures and policies
- Teaching seminars for nursing and medical staff

Perinatal Outreach Education

Design and coordination of a program for perinatal outreach education should be provided jointly by neonatal/obstetric physicians and neonatal/obstetric APNs. Responsibilities should include assessing educational needs; planning curricula; teaching, implementing, and evaluating the program; collecting and using perinatal data; providing patient follow-up information to referring community personnel; writing reports; and maintaining informative working relationships with community personnel and outreach team members.

Ideally, a maternal–fetal medicine specialist, a certified nurse–midwife, an obstetric nurse, a neonatologist, and a neonatal nurse should be members of the perinatal outreach education team. Other professionals (eg, a social worker, respiratory therapist, occupational and physical therapist, or nutritionist) may also be assigned to the team. Each member should be responsible for teaching, consulting with community professionals as needed, and maintaining communication with the program coordinator and other team members.

Each subspecialty care center in a regional system is responsible for organizing an education program that is tailored to meet the needs of the perinatal health professionals and institutions within the network. The various educational strategies that have been found to be effective include a series of seminars, audiovisual/media programs, self-instruction booklets, and clinical practice rotations. Perinatal outreach education meetings should be held at a routine time and place to promote standardization and continuity of communication among community professionals and regional center personnel. As mandated by the subspecialty boards, a subspecialty care center that has a fellowship training program should have an active research program.

Physical Facilities

The physical facilities in which perinatal care is provided should be conducive to care that meets the unique physiologic and psychosocial needs of mothers, neonates, fathers, and families (see Chapter 1). Special facilities should be available when deviations from the norm require uninterrupted physiologic, biochemical, and clinical observation of patients throughout the perinatal period. Labor, delivery, and newborn care facilities should be located in as close proximity to each other as possible. When these facilities are distant from each other, provisions should be made for appropriate transitional areas.

The following recommendations are intended as general guidelines and should be interpreted with consideration given to local needs. It is recognized that individual limitations of physical facilities for perinatal care may impede strict adherence to these recommendations. Furthermore, every facility will not have each of the functional units described. Provisions for individual units should be consistent with a regional perinatal care system and state and local public health regulations.

Obstetric Functional Units

The patient's personal needs, as well as those of her newborn and family, should be considered when obstetric service units are planned. The service should be consolidated in a designated area that is physically arranged to prohibit unrelated traffic through the service units. The obstetric service should have facilities for the following functional components:

- Antepartum care for patient stabilization or hospitalization before labor
- Fetal diagnostic testing (eg, nonstress and contraction stress testing, biophysical profile, amniocentesis, and ultrasound examinations)
- Labor observation and evaluation for patients who are not yet in active labor or who must be observed to determine whether labor has actually begun; hospital obstetric services should develop a

casual, comfortable area ("false-labor lounge") for patients in prodromal labor

• Labor

• Delivery

• Postpartum care

Patient volume and patient care resources may allow for some of the functional components to be combined in close proximity or in a single room. For example, an admission or examination room may also serve as a labor room or a recovery room, or a family waiting room may be used for sibling visitation. To maximize economy and flexibility of staff and space, many hospitals have successfully combined functions into single areas called labor–delivery–recovery (LDR) rooms. Some institutions have developed a separate birthing center within the hospital that is self-governing and is regulated separately (see Chapter 5, "Intrapartum Care").

In planning for antepartum, intrapartum, and postpartum beds, an analysis of the present patterns of care should be reviewed and consideration given to the following types of information:

• Projected birth rate

• Projected cesarean birth rates

• Occupancy projections that address "peaks and valleys" in the census

• Present (and projected) number of women in the unit during peak periods, as well as the length of the peak periods

• Numbers and types of high-risk births

• Anticipated lengths of stay for women during labor, delivery, and recovery

The following facilities should be available to both antepartum and postpartum units and, in appropriate circumstances, may be shared:

• Unit director/head nurse's office

• Nurses' station

- Physician and nurse charting area
- Conference room
- Patient education area
- Staff lounge, locker rooms, and on-call sleep rooms
- Examination and treatment room(s)
- Secure area for storage of medications
- Instrument cleanup area
- Area and equipment for bedpan cleansing
- Sitz bath facilities
- Kitchen and pantry
- Workroom and storage area
- Sibling visiting area

Nonobstetric Patients

The labor and delivery area should be used for nonobstetric patients only during periods of low occupancy. The obstetric department, in conjunction with the hospital administration, should establish written policies according to state and local regulations indicating which nonobstetric patients may be admitted to the labor and delivery suite. Under all circumstances, however, labor and delivery patients must take precedence in this area over nonobstetric patients. Clean gynecologic operations may be performed in the delivery rooms if patients are adequately screened to eliminate infectious cases and if enough personnel are present to prevent any compromise in the quality of obstetric care.

Labor

In a traditional setting, the room provided for patients in labor should include a comfortable chair. Partitions or curtains are essential to provide privacy in multibed rooms. Each patient should have direct access to toilet and hand-washing facilities, either in or immediately adjacent to each room. Toilet facilities may be shared with an adjoining room.

Areas used for women in labor should be equipped with the following components:

- Sterilization equipment (if there is no central sterilization equipment)
- X-ray view box
- Stretchers with side rails
- Equipment for pelvic examinations
- Emergency drugs
- Suction apparatus, either operated from a wall outlet or portable equipment
- Cardiopulmonary resuscitation cart
- Protective gear for personnel exposed to body fluids
- Warming cabinets for solutions and blankets
- A labor or birthing bed and a footstool
- A storage area for the patient's clothing and personal belongings
- Sufficient work space for information management systems
- One or more comfortable chairs
- Adjustable lighting that is pleasant for the patient and adequate for examinations
- An emergency signal and intercommunication system
- Adequate ventilation and temperature control
- A sphygmomanometer and stethoscope
- Mechanical infusion equipment
- Fetal monitoring equipment
- Oxygen outlets
- Access to at least one shower for use by patients in labor
- A writing surface for charting
- Storage facilities for supplies and equipment

The room should have adequate space for support persons, personnel, and equipment. Although local regulations concerning the occupancy and size of labor rooms vary, single-bed or two-bed rooms require a minimum of 100 net square feet per bed. Labor rooms used for intensive care of high-risk patients in hospitals with no designated high-risk units should be planned with a minimum of 160 net square feet and should have at least two oxygen and two suction outlets. Design or renovation should include planning for information management systems at bedside and at work stations and for computer management of medical information.

Patients with significant medical or obstetric complications should be cared for in a room that is specially equipped with cardiopulmonary resuscitation equipment and other monitoring equipment necessary for observation and special care. This room is best located in the labor and delivery area and should meet the physical standards of any other intensive care room in the hospital. When patients with significant medical or obstetric complications receive care in the labor and delivery area, the capabilities of the unit should be identical to those of an intensive care unit.

Delivery

The delivery rooms should be close to the labor rooms to afford easy access and to provide privacy to women in labor. A comfortable waiting area for families should be adjacent to the delivery suite, and restrooms should be nearby.

Traditional delivery rooms and cesarean birth rooms are similar in design to operating rooms. Vaginal deliveries can be performed in either room, whereas cesarean birth rooms are designed especially for that purpose and are thus larger. The traditional delivery room should be 350 net square feet with a 9-foot ceiling. A cesarean birth room should be 400 net square feet. Each room should be well lighted and environmentally controlled to prevent chilling of mother and neonate. Cesarean deliveries should be performed in the obstetric unit, and postpartum sterilization capabilities should be available in that area when appropriate.

Each delivery room should be maintained as a separate unit that has the equipment and supplies necessary for normal delivery and for the management of complications:

- Delivery/operating table that allows variations in position for delivery

- Instrument table and solution basin stand
- Instruments and equipment for vaginal delivery, repair of lacerations, cesarean delivery, and emergency laparotomy or hysterectomy
- Solutions and equipment for the intravenous administration of fluids
- Equipment for administration of all types of anesthesia, including equipment for emergency resuscitation of the mother
- Individual oxygen, air, and suction outlets for mother and neonate
- An emergency call system
- Mirrors for patients to observe the birth (optional)
- Wall clock with a second hand
- Equipment for fetal heart rate monitoring
- Neonatal resuscitation/stabilization unit (as defined under "Neonatal Functional Units" in this chapter)
- Scrub sinks strategically placed to allow observation of the patient

Trays containing drugs and equipment necessary for emergency treatment of both mother and neonate should be kept in the delivery room area. Equipment necessary for the treatment of cardiac arrest should also be easily accessible.

A workroom should be available for washing instruments. Instruments should be prepared and sterilized in a separate room; alternatively, these services may be performed in a separate area or by a central supply facility. There should also be a room for the storage and preparation of anesthetic equipment.

Postpartum Care

The postpartum unit should be flexible enough to permit the comfortable accommodation of patients when the patient census is at its peak and allow the use of beds for alternate functions when the patient census is low. Ideally, single-occupancy rooms should be provided; however, not more than two patients should share one room. Each room in the postpartum unit should have a hand-washing sink and, if possible, a toilet and shower. When this is not possible and it is necessary for patients to use common facilities, patients should be able to reach them without entering a general corridor. When the newborn rooms with the mother, the room should have a hand-washing sink, a mobile bassinet unit, and supplies necessary for the care of the newborn. Siblings may visit in the mother's room or in a designated space in the antepartum or postpartum area.

Larger services may have a specific recovery room for postpartum patients and a separate area for high-risk patients. The equipment needed is similar to that needed in any surgical recovery room and includes equipment for monitoring vital signs, suctioning, administering oxygen, and infusing fluids intravenously. Cardiopulmonary resuscitation equipment must be immediately available. Equipment for pelvic examinations should be available.

Combined Units

Comprehensive obstetric and neonatal care can be provided to both low-risk and high-risk women in labor and their infants in a single room. During the labor, delivery, and recovery phases, care can be provided in an LDR room. Registered nurses who are cross-trained in antepartum care, labor and delivery, postpartum care, and neonatal care should staff this unit, increasing the continuity and quality of care. The LDR room should be located in or close to the intrapartum area and should contain the equipment recommended for separate units.

Each LDR room is a single-care room containing a toilet and shower with optional tub. A lavatory should be located in each room for scrubbing, hand-washing, and infant bathing. A window with an outside view is desirable in the LDR room. Each room should contain a birthing bed that is comfortable during labor and can be readily converted to a delivery bed and transported to the cesarean delivery room when necessary. Separate oxygen, air, and suction facilities should be provided in two separate locations for the mother and the neonate. Gas outlets and wall-mounted equipment should be easily accessible but may be covered with a panel. Either a ceiling mount or a portable delivery light may be used, depending on the preference of the medical staff.

Proper care of the mother requires sufficient space for a sphygmo-manometer, stethoscope, fetal monitor, infusion pump, and regional anesthesia administration, as well as resuscitation equipment at the head of the bed. Proper care requires access to the infant from three sides and quick transport to the nursery should the need arise. The family area should be farthest from the entry to the room, and there should be a comfortable area for the support person.

An enclosed equipment-holding area should be provided in each room and may be shared between two rooms. Ideally, for ease of movement, equipment should be located below the foot of the bed. Standard major equipment held in this area for delivery should include a fetal monitor, delivery case cart, linen hamper, and portable examination lights. A unit equipped for neonatal stabilization and resuscitation (described in "Neonatal Functional Units," this chapter) should be available during delivery.

The workable size of an LDR room is 256 net square feet with room dimensions of 16 × 16 feet, excluding the toilet and/or shower. This room would be able to accommodate six to eight people comfortably during the childbirth process. A minimum 5-foot clear space at the foot of the bed should be available for the providers to occupy during delivery.

Bed Need Analysis

Historically, the calculation of the number of patient rooms needed for all phases of the birth process was based on a simple ratio involving the number of births, the average lengths of stay, and the accepted occupancy levels. To best estimate needs, each birth service should thoroughly analyze functions, philosophies, and projections that will determine the types and quantities of rooms needed.

One planning method is to analyze carefully the activities that will occur in each type of room. For example, LDR rooms should not routinely be used to accommodate care such as outpatient testing when another room would provide a more appropriate setting. Rooms that allow adequate privacy are recommended for the entire birth process, from labor through discharge.

In planning the number of LDR rooms, many questions should be addressed, including the following:

- Will mothers scheduled for cesarean delivery use LDR rooms or other types of patient rooms for their preoperative, recovery, and postpartum stays?

- What is the maximum projected number of annual births that will be accommodated?
- What is the length of stay for all antepartum, intrapartum, postpartum, and ambulatory patients?
- Are the LDR rooms to be used for other purposes, such as triage or short-term observation for false labor or antepartum admission? If so, the length of stay and volume of all these activities must be used in the calculation of bed need.
- What are the current and projected rates for cesarean births—both scheduled and unscheduled?
- What are the acceptable occupancy rates for all levels of patient rooms?
- What are the expected peak census and frequencies of peak occupancy?

Once the data have been accumulated, the following normative formula can be used to calculate the number of rooms needed by type of room (note that patient episodes—cases or activities—is used rather than the number of births):

$$\frac{\text{Number of patient episodes (considering all activities such as admission, observation, and transitional care in this room)}}{365 \text{ days} \times \text{occupancy for the room type}} \times \text{mean overall length of stay}$$

Neonatal Functional Units

A neonatal service should have facilities available to perform the following functions:

- Resuscitation and stabilization
- Admission and observation
- Normal newborn nursery care
- Continuing care

• Intermediate care
• Intensive care
• Isolation
• Visitation
• Supporting service areas

Physically separate neonatal intensive, intermediate, and continuing care areas are a common alternative in nursery design. Primary care nursing and staffing efficiency may be enhanced by having a mix of neonatal patients in a single area. Local circumstances should be considered in the design and management of these care areas.

Resuscitation and Stabilization

The resuscitation area should be illuminated to at least 100 footcandles at the neonate's body surface and should contain the following items:

• Overhead source of radiant heat that can be regulated by the infant's skin temperature
• Noncompressible resuscitation and examination mattress that allows access on three sides
• Wall clock
• Flat working surface for charting
• Table or flat surface for trays and equipment
• Equipment and medications
• Oxygen, compressed air, suction catheters, dry towels, bulb syringe, and vascular access catheters
• Equipment for examination, immediate care, and identification of the neonate
• Resuscitation equipment, including laryngoscope, endotracheal tubes, meconium aspirator, and ventilation bags and masks for full-term and preterm neonates
• Protective gear for exposure to body fluids

The resuscitation area is usually within the delivery or LDR room, although it may be in a designated, contiguous separate room. If resuscitation takes place in the delivery or LDR room, the area should be large enough to allow for proper resuscitation of the infant without interference with the care of the mother. The room temperature should be higher in the area for resuscitation or operating suites than is customary for patient rooms. After the neonate has been stabilized, if the mother wishes to hold her newborn, a radiant heater or pre-warmed blankets should be available to keep the neonate warm. Although some infants requiring resuscitation may remain with their mothers after stabilization, they will require increased vigilance for abnormal temperature, cardiorespiratory instability, hypoglycemia, apnea, and cyanosis. Nursing protocols addressing these issues are required. Qualified nursing staff should be available to monitor the newborn during this period.

A resuscitation area should be allotted a minimum of 40 net square feet of floor space if it is within a delivery or LDR room. A separate resuscitation room should have approximately 150 net square feet of floor space. The area should have adequate suction, oxygen, and compressed-air outlets to accommodate simultaneous resuscitation of twins and should contain at least six electrical outlets. A separate resuscitation room should also have an electrical outlet to accommodate a portable X-ray machine, if needed. Electrical outlets should conform to regulations for areas in which anesthetic agents are administered.

Admission and Observation (Transitional and/or Stabilization Care)

The admission and observation area (for evaluating the neonate's condition in the first 4–8 hours of life) should be near or adjacent to the delivery and cesarean birth room and preferably part of a recovery room, LDR room, or other area for maternal recovery. Physical separation of the mother and newborn during this period should be avoided. This evaluation may take place within one or more areas, including the room in which the mother is recovering, the LDR room, or the newborn nursery. In some hospitals, the newborn nursery is the primary area for transitional care, both for neonates born within the hospital and for those born outside the hospital. No special or separate isolation facilities are required for neonates born at home or in transit to the hospital. An estimated 40 net square feet of floor space is needed for each neonate in the admission and observation area. The capacity required depends on the size of the delivery service and the duration of close observation. The number of observation stations required depends on the birth rate and the length of stay in the observation area. There should be a minimum of two observation stations. The admission and observation area should be well lighted and should contain a wall clock and emergency resuscitation equipment similar to that in the designated resuscitation area. Outlets should also be similar to those in the resuscitation area.

The physician's and nurse's assessment of the neonate's condition determines the subsequent level of care. Most neonates are taken from the admission and observation area to the newborn nursery or to the postpartum area for rooming-in. Some neonates require transfer to an intermediate or intensive care area.

Newborn Nursery

Routine care of apparently normal full-term or some preterm neonates (usually those weighing $\geq$2,000 g) who have demonstrated successful adaptation to extrauterine life may be provided either in the newborn nursery or in the area where the mother is receiving postpartum care. The nursery should be close to the postpartum area. In a multifloor maternity unit, there should be a newborn nursery on each floor.

The number of bassinets in the newborn nursery should exceed the number of obstetric beds to accommodate multiple births, extended neonatal hospitalization, maternal illness, cesarean birth, and fluctuations in demand. The bed requirement for the newborn nursery should be estimated by using data on the mean length of stay and annual number of liveborn, normal, full-term neonates. The use of combination LDR rooms and rooming-in of infants with mothers may substantially alter nursery bed requirements.

Because relatively few staff members are needed to provide care in the newborn nursery and because no bulky equipment is needed, 30 net square feet of floor space for each neonate should be adequate. Bassinets should be at least 3 feet apart in all directions, measured from the edge of one bassinet to the edge of the neighboring bassinet. The newborn care area may be one room (in a small hospital) or one or more rooms (in larger hospitals). Because one nursing staff member is recommended for each 6–8 neonates, individual rooms should have accommodations for 6–8, 12–16, or 18–24 neonates (Table 2–1). This 1:6–8 nurse/patient ratio reflects traditional newborn nursery care. A registered nurse should be available at all times, but only one may be necessary because most infants will not be physically present in the nursery. Direct care of those infants in the nursery may be provided by ancillary personnel under the registered nurse's direct supervision.

The newborn nursery should be well lighted, have a large wall clock, and be equipped for emergency resuscitation. One pair of wall-mounted electrical outlets is recommended for each two neonatal stations; one oxygen outlet, one compressed-air outlet, and one suction outlet are recommended for each four neonatal stations. Cabinets and counters should be available within the newborn care area for storage of routinely used supplies, such as diapers, formula, and linens. If circumcisions are performed in the nursery, an appropriate table with adequate lighting is required. Electrical outlets to power portable X-ray machines are highly recommended.

Continuing Care

Low-birth-weight neonates who are not ill but require frequent feeding, as well as those who require more hours of nursing than do normal neonates, should be taken to the continuing care area. This area should be close to the intermediate and intensive care areas so that neonates who have received intermediate or intensive care, but no longer require these levels of care, may be transferred to the continuing care area for convalescence. This area is also used for convalescing babies who have returned to specialty facilities from an outside intensive care unit.

Because the care of neonates in this area requires appropriate equipment as well as more personnel than are needed in the newborn nursery, more space is needed per patient unit. There should be 50 net square feet of floor space for each patient station, with approximately 4 feet between bassinets or incubators.

As in the resuscitation and stabilization area and the admission and observation area, equipment for emergency resuscitation is required in the neonatal continuing care area. It may be most conveniently kept on an emergency cart or in a cabinet, but it should be readily available. Each neonatal station should have six electrical outlets, one oxygen outlet, one compressed-air outlet, and one suction outlet. In addition, the equipment and supplies required in the newborn nursery should be available in the continuing care area. Provisions should be made for the comfort of parents or personnel who feed neonates in both incubators and bassinets.

Intermediate Care

Sick neonates who do not require intensive care but require 6–12 hours of nursing time each day should be taken to the intermediate care area. Infants requiring complex care, such as assisted ventilation, for more than several hours should be moved to an intensive care area.

The neonatal intermediate care area should be close to the delivery and cesarean birth room and the intensive care area, and away from general hospital traffic. It should have radiant heaters or incubators for maintaining body temperature, as well as infusion pumps, cardiopulmonary monitors, and equipment for ventilatory assistance.

At least 100–120 net square feet per infant is suggested for subspecialty patients, but for intermediate care this space may be less. Space needed for other purposes (eg, for desks, counters, cabinets, corridors, and treatment rooms) should be added to the space needed for patients. There should be at least 4 feet between incubators, bassinets, or radiant heaters in intermediate care areas. Aisles should be 5 feet wide.

Neonates receiving intermediate care may be housed in a single large room or in two or more smaller rooms. In the latter case, each room should accommodate some multiple of four to six infant stations, because one nursing staff member is generally required for every three to four neonates who require intermediate care. Large rooms allow greater flexibility in the use of equipment and assignment of personnel, but less privacy for parental involvement in infant care.

Eight electrical outlets, two oxygen outlets, two compressed-air outlets, and two suction outlets should be provided for each patient station. In addition, the area should have a special outlet to power the neonatal unit's portable X-ray machine. All electrical outlets for each patient station should be connected to both regular and auxiliary power. An oxygen tank for emergency use should be stored but readily available for each infant receiving wall-supplied oxygen. All equipment and supplies for resuscitation should be immediately available within the intermediate care unit. These items may be conveniently placed on an emergency cart.

Intensive Care

Constant nursing and continuous cardiopulmonary and other support for severely ill infants should be provided in the intensive care area. Because emergency care is provided in this area, laboratory and radiologic services should be readily available 24 hours a day. The results of blood gas analyses should be available shortly after sample collection. In many centers, a laboratory adjacent to the intensive care unit provides this service.

The neonatal intensive care area should be near the delivery and cesarean birth room and should be easily accessible from the hospital's ambulance entrance. It should be located away from routine hospital traffic. Intensive care may be provided in a single area or in two or more separate rooms.

The number of nursing, medical, and surgical personnel required in the neonatal intensive care area is greater than that required in other perinatal care areas. In addition, the amount and complexity of equipment required are also considerably greater. Therefore, incubators or overhead warmers should be separated by at least 6 feet, and aisles should be 8 feet wide. The area should have 150 net square feet of floor space for each neonate, plus space for desks, cabinets, and corridors. In addition, the educational responsibilities of a subspecialty facility require that the design of its neonatal intensive care area include space for instructional activities and office space for files on the region's perinatal experience.

Each patient station needs 16–20 electrical outlets, 3–4 oxygen outlets, 3–4 compressed-air outlets, and 3–4 suction outlets. Like those in the intermediate care area, all electrical outlets for each patient station should be connected to both regular and auxiliary power. In addition, each room should have a special outlet to power the portable X-ray machine housed in the NICU. An oxygen tank for emergency use should be stored but readily available for each infant receiving wall-supplied oxygen.

Equipment and supplies in the intensive care area should include all those needed in the resuscitation and intermediate care areas. Immediate availability of emergency oxygen is essential. In addition, equipment for long-term ventilatory support should be provided. Respirators should be equipped with nebulizers or humidifiers with heaters. Continuous on-line monitoring of oxygen concentrations, body temperature, heart rate, respiration, oxygen saturation, transcutaneous oxygen tension, transcutaneous carbon dioxide tension, and blood pressure should be available. Supplies should be kept close to the patient station so that nurses are not away from the neonate unnecessarily and may use their time and skills efficiently. A central modular supply system can enhance efficiency.

In some cases, certain surgical procedures (eg, ligation of a patent ductus arteriosus) are performed in an area in or adjacent to the NICU. Specific procedures addressing preparatory cleaning, physical preparation of the unit, presence of other infants, venting of volatile anesthetics, and quality assessment should be documented in writing. Equipment, facilities, and supplies for this area, as well as procedures, must conform to or be comparable to those required for similar procedures in the surgical department of the hospital. The latter includes adequate air exchange (at least six air changes per hour).

Isolation

Although most neonates with closed-space infections need not be removed from the newborn nursery, provisions should be made for isolating those neonates who may be harboring certain highly contagious agents (eg, varicella–zoster and herpes simplex viruses; see Chapter 9). Because placing an infected infant in an incubator does not protect other infants in the nursery, an incubator is not adequate isolation. Because of the inefficiency associated with the use of personnel and space for isolation rooms, neonatal units in smaller hospitals may consider sharing isolation space with another unit of the pediatric service.

Visitation

Parents should have access to their newborns 24 hours a day at all levels of care within all functional units and should be encouraged to participate in the care of their newborns (see Chapter 7). Generally, parents can be with their newborns in the mother's room.

Special provisions may be necessary when neonates are in special care units (ie, continuing, intermediate, or intensive care units). In these situations, mothers are often discharged from the hospital before their newborns and sometimes must travel long distances to be with them. Several systems have been developed to meet the needs of parents and their newborns under these circumstances (eg, rooms for parents in the hospital, adjacent facilities outside the hospital provided by the hospital, or other lodgings nearby). A period of mother–newborn rooming-in prior to discharge is highly desirable when special care is needed. In addition, intensive and intermediate care units require special areas that are appropriately furnished for the counseling of parents, the breastfeeding of infants; and the support of grieving mothers and families.

Supporting Service Areas

Utility Rooms. Both clean and soiled utility rooms are needed in neonatal care areas. A clean utility room is used for storing breast milk and storing and preparing formulas, medications, and supplies frequently needed for the care of neonates in all functional units. The use of ready-mixed formulas, unit-dose medications, and disposable supplies and equipment has lessened the need for clean utility rooms, however, and they may be replaced by storage areas and clean working surfaces within each functional unit. Utility rooms should be away from direct lighting sources because some of the formulas, medications, and supplies may be light sensitive.

A utility room is required for storing used and contaminated material before it is removed from the care area. It should have negative air pressure, with 100% of its air exhausted to the outside. There should be a two-door zone, one providing direct access from within the unit, and another from outside the unit. This room should contain a countertop and a sink with hot and cold running water that is turned on and off by knee or foot controls, soap and paper towel dispensers, and a covered waste receptacle with foot control. A separate deep sink with hot and cold running water should be available for cleaning equipment prior to its return to the central service department for resterilization. Contaminated equipment may be decontaminated in the soiled utility area and transported to the central service department in plastic bags or containers. Contaminated materials should be removed from the care area regularly. Contaminated linen should not be stored in the soiled utility area but should be taken directly from the care area, in plastic or other nonporous containers, to appropriate hospital facilities.

Storage Areas. A three-level storage system is desirable. The first storage area should be the central supply department of the hospital. The second storage area should be adjacent to or within the patient care areas. In this area, routinely used supplies, such as diapers, formula, linen, cover gowns, charts, and information booklets, may be stored. Generally, space is required in this area only for the amount of each item used between deliveries from the hospital's central supply department (eg, daily or three times weekly). The third area is needed for storage of items frequently used at the neonate's bedside.

The bedside cabinet storage area should be approximately 8 net cubic feet for each bed patient unit in the newborn nursery, 16 net cubic feet for each bed patient unit in the intermediate care area, and 24 net cubic feet for each bed patient unit in the intensive care area. The newborn nursery requires approximately 3 net cubic feet per patient for secondary storage of items such as linen and formula. In the resuscitation and stabilization area, the admission and observation area, and the continuing, intermediate, and intensive care areas, there should be approximately 8 net cubic feet per patient for secondary storage of syringes, needles, intravenous infusion sets, and sterile trays needed in procedures such as umbilical vessel catheterization, lumbar puncture, and thoracotomy.

Large equipment items (eg, bassinets, warmers, radiant heaters, phototherapy units, and infusion pumps) should be stored in a clean, enclosed storage area in close proximity to, but not within, the immediate patient care area. Approximately 6 net square feet of floor space for equipment is required for each patient in the newborn nursery, 18 net square feet for each patient in the intermediate care area, and 30 net square feet for each patient in the intensive care area. Easily accessible electrical outlets are desirable in this area.

Treatment Rooms. Many facilities have developed areas for resuscitation and stabilization, admission and observation, intermediate care, and intensive care, in which each patient station constitutes a treatment area. This has largely eliminated the need for a separate treatment room for procedures such as lumbar punctures, intravenous infusions, venipuncture, and minor surgical procedures. A separate treatment area may be necessary, however, if neonates in the newborn nursery or continuing care area or the postpartum new family unit are to undergo certain procedures (eg, circumcision). The facilities, outlets, equipment, and supplies in the treatment area should be similar to those of the resuscitation area. The amount of space required depends on the procedures performed.

Scrub Areas. At the entrance to each nursery, there should be a scrub area that can accommodate all personnel entering the area. It should have a sink that is large enough to prevent splashing, with faucets operated by foot or knee controls. A backsplash should be provided to prevent standing or retained water. Sinks for hand-washing should not be built into counters used for other purposes. The scrub areas should also contain racks, hooks, or lockers for storing clothing and personal items, as well as cabinets for clean gowns, a receptacle for used gowns, and a large wall clock with a sweep second hand for timing hand-washing.

Scrub sinks should have foot-operated, knee-operated, or photo-electric-operated faucets and should be large enough to control splashing and to prevent retained water. These sinks should be provided at a minimum ratio of one for at least every six to eight patient stations in the newborn nursery and one for every three to four patient stations in the intermediate or intensive care area. In addition, one scrub sink is needed in the resuscitation and stabilization area, and one is needed for every three to four patient stations in the admission and observation area and in the continuing care area.

Nursing Areas. Space should be provided at the bedside, not only for patient care, but also for instructional and charting activities. A flat writing surface (eg, a clipboard) is needed.

A nurses' charting area or desk for tasks such as compiling more detailed records, completing requisitions, and handling specimens is useful. Physicians may also perform charting and clerical activities in this area. Charting should be considered an unclean procedure, and personnel who have been charting should wash their hands before they have further contact with a neonate.

The unit director or head nurse should have an office close to the newborn care areas. Nurses' dressing rooms preferably should be adjacent to a lounge and should contain lockers, storage for clean and soiled scrub attire, toilets, and showers.

Education Areas. A conference room suitable for educational purposes is highly desirable, particularly for specialty and subspecialty facilities. It should be in or adjacent to the maternal–newborn areas.

Clerical Areas. The control point for patient care activities is the clerical area. It should be located near the entrance to the neonatal care areas so that personnel can supervise traffic and limit unnecessary entry into these areas. It should have telephones and communication devices that connect to the various neonatal care areas and the delivery suite. In addition, patients' charts, computer terminals, and hospital forms may be located in the clerical area.

General Considerations

Infant Security

Security devices should be part of an overall security program to protect the physical safety of infants, families, and staff. Both the NICU and normal nurseries should be designed to minimize the risk of infant abduction.

Evacuation Plan

An evacuation policy should be developed for each perinatal care area (ie, antepartum care, labor and delivery, postpartum care, the normal newborn nursery, intermediate care, and intensive care). The policy should specify (1) who orders the evacuation and destination, (2) who designates the assignments, (3) the roles and responsibilities of the staff, and (4) what equipment is needed. A floor plan that indicates designated evacuation routes should be posted in a conspicuous place in each unit. The policy and floor plan should be reviewed with the staff at least annually.

Safety and Environmental Control

Because of the complexities of environmental control and monitoring, a hospital environmental engineer must ensure that all electric, lighting, air composition, and temperature systems function properly and safely. A regular maintenance program should be specified to ensure that systems continue to function as designed after initial occupancy.

The environmental temperature in newborn care areas should be independently adjustable, and control should be sufficient to prevent hot and cold spots, particularly when heat-generating equipment (eg, a radiant warmer) is in use. The air temperature should be kept at 23.8–26.1°C (75–79°F). Humidity should be kept between 30–60% and should be controlled through the heating and air-conditioning system of the hospital. Condensation on wall and window surfaces should be avoided.

A minimum of six air changes per hour is recommended, and a minimum of two changes should be outside air. The ventilation pattern should inhibit particulate matter from moving freely in the space, and intake and exhaust vents should be placed as to minimize drafts on or near the patient beds. Ventilation air delivered to the NICU should be filtered at 90% efficiency.

Fresh-air intake should be located at least 25 feet from exhaust outlets of ventilating systems, combustion equipment stacks, medical or surgical vacuum systems, plumbing vents, or areas that may collect vehicular exhausts or other noxious fumes.

Radiation exposure to infants, families, and staff is another safety concern. Radiation exposure to personnel is negligible at a distance of more than 1 foot lateral to the primary vertical roentgen beam. Care should be taken to ensure that only the patient being examined is in the primary beam. It is unnecessary for families or personnel to leave the area during the roentgen exposure.

Illumination

Ambient lighting levels in newborn intensive care rooms should be adjustable through a range of at least 10–600 lux (approximately 1–60 ft-c), as measured at each bedside. Both natural and artificial light sources should have controls that allow immediate darkening of any bed position sufficient for transillumination when necessary. Artificial light sources should have a visible spectral distribution similar to that of daylight but should avoid unnecessary ultraviolet or infrared radiation by the use of appropriate lamps, lenses or filters.

Appropriate general lighting levels for NICUs have not been established. In the past, relatively high levels (60–100 ft-c) have been recommended to allow evaluation of an infant's skin color and perfusion at any spot in the NICU.

Newly constructed or renovated NICUs should also be able to provide ambient lighting at levels recommended by the Illuminating Engineering Society (10–20 ft-c). In most cases, these levels are adequate.

Studies have demonstrated benefits to some NICU patients exposed to diurnal variation in ambient lighting that reduces nighttime levels to as low as 0.5 ft-c. If these preliminary studies are confirmed and problems surrounding evaluation of skin color and perfusion under low-light conditions can be adequately resolved, newly designed units should also possess the capability to reduce general lighting to a similar degree.

Nurseries should have the capability for adjustable illumination. Multiple switching can be helpful in this regard, but unless a master switch is also provided, this method can pose serious difficulties when rapid darkening of a room is required to permit transillumination.

Because perception of skin tones is critical in the NICU, light sources must be as balanced and as free of glare or veiling reflections as possible. Although harmful in high doses, ultraviolet radiation might be useful in small doses because of photobiologic effects in the skin. The magnitude of both harmful and beneficial doses for the newborn have not yet been defined.

Until better data are available, the output of ultraviolet radiation by fluorescent fixtures in patient care areas should be minimized by plastic or glass shields that filter out most ultraviolet radiation. Separate procedure lighting that provides no more than 1,000–1,500 lux (100–150 ft-c) of illumination to the patient bed should be available at each patient care station.

Lighting should minimize shadows and glare, and it should be controlled with a rheostat so that it can be provided at less than maximal levels whenever possible. Light should be highly framed so that infants at adjacent bed stations will not experience any increase in illumination. Temporary increases in illumination necessary to evaluate an infant or to perform a procedure should be possible without increasing lighting levels for other infants in the same room.

High levels of light to perform a procedure may represent a danger to the developing retina. Given the lack of safety standards, it may be prudent to design directable lighting, where the procedure light can be framed away from the eyes of patients during use.

Illumination of support areas within the NICU, including charting areas, medication preparation area, reception desk, and handwashing areas, should conform to specifications of the Illuminating Engineering Society. Illumination should be adequate in the areas of the NICU where staff perform important or critical tasks. In locations where these functions overlap with patient care areas (eg, close proximity of the nurse charting area to patient beds), the design should nevertheless permit separate light sources with independent controls so that the very different needs of sleeping infants and working nurses can be accommodated to the greatest possible extent.

Windows

Windows provide an important psychologic benefit to staff and families in the NICU. Properly designed natural light is the most desirable illumination for nearly all nursing tasks, including charting and evaluation of infant skin tone. However, placing infants too close to external windows can cause serious problems with temperature control and glare, so provision of windows in the NICU requires careful planning and design. At least one source of natural light should be visible from each patient care area. External windows in patient care rooms should be glazed with insulating glass to minimize heat gain and loss. They should be situated at least 2 feet away from any part of a patient bed to minimize radiant heat loss from the infant. All external windows should be equipped with shading devices that are easily controlled to allow flexibility at various times of day. These shading devices should be either contained within the window or easily cleanable.

Interior Finish

Off-white or pale-beige walls minimize distortion of staff's color perception in patient care areas. This advantage can be nullified by the use of inappropriate fluorescent lighting. Brighter colors may be used elsewhere. Windows in neonatal care areas should have opaque shades that make it possible to darken the area for procedures such as transillumination.

Oxygen and Compressed-Air Outlets

Newborn care areas should have oxygen and compressed air piped from a central source at a pressure of 50–60 pounds per square inch (psi). An alarm system that warns of any critical reduction in line pressure should be installed. Reduction valves and mixers should produce adjustable concentrations of 21–100% oxygen at atmospheric pressure for head hoods and 50–60 psi for mechanical ventilators.

Acoustic Characteristics

The ventilation system, monitors, incubators, suction pumps, mechanical ventilators, and staff produce considerable noise, and the noise level should be monitored intermittently. The construction and redesign of neonatal care areas should include acoustic absorption units or other means to ensure that the peak sound intensity does not exceed 90 decibels (dB) and preferably remains below that level. Background noise mean level should not exceed 70 dB. Staff members should take particular care to avoid noise pollution in enclosed patient spaces (eg, incubators). Care should be taken to avoid spaces shaped so as to focus or amplify sound levels, thus creating "hot spots" that exceed the maximum recommended noise levels.

Electrical Outlets and Electrical Equipment

All electrical outlets should be attached to a common ground. All electrical equipment should be checked for current leakage and grounding adequacy when first introduced into the neonatal care area, after any repair, and periodically while in service. Current leakage allowances, preventive maintenance standards, and equipment quality should meet the standards developed by the Joint Commission on Accreditation of Healthcare Organizations. Personnel should be thoroughly and repeatedly instructed on the potential electric hazards within the neonatal care areas.

Bibliography

American Academy of Pediatrics, Committee on Fetus and Newborn. Advanced practice in neonatal nursing (RE9257). AAP News 1992;8:17 (reaffirmed 1995)

Graven SN, Bowen FW Jr, Brooten D, Eaton A, Graven MN, Hack M, et al. The high-risk infant environment. I. The role of the neonatal intensive-care unit in the outcome of high-risk infants. J Perinatol 1992;12:164–172

Graven SN, Bowen FW Jr, Brooten D, Eaton A, Graven MN, Hack M, et al. The high-risk infant environment. II. The role of caregiving and the social environment. J Perinatol 1992;12:267–275

March of Dimes Birth Defects Foundation, Committee on Perinatal Health. Toward improving the outcome of pregnancy: the 90s and beyond. White Plains, New York: March of Dimes Birth Defects Foundation, 1993

National Association of Neonatal Nurses. Neonatal nursing standards, guidelines, and related documents: annotated bibliography. Petaluma, California: National Association of Neonatal Nurses, 1993

National Association of Neonatal Nurses. Standards of care for neonatal nursing practice. Petaluma, California: National Association of Neonatal Nurses, 1993

Smith JA. The family birthplace: planning and designing today's obstetric facilities. Chicago, Illinois: American Hospital Association, 1995

Chapter 3

Interhospital Care of the Perinatal Patient

Interhospital transport of pregnant women and neonates is an essential component of regional perinatal care. The goal is to care for high-risk mothers and neonates in facilities that provide the required level of specialized care. Mothers who are at risk for complications that affect perinatal outcome or whose neonates are likely to require intensive support should be referred during the antepartum period or transferred prior to delivery. Neonates born to women transported during the antepartum period have better survival rates and lower risks of long-term sequelae than those who are transferred after birth.

Interhospital transport of a pregnant woman is recommended if appropriate services and staff are not available for either the woman or her neonate at the referring facility. Both the facilities and the professionals providing health care to pregnant women need to understand their obligations under the law for patient transfer.

Federal law requires all Medicare-participating hospitals to provide an appropriate medical screening examination for any individual seeking medical treatment at an emergency department to determine whether the patient has an emergency medical condition. It also places strict requirements on the transfer of these patients. A woman having contractions is not considered to be having an emergency medical condition if there is adequate time for her safe transfer before delivery or if the transfer will not pose a threat to the health or safety of the mother or fetus. Some states have similar statutory requirements. For detailed information about federal requirements for patient screening and transfer, see Appendix D.

Program Components

There are three types of perinatal patient transport between facilities:

1. Maternal transport: A pregnant woman is transferred during the antepartum or intrapartum period for special care of the mother or neonate.

2. Neonatal transport:
   - A team is sent from the receiving hospital to evaluate and stabilize the condition of a neonate at the referring hospital and then transport the neonate to the receiving hospital for specialized or intensive support.
   - A team is sent from the referring hospital with a neonate who is being transferred to another hospital for specialized or intensive support.

3. Return transport: A mother or her neonate, after receiving intensive or specialized care at a referral center, is returned to the original referring hospital or to a local hospital for continuing care after the problems that required transferral have been resolved. This should be done in consultation with the referring physician.

To ensure optimal care of high-risk patients, the following components should be a part of a regional referral program:

- Formal transfer agreements between participating hospitals
- Risk identification and assessment of problems that are expected to benefit from consultation and transport
- Resource management
- Adequate financial and personnel support
- A reliable, accurate, and comprehensive communication system between participating hospitals

An interhospital transport program should provide 24-hour service. It should include a receiving or program center responsible for ensuring that high-risk patients receive the level of care they need, a dispatching unit to coordinate the transport of patients between facilities, an appropriately equipped transport vehicle, and a specialized transport team. The program should also encompass a system for providing a continuum of care by various providers, including the personnel and equipment required for the level of care needed, as well as outreach education and program evaluation.

Responsibilities

Each of the functional components of an interhospital transport program has specific responsibilities. If the transport is done by the referring hospital, the referring physician and hospital retain responsibility until the transport team arrives with the patient at the receiving hospital. If the transport team is sent by the receiving hospital, the receiving physician or designee assumes responsibility for patient care from the time the patient leaves the referring hospital. Regardless of the site of origin of the transport team, qualified medical and nursing staff should accompany the patient to the receiving hospital.

Medical–Legal Aspects

Many legal details of perinatal transport are not well defined. However, all involved parties (eg, the referring hospital and personnel, the receiving hospital and personnel, and the transportation carriers or corporations) assume a number of responsibilities for which they are accountable:

- Each transport system must comply with the standards and regulations set forth by local, state, and federal agencies.
- Informed consent for transfer, transport, and admission to and care at the receiving hospital should be obtained before the transport team moves the patient. All federal and state laws regulating patient transfer must be followed.
- Formal agreements between hospitals should be developed to outline procedures for transport and responsibilities for patient care.
- Relevant personal identification and information must be provided for the patient to wear during transport.

• Patient care guidelines, standing orders, and verbal communication with the designated transport physician are to be used to initiate and maintain patient care interventions during transport.

The professional qualifications and actions of the transport team are the responsibility of the institution that employs the team. Insurance must be adequate to protect both patients and transport team members.

Director

The director of the transport program should be either a subspecialist in maternal–fetal medicine or neonatology or an obstetrician–gynecologist or pediatrician with special expertise in these subspecialty areas. The program director's responsibilities include the following:

• Training and supervising staff
• Reviewing the transport records of all transported patients
• Developing and implementing patient care protocols
• Developing and maintaining records and data collection systems for analysis
• Identifying trends and effecting improvements in the transport system by regularly reviewing the following:
  — Operational aspects of the program, such as response times, effectiveness of communications, and equipment issues
  — Evaluation forms prepared by the referring and receiving hospitals soon after each transport

Referring Hospital

Referring physicians should understand the transport system, including how to gain access to and appropriately use its services. The referring physician is responsible for evaluating and stabilizing the patient's condition before transfer.

When transferred, each patient should be accompanied by a maternal or neonatal transport form. This form should contain general information about the patient, including the reason for referral,

the transport mode, and any additional information that may enhance understanding of the patient's needs. Also provided should be relevant neonatal medical information that maximizes the opportunity for appropriate and timely care and minimizes duplication of tests and diagnostic procedures at the receiving hospital.
Items that should be sent with a neonate include the following:

• Properly labeled, red-topped tubes of clotted maternal and cord blood

• Copies of all relevant maternal antepartum, intrapartum, and postpartum records

• All recent or new diagnostic or clinical information on the neonate, including imaging studies

Responsibility for care of the newborn should be delineated between the referring team and the transport team. Parental consent should be obtained for transfer to and treatment of the neonate at the receiving hospital. A report on the neonate's care should be provided by the referring hospital's nursing staff to the appropriate transport team member.

Receiving Center

The receiving center is responsible for the overall coordination of the regional program. It should ensure that interhospital transport is organized in a way that ensures that patients will receive the appropriate level of care.

Contingency plans should be in place to avoid a shortage of beds for patients needing tertiary care. Plans should include provisions for accepting or transferring patients among the cooperating centers or to an alternate receiving center, rather than only the receiving center affiliated with the referral center, when special circumstances warrant (eg, patient census or need for specialized services such as extracorporeal membrane oxygenation).

The receiving center is responsible for providing referring physicians with the following:

• Access by telephone on a 24-hour basis to communicate with receiving obstetric and neonatal units

- Follow-up reports describing the patient's condition, events of the transport, and planned therapy
- A complete summary, including diagnosis, an outline of the hospital course, and recommendations for ongoing care for each patient at discharge
- Ongoing communication and follow-up

Dispatching Units

Dispatching units are responsible for the following activities:

- Providing rapid coordination of vehicles and staff
- Serving as a communication link between the transport team and the referring and receiving hospitals
- Communicating the transport team's estimated time of arrival at the referring hospital to pick up the patient so that any planned therapeutic or diagnostic interventions can be completed in time
- Communicating the patient's estimated time of arrival at the receiving center so that all resources can be mobilized and ready
- Coordinating any connections that need to be made between air transport and ground ambulances

Personnel

The transport team collectively should have the expertise necessary to provide supportive care for a wide variety of emergency conditions that can arise with high-risk mothers and neonates. Team members may include physicians, neonatal nurse practitioners, registered nurses, respiratory therapists, and emergency medical technicians. The composition of the transport team should be consistent with the expected level of medical need of the patient being transported. Transport personnel should also be thoroughly familiar with the transport equipment to ensure that any malfunction en route can be handled without the assistance of hospital maintenance staff.

Equipment

Safe and successful patient transfer depends on the equipment available to the transport team. The kinds and amounts of equipment, medications, and supplies needed by the transport team depend on the type of transport (maternal or neonatal), the distance of the transfer, the type of transport vehicle used, and the resources available at the referring medical facility. The transport equipment and supplies should be based on the needs of the most seriously ill patients to be transported and should include essential medications and special supplies needed during stabilization and transfer.

The following items are generally necessary for the transport team to perform its functions:

- Equipment for monitoring physiologic functions (heart rate, blood pressure [invasive or noninvasive], temperature [skin or axillary], respiratory rate, noninvasive pulse oximetry, and transcutaneous oxygen or carbon dioxide)

- Resuscitation and support equipment (intravenous pumps, suction apparatus, mechanical ventilators, and infant incubators)

- Portable medical gas tanks attached to a flowmeter, with or without a blender, that can be easily integrated with vehicle or building sources of pressurized gas during transport if ventilator-dependent patients are transported

- Electrical equipment that is capable of alternating-current or extended direct-current operation, or both, and is compatible with the sources in the transport vehicle or medical facility

The performance characteristics of transport equipment should be tested for the most severe environmental conditions of air or ground transport that may be encountered. Equipment performance may be altered by a harsh electromagnetic environment, altitude changes, vibration, forces of acceleration, or extremes of temperature and humidity. Hospital-based equipment may cause electromagnetic interference with aircraft navigation or communication systems. Altered performance of medical or aircraft systems could affect the safety of the transport team and the patient.

All equipment should be tested to ensure accuracy and safety in flight. The Federal Aviation Administration and the U.S. Food and Drug Administration have no comprehensive testing guidelines. The comprehensive testing programs of the U.S. Department of Defense have discovered flaws in hospital-based medical equipment that could affect safety when used in air transport. The U.S. Army Aeromedical Research Laboratory at Fort Rucker, Alabama, has tested medical equipment for rotorcraft use, and the Armstrong Laboratory at Brooks Air Force Base in Texas has tested equipment for fixed-wing aircraft. These laboratories can report on completed equipment tests or conduct new evaluations. The following organizations can also offer assistance in choosing medical equipment suitable for use in aircraft:

- Association of Air Medical Services, Pasadena, California
- Professional Aeromedical Transport Association, Bonsall, California
- National Aeronautics and Space Administration, Washington, DC
- Federal Aviation Administration, Washington, DC
- Emergency Care Research Institute, Plymouth Meeting, Pennsylvania

Several factors should be considered in selecting vehicles for an interhospital transport system. Ground transportation is most appropriate for short-range transport. The use of fixed-wing aircraft facilitates coverage of a large referral area but is more expensive, requires skilled operators and specially trained crews, and may actually prolong the time required for response and transport over relatively short distances because of the time needed to prepare for flight. Helicopters can shorten response and transport time over intermediate distances or in highly congested areas but are very expensive to maintain and operate.

The decision to use aircraft in a patient transport system requires special commitments from the director and members of the transport team. During air transport, the pilot should be considered an integral part of the transport team. Therefore, the pilot should be included in appropriate decision making and should have the authority to change, modify, or cancel the mission for safety reasons.

Transport Procedure

Interhospital transport should be considered if the necessary resources or personnel for optimal patient outcomes are not available at the facility currently providing care. The resources available at both the referring and the receiving hospitals should be considered. The risks and benefits of transport, as well as the risks and benefits associated with not transporting the patient, should be assessed. Transport may be undertaken if the physician has determined that the well-being of either the mother or the fetus would not be adversely affected or that the benefits of transfer outweigh the foreseeable risks. As soon as the need for transport of a neonate is considered, the referring hospital should request assistance and coordination. This will help the transport team to prepare in advance to minimize the time spent at the referring hospital.

Transportation of patients to an alternate receiving center solely because of third-party payer issues (eg, conflicts between managed-care plans and referring and receiving hospital affiliations) should be strongly discouraged and may even be illegal in certain situations. All transfers should be based on medical need.

If the patient to be transferred is a neonate, the family should be given an opportunity to see and touch the baby beforehand. A transport team member should meet with the family to explain what the team will be doing en route to the receiving hospital. The patient, personnel, and all equipment should be safely secured inside the transport vehicle.

Patient Care and Interactions

Following are important components of patient care during transport:

- Patients should be observed continuously.
- Vital signs should be monitored and charted.

- Ventilator pressures and inspired oxygen percentage should be monitored.
- Uterine activity of maternal patients and fetal heart rate should be monitored.
- Neonatal patients should be kept in a neutral thermal environment and should receive appropriate respiratory support and additional monitoring, such as assessment of blood gases, oxygen saturation, and blood glucose, as clinically indicated.
- Intravenous fluids and medications should be given, monitored, and recorded as required.
- The team should be prepared to perform life-saving invasive procedures, such as placement of a chest tube and intubation, on neonatal patients.

On arrival at the receiving hospital, the following activities are recommended:

- The receiving staff should be prepared to address any unresolved problems or emergencies involving the transported patient.
- The transport team should report the patient's history and clinical status to the receiving providers.
- The receiving staff should inform the patient's family, as well as the referring physician and staff at the referring hospital, of the condition of the patient upon arrival to the receiving hospital and periodically thereafter.
- Upon completion of the patient transfer, the transport team or other designated personnel should immediately restock and re-equip the transport vehicle in anticipation of another call.

Return Transport

The transport team should call the referring hospital and the child's parents to inform them that the transport is completed and to report the child's condition. Return transport should be considered if the patient's condition permits. Transfer is best done after careful communication between physicians at both hospitals and between both nursing services concerning the patient's needs. If special equipment or treatment is required at the return transfer facility, these arrangements should be made before the patient is transferred. To ensure optimal care during a return transfer, the following guidelines are recommended:

- The patient's (or parents') informed consent should be obtained.
- Return transfer should be accomplished via an adequately equipped vehicle with trained personnel so that the level of care received by the patient is unaltered during transport.
- Staffing at both hospitals should be adequate to ensure a safe transition of care.
- The family should be notified of the transfer so that they may be present at the accepting facility when transfer occurs.
- Appropriate records, including an outline of the treatment plan and current and other recommended follow-up care, should accompany the patient.
- The center that provided the higher level of care should provide consultation on current or new problems to physicians at the return transfer facility.

Outreach Education

Critical to the appropriate use of a regional referral program is a program to educate the public and users about its capabilities. The receiving center and receiving hospitals should participate in efforts to educate the public about the kinds of services available and their accessibility.

Outreach education should reinforce cooperation between all persons involved in the interhospital care of perinatal patients. Receiving hospitals should provide all referring hospitals with information about their response times and clinical capabilities and should ensure that providers know about the specialized resources that are available through the perinatal care network. Primary physicians should be informed as changes occur in indications for consultation and referral of high-risk perinatal patients and for the stabilization of their conditions. Each receiving hospital should also provide continuing education and information to referring physicians about current treatment modalities for high-risk situations.

Program Evaluation

Ideally, the director of a regional program should coordinate program evaluation based on patient outcome data and logistic information. Program monitoring should include the following information:

- Unexpected neonatal mortality or morbidity (eg, hypothermia or tension pneumothorax) during transport
- Mortality or morbidity of patients at the receiving unit
- Frequency with which the referring hospital fails to transfer patients generally considered to require tertiary care (eg, infants born at <32 weeks of gestation)
- Availability of all the services that may be needed by the perinatal patient
- Accessibility of services; capability to connect the patient quickly and appropriately with the services needed, and knowledge by those who need services about where to get them

These data should be tracked as part of the transport team's and the receiving hospital's ongoing quality assessment programs.

Bibliography

American Academy of Pediatrics, Task Force on Interhospital Transport. Guidelines for air and ground transport of neonatal and pediatric patients. Elk Grove Village, Illinois: American Academy of Pediatrics, 1993

American College of Critical Care Medicine, Guidelines Committee; Society of Critical Care Medicine; and American Association of Critical-Care Nurses Transfer Guidelines Task Force. Guidelines for the transfer of critically ill patients. Crit Care Med 1993;21:931–937

American College of Obstetricians and Gynecologists. Guidelines for women's health care. Washington, DC: ACOG, 1996

March of Dimes Birth Defects Foundation, Committee on Perinatal Care. Toward improving the outcome of pregnancy: the 90s and beyond. New York: March of Dimes Birth Defects Foundation, 1993

Chapter 4

Antepartum Care

A comprehensive antepartum care program involves a coordinated approach to medical care and psychosocial support that optimally begins before conception and extends throughout the antepartum period. Health care professionals should integrate the concept of family-centered care into antepartum care (see "Family-Centered Care," Chapter 1). Care should include assessment of the parents' attitudes toward the pregnancy, the support systems available, and the need for parenting education. Couples should be encouraged to participate in developing a birthing plan and in making decisions about pregnancy, labor, delivery, and the postpartum period.

Preconception Care

Preconception care includes identifying those conditions that could affect a future pregnancy but may be ameliorated by early intervention, such as hypertension, diabetes mellitus, or other metabolic and inherited disorders. For example, adverse effects on the fetus from maternal phenylketonuria or uncontrolled diabetes mellitus can be reduced if strict metabolic control is achieved before conception and continued throughout pregnancy; establishing metabolic control later in pregnancy is believed to be of less benefit.

When contemplating pregnancy, prospective parents should be evaluated for conditions that may affect a future pregnancy. All health encounters during a woman's reproductive years, particularly those that are a part of preconception care (see Chapter 1), should include counseling on appropriate behavior to optimize pregnancy outcomes.

The following maternal assessments may serve as the basis for counseling:

- Family history
- Genetic history (both maternal and paternal)
- Medical history
- Current medications (prescription and nonprescription)
- Substance use, including alcohol, tobacco, and illicit drugs
- Physical abuse
- Nutrition
- Environmental exposures
- Obstetric history
- General physical examination

Immunization should be offered to women at risk, including rubella vaccination for women demonstrated to be susceptible and hepatitis B virus vaccination for those at risk of acquiring this infection. Screening or diagnostic studies are recommended or offered during the preconception evaluation. Screening for human immunodeficiency virus (HIV) infection should be recommended. A number of tests can be performed for specific indications:

- Screening for sexually transmissible infections, based on risk assessment
- Testing to assess recurrent pregnancy loss
- Testing for maternal diseases based on medical or reproductive history
- Mantoux skin test with purified protein derivative for tuberculosis
- Screening for genetic disorders based on racial and ethnic background:
  — Sickle hemoglobinopathies
  — β-thalassemia
  — α-thalassemia
  — Tay–Sachs disease

- Screening for other genetic disorders on the basis of family history (eg, cystic fibrosis, fragile X for family history of nonspecific mental retardation, Duchenne muscular dystrophy)

Patients should be counseled on the benefits of the following activities:

- Preventing HIV infection and testing for it during pregnancy
- Determining the time of conception by an accurate menstrual history
- Abstaining from tobacco and alcohol use during pregnancy
- Consuming folic acid, 0.4 mg per day, while attempting pregnancy and during the first trimester for prevention of neural tube defects (NTDs); women with a history of a previous conception with an NTD should consume 4 mg of folic acid daily for 1 month prior to conception and during the first trimester to reduce the risk of NTDs (see Chapter 11)
- Maintaining good control of any preexisting medical conditions (eg, diabetes, hypertension)

Routine Antepartum Care

Women who receive early and regular prenatal care are more likely to have healthier babies. The early diagnosis of pregnancy is important in establishing a management plan. This plan of care should take into consideration the medical, nutritional, psychosocial, and educational needs of the patient and her family, and it should be periodically reevaluated and revised in accordance with the progress of the pregnancy.

All pregnant women should have access in their community to readily available and regularly scheduled obstetric care, beginning in early pregnancy and continuing through the postpartum period. Pregnant women should also have access to readily available unscheduled or emergency visits on a 24-hour basis; ready availability is considered to be from 1 hour to 24 hours or more, depending on the nature of the problem.

Patient Education

Patient education is an essential element of prenatal care. The physician or other providers participating in antepartum care should discuss the following information with each patient:

- Scope of care that is provided in the office
- Laboratory studies that may be performed
- Expected course of the pregnancy
- Signs and symptoms to be reported to the physician (eg, bleeding or rupture of membranes)
- Anticipated schedule of visits
- Practices to promote health maintenance (eg, use of safety belts)
- Educational programs available
- Options for intrapartum care
- Planning for discharge and child care

Each patient should be provided with information about balanced nutrition, as well as ideal caloric intake and weight gain. Daily supplements of vitamins and minerals, including iron, may be needed if there are doubts about the adequacy of the patient's diet or if she is at high risk for vitamin deficiency (see Chapter 11). Women should be cautioned about keeping these supplements and any other medications out of the reach of children.

Women should be made aware of the safety of exercise and daily activity but cautioned that a sensation of extreme fatigue suggests that activity has been excessive. The gestational period is not the time for dangerous sports or the acquisition of new athletic skills.

Tobacco and alcohol consumption should be strongly discouraged, and information regarding cessation programs should be provided. Patients should be cautioned about the use of drugs, particularly illicit drugs, that can have a significantly detrimental effect on the fetus. They should also be advised to consult with their health care provider before using nonprescription drugs.

The roles of the various members of the health care team, office policies (including emergency coverage), and alternate physician coverage should also be explained. Specific information regarding costs should be provided.

Couples should be referred to appropriate educational literature and urged to attend childbirth education classes. These education classes provide an excellent opportunity for women to obtain specific information about labor, pain relief, delivery, breastfeeding, normal infant care, and postpartum adjustment. Other family members should also be encouraged to participate in childbirth education programs. Adequate preparation of family members may benefit the mother, the neonate, and, ultimately, the family unit. Many hospitals, community agencies, and other groups offer such educational programs. The participation of physicians, certified nurse–midwives, and hospital obstetric nurses in educational programs is desirable to ensure continuity of care and consistency of instruction.

At some time during the prenatal period, parents should identify a pediatrician and may benefit from a consultation regarding newborn and pediatric care. By early in the third trimester, patient education should include information about the following points:

- Plans for hospital admission and labor, delivery, and anesthesia services
- What to do when labor begins, when membranes rupture, or if bleeding occurs
- The consequences of ingesting solid food after the onset of labor, given that a general anesthetic could be required for the delivery
- Aspects of maternal postpartum care, including postpartum contraception and sterilization
- Plans for infant feeding
- Available lactation support services
- Aspects of newborn care, such as cord care, physiologic jaundice, and circumcision of male neonates
- Timing of discharge from the hospital and any necessary preparations, such as obtaining an infant car seat
- Resources available for home health services after discharge

A woman with an uncomplicated pregnancy can usually continue to work until the onset of labor. Women with medical or obstetric complications of pregnancy may need to make adjustments based on the nature of their activities, occupation, and specific complications.

Most women can plan to return to work several weeks after an uncomplicated vaginal delivery. Although a period of 4–6 weeks is generally required for a woman's physiologic condition to return to normal, the patient's individual circumstances should be considered when recommending resumption of full activity. (See also "Maternal Considerations" in Chapter 7.) It is also important for the development of children and the family unit that adequate family leave be available for fathers and mothers to be able to participate in early childrearing. The federal Family and Medical Leave Act and state law should be consulted for information on family and medical leave.

Psychosocial Services

Confronting psychologic and social problems, such as fear of pregnancy, guilt associated with an unintended pregnancy, financial concerns, and marital or other family conflicts, may be the most distressing aspect of a woman's pregnancy. A woman with negative feelings about her pregnancy should receive additional support from the health care team, and she may need professional advice on the alternatives to completing the pregnancy and keeping the baby. Family members and their interactions with the pregnant woman should be considered in whatever recommendations are made. To ensure the early detection and effective management of emotional problems, the obstetrician should be alert to the stresses that may arise from the pregnant woman's psychologic and social conflicts. Physicians should be aware of individuals and community agencies to which patients can be referred for additional counseling and assistance when necessary.

Adolescent Pregnancy

The physician should be prepared to assist the pregnant adolescent with conflicts that may arise, especially if the pregnancy is unplanned. The adolescent, her family, and her partner may have strong feelings about the pregnancy that seriously disturb family and social relationships. The physician can do much to ease tensions through counseling, education, and the use of community and social resources.

Once pregnancy has been confirmed in an adolescent, the physician should explore with the patient her feelings about the pregnancy and the options available to her. Late diagnosis of pregnancy, however, may complicate these considerations and sometimes limit the options for management. The adolescent should take an active role in the decision-making process, and the physician should direct recommendations specifically toward her needs. Sensitive, perceptive, and in-depth discussions with the adolescent may be necessary. Many states have laws regarding adolescent rights, and the physician should be aware of these state laws in order to make health care decisions.

Domestic Violence

Risk assessment during pregnancy should routinely include identification of women who are victims of domestic violence. It has been reported that one in four women in the United States will be physically abused at some time during her life and that pregnancy is a risk factor for abuse. For women in an ongoing abusive relationship, violence typically does not abate during pregnancy and may increase. There may be no pathognomonic signs or symptoms of battering. Unfortunately, most abuse is not discussed by patients.

The physician's role is to encourage the patient to acknowledge that abuse is unacceptable, and to provide information about community resources. These resources include emergency housing (usually in shelters), peer group and individual counseling, and legal and social service advocacy. Most communities have agencies and programs to help battered women and families to seek viable alternatives. The health care provider may need to reinforce to victims that they have done nothing to deserve a beating or other abusive behavior.

Substance Use

Large numbers of women of childbearing age abuse potentially addictive and mood-altering drugs. The two most commonly used substances are alcohol and nicotine. Use of these substances, as well as cocaine, marijuana, diazepam, and other prescription drugs, and approximately 150 other substances, can lead to chemical dependency in susceptible individuals. Depending on geographic location, it is estimated that 1–40% of pregnant women have used one of these substances during pregnancy. Empirical data suggest that approximately 1 in 10 infants is exposed to one or more mood-altering drugs during pregnancy; the number varies only slightly for public versus private practices.

Chemical dependency is likely to be a chronic, relapsing, and progressive disease. Many drug-dependent pregnant women do not seek early prenatal care and therefore are at increased risk for medical and obstetric complications. Drug-exposed infants often go unrecognized and are discharged from the newborn nursery to homes where they are at increased risk for a complex of medical and social problems, including abuse and neglect.

Maternal alcohol use has been recognized to pose a significant perinatal risk of mental retardation and teratogenic effects expressed as fetal alcohol syndrome. Heavy smokers have more frequent occurrences of spontaneous abortion, abruptio placentae, premature rupture of membranes, preterm delivery, and babies with lower birth weights. Opiates in large amounts can cause chemical dependency in the fetus and withdrawal in the neonate.

Recently, cocaine use during pregnancy has also been demonstrated to pose a major perinatal risk. Cocaine-exposed infants appear to have an increased incidence of premature birth, restricted fetal growth, and neonatal seizures. Although a specific cocaine withdrawal syndrome in the neonate has not been defined, signs of irritability and tremulousness, lethargy, and an inability to respond appropriately to stimulation may occur. Because most published studies of cocaine's effect on pregnancies and infants have focused on recognized substance-abusing populations, little information is available regarding the effects of low doses of cocaine. In addition, interpretations of clinical studies are complicated by the fact that patients typically abuse multiple drugs.

All pregnant women should be questioned at the time of the first prenatal visit about their past and present use of alcohol, nicotine, and other drugs. Use of specific screening questionnaires may improve detection rates. A woman who acknowledges the use of alcohol, nicotine, cocaine, or other mood-altering drugs should be carefully counseled about the perinatal implications of their use during pregnancy and offered referral to an appropriate drug-treatment program if chemical dependence is suspected.

To reinforce and encourage continued abstinence, periodic questioning or testing may be desirable for a pregnant woman who reports substance use before or during pregnancy. Because positive test results have implications for patients that transcend their health, patients should give informed consent prior to testing. The requirements for consent vary from state to state, and practitioners should be familiar with testing and reporting requirements in their states.

Testing of the mother or the neonate or both may be useful in some clinical situations, even when substance use has not been suspected previously. Such circumstances include the presence of unexplained intrauterine growth restriction, third-trimester stillbirth, unexpected prematurity, or abruptio placentae in a woman not known to have hypertensive disease. Meconium testing for cocaine may offer another screening method; however, its specificity has not been clarified in population studies. Screening of all patients at the time of delivery is not recommended. Screens are likely to be negative when drugs were used early in pregnancy and can be negative even when women have taken some drugs during the 48 hours before delivery. Because the components of urine toxicology screens vary among laboratories, physicians should verify with their laboratory which metabolites are included in its screen. To identify drug-exposed infants, pediatricians should obtain a thorough maternal history from all pregnant women in a nonthreatening, organized manner. Practitioners should also be aware that laws in some states consider in utero drug exposure to be a form of child abuse or neglect and require reporting of positive drug tests in pregnant women or their newborns to the state's child protection agency.

Antepartum Surveillance

Antepartum surveillance begins with the first prenatal visit, at which time the physician or nurse begins to compile an obstetric data base. Appendix A contains a format for documenting information and the data base recommended by the American College of Obstetricians and Gynecologists (ACOG).

The frequency of follow-up visits is determined by the individual needs of the woman and an assessment of her risks. The frequency and regularity of scheduled prenatal visits should be sufficient to enable providers to accomplish the following activities:

- Monitor the progression of the pregnancy
- Provide education and recommended screening and interventions
- Reassure the mother
- Assess the well-being of the fetus and mother
- Detect medical and psychosocial complications and institute indicated interventions

Generally, a woman with an uncomplicated pregnancy is examined every 4 weeks for the first 28 weeks of pregnancy, every 2–3 weeks until 36 weeks of gestation, and weekly thereafter. Women with medical or obstetric problems, as well as younger adolescents, may require closer surveillance; the appropriate intervals between scheduled visits are determined by the nature and severity of the problems.

During each regularly scheduled visit, the health care provider should evaluate blood pressure, weight, urine protein and glucose, uterine size for progressive growth and consistency with estimated date of delivery, and fetal heart rate. After the patient reports quickening and at each subsequent visit, she should be asked about fetal movement, contractions, leakage of fluid, or vaginal bleeding.

Estimated Date of Delivery

Management of pregnancy requires establishing an estimated date of delivery. Problems such as intrauterine growth restriction, preterm labor, and postterm pregnancy are managed most effectively when an accurate estimated date of delivery is known. In addition, accurate gestational dating is important for the application and interpretation of certain antepartum tests (eg, maternal serum alpha-fetoprotein [MSAFP] or assessment of fetal maturity).

If there is a size–date discrepancy or if menstrual dates are uncertain, an ultrasound examination is indicated for the purpose of dating. Such an examination is most accurate when performed before 20 weeks of gestation. Ultrasound is considered to be consistent with menstrual dates if there is gestational age agreement to within 1 week by crown–rump measurement obtained at 6–11 weeks, or within 10 days by the average of multiple measurements obtained at 12–20 weeks.

Routine Testing

Certain laboratory tests should be performed routinely in pregnant women. The following tests are performed early in pregnancy, as appropriate, and the results are made available to the physician responsible for care of the newborn:

- Hematocrit or hemoglobin
- Urinalysis, including microscopic examination
- Urine testing to detect asymptomatic bacteriuria
- Determination of blood groups and CDE (Rh) type
- Antibody screen
- Determination of immunity to rubella virus
- Syphilis screen
- Cervical cytology (as needed)
- Antibodies to hepatitis B virus surface antigen

All pregnant women should receive education and counseling about preventing HIV infection as part of their regular prenatal care. Testing for HIV is recommended for all pregnant women, with their consent. Refusal of testing should be documented. In some states, it is necessary to obtain the mother's written authorization prior to disclosing her HIV status to health care providers who are not members of her health care team.

Recommended intervals for additional tests that are indicated after the first prenatal visit are detailed on the ACOG Antepartum Record (see Appendix A). Additional laboratory evaluations, such as testing for sexually transmissible infections, genetic disorders, and tuberculosis, are recommended or offered on the basis of the patient's history and physical examination or in response to public health guidelines. Pregnancy is not a contraindication for Mantoux skin test with purified protein derivative for tuberculosis and may be indicated in high-risk areas or for health care workers. Tests for sexually transmissible infections may be repeated at 32–36 weeks of gestation if the woman has specific risk factors for these diseases. Early in the third trimester, measurement of hemoglobin or hematocrit levels should be repeated. Although ultrasound is not recommended routinely, it may be used for specific indications at various gestational ages, such as at 16–18 weeks of gestation for mothers with diabetes mellitus or at 32–34 weeks of gestation to assess fetal growth restriction for women at high risk. In some instances, repeated or planned serial ultrasound examinations may be indicated, such as for women with D (Rh) isoimmunization or other causes of fetal hydrops.

Risk Assessment and Management

Identification of risk factors is critical in order to minimize maternal and neonatal morbidity and mortality. Although a correlation can be seen between antenatal risk factors and the development of problems, a significant percentage of intrapartum and neonatal problems occur in patients without identified antenatal risk factors. Appendixes B and C provide essential data important for early and ongoing risk assessment.

In many instances, special obstetric problems require a multidisciplinary approach to antepartum care. Some conditions may require the involvement of a maternal–fetal medicine subspecialist, geneticist, pediatrician, neonatologist, anesthesiologist, or other medical specialist in the evaluation, counseling, and care of the patient.

Antibody Testing

Antibody tests should be repeated in an unsensitized, D-negative patient at approximately 28 weeks of gestation. She should also receive D (Rho[D]) immune globulin prophylactically at that time. In addition, any unsensitized, D-negative patient should receive D immune globulin if she has had one of the following:

- Ectopic gestation
- Abortion (either spontaneous or induced)
- Procedure associated with possible fetal-to-maternal bleeding, such as chorionic villus sampling (CVS) or amniocentesis

- Condition associated with fetal–maternal hemorrhage (eg, abdominal trauma, abruptio placentae)
- Delivery of a D-positive infant

Diabetes Screening

Obstetric providers should develop a plan for screening pregnant patients for gestational diabetes. Depending on the care setting and population, either universal or selective screening can be used and should be performed at 24–28 weeks of gestation. For selective screening, the following risk factors may be used:

- Family history of diabetes
- Previous birth of a macrosomic, malformed, or stillborn baby
- Hypertension
- Glycosuria
- Maternal age of 30 years or older
- Previous gestational diabetes

Teratogens

Major birth defects are apparent in about 2–3% of the general population at birth, although the actual incidence could be greater. Many patient inquiries concern environmental or teratogenic exposure about which there is little scientifically valid information for determining the exposure risk, if any, in human pregnancy. These are valid concerns. Patients should be counseled that relatively few agents have been identified that are known to cause malformations in a high percentage of exposed pregnancies. The background rate of birth defects (2–3%) and the possibility of no risk or a low increase in risk based on exposure can be discussed.

Relatively few patients will have been exposed to agents that are known to be associated with significantly increased risk for fetal malformation and mental retardation. The physician may wish to consult with or refer such a patient to a health professional with special knowledge or experience in teratology and birth defects.

Many patients raise questions about methods of detecting birth defects related to drug exposure. Amniocentesis for chromosome analysis is not appropriate for the diagnosis of birth defects caused by teratogens. Methods used for prenatal genetic diagnosis may not be appropriate for the evaluation of birth defects caused by teratogens.

Diagnostic Imaging. Imaging modalities used for diagnosis during pregnancy include X-ray, ultrasound, and magnetic resonance imaging. The imaging modality that causes the most anxiety for both obstetrician and patient is X-ray or ionizing radiation. Much of this anxiety is secondary to a general misperception that any radiation exposure is harmful and may result in injury to or anomaly of the fetus. This anxiety may lead to inappropriate therapeutic abortion. In fact, most diagnostic X-ray procedures are associated with few, if any, risks to the fetus. Moreover, according to the American College of Radiology, no single diagnostic X-ray procedure results in radiation exposure to a degree that would threaten the well-being of a developing preembryo, embryo, or fetus. Thus, diagnostic X-ray during pregnancy is not an indication for therapeutic abortion.

Some women are exposed to X-rays before pregnancy is diagnosed. Occasionally, X-ray procedures are indicated during pregnancy for significant medical problems or trauma. Concern about radiation exposure during pregnancy should not prevent medically indicated diagnostic X-ray studies when these are important for the care of the mother. When such a study is indicated, the radiologist should be consulted to minimize the extent of exposure of the fetus. There is no contraindication to a diagnostic X-ray that is likely to be beneficial in the diagnosis and treatment of a pregnant woman. Patients concerned about previously performed or planned diagnostic studies should have counseling to allay these concerns.

Ultrasound and magnetic resonance imaging do not involve radiation exposure. These types of imaging studies are increasingly being used to provide diagnostic information and to avoid the use of X-ray studies. Ultrasound and magnetic resonance imaging are not associated with known adverse fetal effects. Until more information is available, however, magnetic resonance imaging is not recommended for use in the first trimester.

Radioisotopes. Most diagnostic studies in which radioisotopes are used are not hazardous to the fetus and incur very low levels of radiation exposure. A typical technetium Tc 99m scan results in a fetal dose of less than 0.5 rads, and a thallium 201 scan also results in a very small dose. Many of these isotopes are excreted in the urine. Therefore, women should be advised to drink plenty of fluids and to void frequently after a radionuclide study.

One important exception is the use of iodine 131 for the treatment of hyperthyroidism. The fetal thyroid gland begins to incorporate iodine actively by the end of the first trimester. Administration of iodine 131 after this time can result in concentration of the radiation within the fetal thyroid and destruction of the fetal thyroid gland. Iodine 131 is therefore contraindicated for therapeutic use during pregnancy.

Maternal Serum Screening

Women who are less than 35 years of age should be offered serum screening to assess the risk of Down syndrome, ideally between 15 and 18 weeks of gestation by menstrual dating. In women age 35 or older (as of the estimated delivery date), multiple marker testing cannot be recommended as an equivalent alternative to cytogenetic diagnosis for detection of Down syndrome. Serum screening for NTDs by MSAFP testing should also be offered to all pregnant women, ideally between 15 and 18 weeks of gestation (optimally at 16 weeks). Samples should be submitted to a clinical laboratory that has a quality-assessment program, has normative data specific to each week of gestational age, and provides interpretations and risk assessment that take into account maternal weight, race, and, for Down syndrome screening, age. The laboratory should be able to confirm that the specific combination of tests and the particular assays performed will yield a detection rate of Down syndrome of at least 55–60% and a positive rate of screening of less than 5% after ultrasound correction of gestational age. Combinations of MSAFP, human chorionic gonadotropin, and unconjugated estriol determinations may be used to achieve this detection rate.

Down Syndrome. A screening result that indicates a midtrimester risk of Down syndrome that is equal to or greater than that of a 35-year-old woman is usually considered positive. This is usually a 1:270 midtrimester risk for the occurrence of Down syndrome. If ultrasound does not reveal an error in gestational dating—or diagnose a fetal disorder—amniocentesis should be offered to analyze fetal karyotype.

Neural Tube Defects. The results of MSAFP may be used to screen for NTDs. The use of a standard screening cutoff (2.5 multiples of the median) will detect approximately 80% of cases of open spina bifida and 90% of cases of anencephaly.

Patients with elevated MSAFP levels are evaluated by ultrasound to detect identifiable causes of false-positive results (eg, fetal death, multiple gestation, underestimation of gestational age) and for targeted study of fetal anatomy for NTDs and other open defects (eg, omphalocele, cystic hygroma). Amniocentesis may be recommended to confirm the presence of open defects and to obtain a fetal karyotype. Amniocentesis may be offered even when ultrasound does not reveal an identifiable defect or cause for the elevated MSAFP level.

Prenatal Diagnosis of Genetic Disorders in Patients at Increased Risk

Prenatal genetic diagnosis should be offered in circumstances in which there is a definable increased risk for a fetal genetic disorder that may be diagnosed by one or more methods. Prenatal genetic screening or diagnosis should be voluntary and informed. In most circumstances, results are normal and provide patients with a high degree of reassurance that a particular disorder does not affect a fetus. Early prenatal genetic diagnosis also affords patients the option to terminate affected pregnancies. Alternatively, a positive diagnosis may allow a patient to prepare for the birth of an affected child and, in some circumstances, may be important in establishing a plan for care during pregnancy, labor, delivery, and the immediate neonatal period.

Risk Assessment and Counseling

Many couples who are at increased risk of having children with a genetic disorder can benefit from genetic counseling. An example of current screening criteria is listed in the ACOG Antepartum Record in Appendix A. The maternal age-adjusted risks for chromosome abnormalities are shown in Table 4–1. Couples at risk of having a child with a genetic disorder may or may not need formal genetic consultation. Sometimes the problem is relatively straightforward. For example, the primary care physician can readily explain the well-known relationship between advanced maternal age and autosomal trisomies. In other cases, referral to a geneticist may be necessitated by the complexities of determining risks, evaluating a family history of such abnormalities, interpreting laboratory tests, or providing counseling. Regardless of the indication, counseling is essential before genetic screening or antenatal diagnostic tests are performed.

Prenatal genetic counseling addresses the risk of occurrence of a genetic disorder in a family. In this process, the primary care physician, a medical geneticist, or other trained person attempts to help the individual or family

- Comprehend the medical facts, including the diagnosis, probable course of the disorder, and available management
- Appreciate the way in which heredity contributes to the disorder and the risk of occurrence or recurrence in specific relatives
- Understand the options for dealing with the risk of recurrence, including prenatal genetic diagnosis
- Choose the course of action that seems appropriate in view of the risk and the family's goals and act in accordance with that decision
- Make the best possible adjustment to the disorder in an affected family member and to the risk of recurrence in another family member

Thus, the key elements in genetic counseling are accurate diagnosis, communication, and nondirective presentation of options. The counselor's function is not to dictate a particular course of action but to provide information that will allow couples to make informed decisions.

Table 4–1. Chromosome Abnormalities in Full-Term, Liveborn Infants*

Maternal Age at Delivery	Risk for Down Syndrome	Total Risk for Chromosome Abnormalities[†]
20	1/1,667	1/526
21	1/1,667	1/526
22	1/1,429	1/500
23	1/1,429	1/500
24	1/1,250	1/476
25	1/1,250	1/476
26	1/1,176	1/476
27	1/1,111	1/455
28	1/1,053	1/435
29	1/1,000	1/417
30	1/952	1/385
31	1/909	1/385
32	1/769	1/322
33	1/602	1/286
34	1/485	1/238
35	1/378	1/192
36	1/289	1/156
37	1/224	1/127
38	1/173	1/102
39	1/136	1/83
40	1/106	1/66
41	1/82	1/53
42	1/63	1/42
43	1/49	1/33
44	1/38	1/26
45	1/30	1/21
46	1/23	1/16
47	1/18	1/13
48	1/14	1/10
49	1/11	1/8

* Because sample sizes for some intervals are relatively small, 95% confidence limits are sometimes relatively large. Nonetheless, these figures are suitable for genetic counseling.

[†] 47,XXX excluded for ages 20–32 years (data not available).

Modified from the following sources: Hook EB, Cross PK, Schreinemachers DM. Chromosomal abnormality rates at amniocentesis and in live-born infants. JAMA 1983;249:2034–2038 (ages 33–49), copyright 1983, American Medical Association; Hook EB. Rates of chromosome abnormalities at different maternal ages. Obstet Gynecol 1981;58:282–285.

Diagnostic Testing

Amniocentesis

Transabdominal amniocentesis is the technique most commonly used for obtaining fetal cells for genetic studies. This well-established, safe, and reliable procedure is usually performed at approximately 16 weeks of gestation. The cells obtained via amniocentesis can be used for blood typing or cytogenetic, metabolic, or other DNA testing. Alpha-fetoprotein can be measured in the supernatant fluid to detect open fetal NTDs, and acetylcholinesterase measurement can be used to discriminate open NTDs from other open defects (eg, gastroschisis). Significant maternal injury from amniocentesis is rare, and the estimated risk of spontaneous abortion due to amniocentesis at 15 weeks or later is 0.5% or less.

Chorionic Villus Sampling

Chorionic villus sampling is a technique for removing a small sample (5–40 mg) of placental tissue (chorionic villi) for performing chromosomal, metabolic, or DNA studies. It is generally performed between 10 and 12 weeks of gestation, either by a transabdominal or a transcervical approach. Chorionic villi, however, cannot be used for the prenatal diagnosis of NTDs, which requires the measurement of alpha-fetoprotein levels in amniotic fluid. Although CVS offers the advantage of first-trimester prenatal diagnosis, the procedure-related risk of pregnancy loss is approximately 0.5–1.0% higher than that for amniocentesis. Until further information is available, CVS should not be performed before 10 weeks of gestation.

The possibility that CVS may cause limb reduction defects remains controversial but should be discussed in counseling. Although further studies are needed to determine whether the risk of transverse digital deficiency increases after CVS at 10–12 weeks of gestation, it is prudent to counsel patients that this is also a possibility and that the estimated risk may be on the order of 1 in 3,000 births. Women who have undergone cytogenetic testing by CVS are offered MSAFP screening, for the detection of NTDs alone, at 15–20 weeks.

Testing D-Negative Women

Because both amniocentesis and CVS can result in fetal-to-maternal bleeding, the administration of D immune globulin is indicated for D-negative, unsensitized women who undergo either of these procedures. Fetal-to-maternal bleeding is more frequent with CVS, and because of the possibility of enhanced sensitization very early in gestation, this procedure is therefore not advisable in D-negative women who are already sensitized.

Tests of Fetal Well-Being

The goals of antepartum fetal surveillance include reducing the risk of fetal demise after 24 weeks of gestation, delaying the need for intervention, and prolonging gestation in pregnancies at risk for preterm delivery. The primary indication for biophysical antepartum tests of fetal well-being is a pregnancy at increased risk for antepartum fetal demise. Some conditions for which testing may be indicated include the following:

• Decreased fetal movement
• Hypertensive disorders
• Insulin-dependent diabetes mellitus
• Oligohydramnios or hydramnios
• Fetal growth restriction
• Postterm pregnancy
• Multiple gestation with discordant fetal growth

The most commonly used tests are assessment of fetal movement (eg, kick counts), the nonstress test, the contraction stress test, and the biophysical profile and its modifications. In most clinical situations, a normal test result indicates that intrauterine fetal death is highly unlikely in the next 7 days. On the other hand, an abnormal result or nonreassuring fetal status is associated with a high rate of false-positive results, which, based on the clinical situation, require additional testing to corroborate or refute.

The most important consideration in deciding when to begin antepartum testing is the prognosis for neonatal survival. In pregnancies with multiple or particularly worrisome high-risk conditions, contraction stress testing and biophysical profile testing can be performed as early as 26–28 weeks of gestation with no alterations in interpretation. The implications of a nonreassuring fetal heart rate at this gestational age, however, are unclear.

When the clinical condition that has prompted testing persists, a reassuring test (reactive nonstress test, negative contraction stress test, or normal biophysical profile) should be repeated periodically until delivery to monitor continued fetal well-being. Allowing an interval of 7 days to elapse between tests has been demonstrated in most studies to result in a false-negative rate of approximately 8/1,000 for various tests of fetal well-being. With some maternal complications, reevaluation at shorter intervals is indicated.

The sequence of tests to determine fetal well-being may vary by practice and protocol. Each test has advantages and disadvantages, and no single test has been shown to be superior to the others in any specific clinical situation. Regardless of which antepartum surveillance test is used, the results and interpretation should be noted in the patient's chart.

Assessment of Fetal Movement

Numerous studies attest to the value of maternal assessment of fetal movement in the evaluation of fetal well-being. Because of its simplicity and effectiveness, women who are at increased risk for antepartum fetal demise should be instructed in the daily assessment of fetal activity, in addition to receiving formal fetal testing. Neither the ideal number of kicks nor the ideal duration for movement counting has been defined, and numerous methods have been used. Perhaps more important than any single quantitative guideline is the mother's perception of a decrease in fetal activity in relation to a previous level.

One approach to assessing fetal movement is to have the woman count distinct fetal movements on a daily basis. The perception of 10 distinct movements in a period of up to 2 hours is considered reassuring. After 10 movements have been perceived, the count can be discontinued for that day. In the absence of a reassuring count, a biophysical means of fetal assessment should be used.

Nonstress Test

For the nonstress test, the fetal heart rate is monitored with an external transducer. The tracing is observed for fetal heart rate accelerations peaking at least 15 beats per minute above the baseline and lasting 15 seconds from baseline to baseline. The testing can be continued for 40 minutes or longer to take into account the typical fetal sleep–wake cycle.

The results of a nonstress test are considered reactive (reassuring) if two or more fetal heart rate accelerations are detected within a 20-minute period, with or without fetal movement discernible by the mother. A nonreactive tracing is one without sufficient fetal heart rate accelerations over a 40-minute period. Acoustic stimulation (lasting 1 second) of a fetus that elicits fetal heart rate accelerations is also reassuring. The use of such stimulation can safely reduce overall testing time. Because fetal heart rate reactivity is a function of fetal maturity, false-positive nonreactive nonstress test results are more common before 28 weeks of gestation.

Contraction Stress Test

For a contraction stress test, the fetal heart rate is obtained using an external transducer, and uterine contraction activity is monitored with a tocodynamometer. A baseline tracing is obtained. If at least three contractions of 40 seconds or more are present in a 10-minute period, uterine stimulation is not necessary. If not, contractions are induced with either nipple stimulation or intravenously administered oxytocin. With nipple stimulation, the patient is instructed to rub one nipple gently through her clothing for 2 minutes or until a contraction begins. Stimulation is then stopped and restarted after 5 minutes if an adequate contraction frequency has not been attained. The cycle is repeated until an adequate contraction pattern is obtained. If the use of oxytocin is preferred by the patient or if nipple stimulation is unsuccessful, an intravenous infusion of low-dose oxytocin can be initiated, usually at a rate of 0.5–1.0 mU/min, and increased every 15–20 minutes until an adequate contraction pattern occurs. The results of the contraction stress test can be categorized as follows:

Negative: No late decelerations

Positive: Late decelerations follow 50% or more of contractions, even if the frequency of contractions is less than three in 10 minutes

Suspicious (equivocal): Intermittent late or variable decelerations

Unsatisfactory: Fewer than three contractions within 10 minutes or poor-quality tracing

Both oxytocin and nipple stimulation can produce hyperstimulation (contractions that occur more frequently than every 2 minutes or exceed 90 seconds in duration). If fetal heart rate decelerations occur in the presence of hyperstimulation, retesting is appropriate to ensure satisfactory interpretation.

Relative contraindications for contraction stress testing generally include the following conditions:

• Preterm premature rupture of membranes
• Classical uterine incision scar
• Placenta previa
• Unexplained vaginal bleeding

Biophysical Profile

Biophysical profile testing consists of a nonstress test with the addition of four observations made by real-time ultrasound. The five components of the biophysical profile are as follows:

1. Reactive nonstress test
2. Fetal breathing movements: One or more episodes of rhythmic fetal breathing movements of 30 seconds or more within 30 minutes
3. Fetal movement: Three or more discrete body or limb movements within 30 minutes

4. Fetal tone: One or more episodes of fetal extremity extension with return to flexion

5. Quantification of amniotic fluid volume: A pocket of amniotic fluid that measures at least 1 cm in two planes perpendicular to each other

With biophysical profile testing, a score of 2 (present) or 0 (absent) is assigned to each of the five observations. A score of 8 or 10 is reassuring, a score of 6 is equivocal and should lead to retesting within 12–24 hours, and a score of 4 or less is nonreassuring and warrants further evaluation and consideration of delivery. Irrespective of the score, more frequent biophysical profile testing or consideration of delivery is warranted when oligohydramnios is present.

Modified Biophysical Profile

As another approach to fetal surveillance, the modified biophysical profile combines the use of a nonstress test as a short-term indicator of fetal status with the assessment of amniotic fluid index as an indicator of long-term placental function. The amniotic fluid index is a semi-quantitative, four-quadrant assessment of amniotic fluid depth, for which ideal cutoff levels for intervention have not been established. The modified biophysical profile is less cumbersome than complete biophysical profile assessment and appears to be as predictive of fetal well-being as other approaches of biophysical fetal surveillance. Another approach is use of the ultrasound component of the biophysical profile alone, without the use of the nonstress test.

Conditions of Special Concern

Prevention of Preterm Labor

Prematurity continues to be the leading cause of perinatal mortality in the United States. Although the survival rate of low-birth-weight neonates has improved, there has been no improvement in the rate of preterm birth for several decades. Risk factors for preterm labor are described in Table 4–2.

Table 4–2. Risk Factors Associated with Spontaneous Preterm Labor and Birth

Pregnancy	Risk Factors
Past	Preterm birth
	Midtrimester spontaneous abortion
	Known uterine anomaly
	Exposure to diethylstilbestrol
	Incompetent cervix
Current	Hydramnios
	Second- or third-trimester bleeding
	Preterm labor
	Preterm premature rupture of membranes
	Multiple gestation
	Preterm cervical dilatation of ≥ 2 cm in a multipara and ≥ 1 cm in a primipara
	Prepregnancy weight <115 pounds
	Age <15 years

Because of the multitude of possible etiologies of preterm birth and the inability to alter many of them, achieving a significant decrease in the preterm birth rate will be difficult. Approximately one quarter of all preterm births are initiated by preterm premature rupture of the membranes, and another one quarter occur in association with maternal obstetric, medical, or surgical complications. Thus, at most only 50% of preterm births occur in women with spontaneous preterm labor.

Risk assessment and patient education about recognizing the signs of preterm labor have not been shown to be effective in preventing preterm birth. The use of home uterine activity monitoring has not been established to add independently to the value, if any, of frequent provider-initiated telephone contact or to result in significantly fewer preterm deliveries.

A more recent and promising strategy to reduce the rate of preterm birth has focused on antimicrobial intervention in women with one or more prior preterm births. The hypothesis tested in these selected populations is that alteration of the flora in the lower genital tract (eg, bacterial vaginosis) is associated with preterm birth. Appropriate maternal antimicrobial therapy in the midtrimester significantly reduced the rate of preterm birth by approximately one third in these populations. These reports need confirmation in more diverse patient populations, as well as in regard to the dosage and duration of treatment and a more precise evaluation of which antimicrobial agents may be most effective. (See "Management of Preterm Birth" in Chapter 6 for additional information.)

Postterm Gestation

Between 3% and 12% of pregnancies extend beyond the start of the 43rd week of gestation (294 days or more from the first day of the last menstrual period) and are considered postterm. Although many apparent cases of postterm pregnancy are the result of an inability to define the time of conception accurately, some patients clearly progress to excessively long gestations that can represent a significant risk to the fetus. Accurate assessment of gestational age may reduce the likelihood of misdiagnosis of postterm gestation.

Antepartum assessments by cervical examination, fetal heart rate testing (nonstress test or contraction stress test), ultrasound evaluation of amniotic fluid volume, biophysical profile, or a combination of these tests should be initiated between 41 and 42 weeks. Assessment should be repeated weekly or more often, depending on the clinical situation. If fetal testing is not reassuring, delivery is usually indicated. Even when fetal testing is reassuring but reliable dating establishes a gestational age of 42 weeks, induction of labor is an acceptable management strategy. In most instances, a patient is a candidate for induction of labor if the pregnancy is at greater than 41 weeks of gestation and the condition of the cervix is favorable.

Antepartum Hospitalization

Pregnant patients with complications who require hospitalization before the onset of labor should be admitted to a designated antepartum area, either inside or near the labor and delivery area. Obstetric patients with serious and acute complications should be assigned to an area where more intensive care and surveillance are available, such as the labor and delivery area or an intensive care unit. An obstetrician–gynecologist or a specialist in maternal–fetal medicine should be involved, either as the primary or the consulting physician, in the care of an obstetric patient with complications. When sufficiently recovered, the pregnant patient should be returned to the obstetric service, provided that her return does not jeopardize her own care or that of other obstetric patients.

Acutely ill obstetric patients who are likely to deliver a neonate requiring intensive care should be cared for in a specialty or subspecialty perinatal center. When feasible, antepartum transfer should be encouraged for these mothers.

Written policies and procedures for the management of pregnant patients seen in the emergency department or admitted to nonobstetric services should be established and approved by the medical staff and must comply with the requirements of federal and state transfer laws. When warranted by patient volume, a high-risk antepartum care unit should be developed to provide specialized nursing care and facilities for the mother and fetus at risk. When this is not feasible, written policies are recommended that specify how the care and transfer of pregnant patients with obstetric, medical, or surgical complications will be handled and where these patients will be assigned.

Whether an obstetric patient is admitted to the antepartum unit or to a nonobstetric unit, her condition should be evaluated soon thereafter by the primary physician or appropriate consultants. The evaluation should encompass a complete review of current illnesses as well as a medical, family, and social history. The condition of the patient and the reason for admission should determine the extent of the physical examination performed and the laboratory studies obtained. A copy of the patient's current prenatal record should become part of the hospital record as soon as possible after admission.

Bibliography

American Academy of Pediatrics, Committee on Genetics. Prenatal genetic diagnosis for pediatricians. Pediatrics 1994;93:1010–1015

American Academy of Pediatrics, Committee on Substance Abuse. Drug-exposed infants. Pediatrics 1995;96:364–367

American College of Obstetricians and Gynecologists. Diabetes and pregnancy. Technical Bulletin 200. Washington, DC: ACOG, 1994

American College of Obstetricians and Gynecologists. Guidelines for diagnostic imaging during pregnancy. Committee Opinion 158. Washington, DC: ACOG, 1995

American College of Obstetricians and Gynecologists. Sexual assault. Technical Bulletin 172. Washington, DC: ACOG, 1992

American College of Obstetricians and Gynecologists. Substance abuse in pregnancy. Technical Bulletin 195. Washington, DC: ACOG, 1994

Briggs GG, Freeman RK, Yaffe SJ. Drugs in pregnancy and lactation: a reference guide to fetal and neonatal risk. 4th ed. Baltimore, Maryland: Williams & Wilkins, 1994

Joint Commission on Accreditation of Healthcare Organizations. Comprehensive accreditation manual for hospitals. Oak Brook Terrace, Illinois: Joint Commission on Accreditation of Healthcare Organizations, 1995

March of Dimes Birth Defects Foundation, Committee on Perinatal Health. Toward improving the outcome of pregnancy: the 90s and beyond. White Plains, New York: March of Dimes Birth Defects Foundation, 1993

Chapter 5

Intrapartum Care

The goal of all labor and delivery units is safe birth for mothers and their newborns. At the same time, staff should attempt to make the patient and her supporters feel welcome, comfortable, and informed throughout the labor and delivery process. Ongoing risk assessment should determine appropriate care for the mother. The father or other primary support person should be encouraged to participate in the labor and delivery experience.

Labor and delivery is a normal physiologic process that most women experience without complications. Obstetric staff can greatly enhance this experience for the woman and her family by exhibiting a caring attitude and helping them understand the process. Efforts to promote healthy behaviors can be as effective during labor and delivery as they are during antepartum care. Physical contact between the newborn and the parents in the delivery room should be encouraged. Every effort should be made to foster family interaction and to support the desire of the family to be together.

Because intrapartum complications can arise, sometimes quickly and without warning, ongoing risk assessment and surveillance of the mother and fetus are essential. The hospital, including a birth center within the hospital complex, provides the safest setting for labor, delivery, and the postpartum period. The collection and analysis of data on the safety and outcome of deliveries in other settings, such as freestanding centers, have been problematic. The development of approved, well-designed research protocols, prepared in consultation with obstetric departments and their related institutional review boards, is appropriate to assess safety, feasibility, and birth outcomes in such settings. Until such data are available, the use of other settings is not encouraged. There may be exceptional situations, however, such as geographically isolated areas in which special programs are required.

Admission

Pregnant women may come to a hospital's labor and delivery area not only for obstetric care but also for treatment of any sign or symptom of illness. A nonobstetric condition may be best treated in another area of the hospital. The obstetric department should establish policies with other hospital units, such as the emergency department, for coordinated care of pregnant women. Departments should agree on which conditions are to be treated in the labor and delivery area and which should be treated in other hospital units. If a medical condition could reasonably be expected to lead to an obstetric consequence, the patient should be assessed in the labor and delivery unit. The obstetric department should also establish policies for the admission of nonobstetric patients according to state regulations (see "Nonobstetric Patients," Chapter 2). Federal and state regulations address the management and treatment of patients in hospital acute care areas, including labor and delivery.

Written departmental policies on triage of patients presenting to a labor and delivery area should be periodically reviewed for compliance with appropriate regulations. A pregnant women presenting to the labor and delivery area should undergo triage within a predetermined reasonable time. Initial evaluation will probably be performed by obstetric nursing staff. Any pregnant woman presenting to a hospital for care should, at a minimum, be assessed for the following:

- Fetal heart rate
- Maternal vital signs
- Uterine contractions

The responsible obstetric caregiver should be informed promptly if any of the following findings are present or suspected:

- Vaginal bleeding
- Acute abdominal pain

- Temperature of 100.4°F or higher
- Preterm labor
- Preterm premature rupture of membranes
- Hypertension

By 36 weeks of gestation, preregistration for labor and delivery at the hospital should be confirmed. A copy of the prenatal record that is on file in the hospital's labor registration area should be sent with information pertaining to the patient's antepartum course, including the results of any additional laboratory and ultrasound tests.

At the time of a patient's admission to the labor and delivery area, pertinent information from the record should be noted in the admission records. Because labor and delivery is a dynamic process, all entries into a patient's record should include the date and time of occurrence. Blood typing and screening tests need not be repeated if they were performed during the antepartum period and no antibodies were present, provided that the report is in the hospital records. If the mother's laboratory values are not known and cannot be obtained, blood typing, D (Rh) type determination, and serologic tests for syphilis should be done on cord blood before discharge. Collection of cord blood may be useful for subsequent testing if the mother is type O. Policies should be developed to ensure expeditious preparation of blood products for transfusion if the need arises or if the patient is at increased risk of hemorrhage. Any patient who is suspected to be in labor or who has rupture of the membranes or vaginal bleeding should be evaluated promptly in an obstetric service area. Whenever a pregnant woman is evaluated for labor, the following factors should be assessed and recorded:

- Blood pressure
- Pulse
- Temperature
- Frequency and duration of uterine contractions
- Fetal heart rate
- Clinical estimation of fetal weight
- Urinary protein and glucose

- Cervical dilatation and effacement, unless contraindicated (eg, placenta previa)
- Fetal presentation and station of the presenting part
- Status of the membranes
- Date and time of the patient's arrival and of notification of the provider

After initial evaluation, if the patient is in prodromal labor and has no complications, admission to the labor and delivery area may be deferred. Patients who have a transmissible infection should be admitted to a site where isolation techniques may be followed according to hospital policy.

If a woman has had prenatal care and a recent examination has confirmed the normal progress of pregnancy, her admission evaluation may be limited to an interval history and physical examination directed at the presenting complaint. Previously identified risk factors should be recorded in the prenatal record. If no new risk factors are found, attention may be focused on the following historical factors:

- Time of onset and frequency of contractions
- Status of the membranes
- Presence or absence of bleeding
- Fetal movement
- History of allergies
- Time, content, and amount of the most recent food or fluid ingestion
- Use of any medication

Serologic testing for hepatitis B virus surface antigen may be necessary as described in Chapter 9. Women who have not had prenatal care or who received such care late in pregnancy are more likely to have sexually transmissible infections and substance use problems. Social problems such as poverty and family conflict may also affect patients' health. A shortened obstetric hospital stay poses even greater problems for patients who have had no prenatal care. Routine obstetric screening tests, social intervention, and additional education may be needed within this limited time.

If no complications are detected during initial assessment in the labor and delivery area and if contraindications have been ruled out, qualified nursing personnel may perform the initial pelvic examination. Once the results of the examination have been obtained and documented, the provider responsible for the woman's care in the labor and delivery area should be informed of her status. A decision regarding her management can be made by the provider. The timing of the provider's arrival in the labor area should be based on this information and hospital policy. If epidural, spinal, or general anesthesia is anticipated, or if risk factors may require rapid institution of an anesthetic, anesthesia personnel should be informed of the patient's presence soon after her admission. If a preterm delivery, infected or depressed infant, or a prenatally diagnosed congenital anomaly is expected, the provider who will assume responsibility for the infant's care should be informed. When the patient has been examined and instructions regarding her management have been given and noted on the record, all necessary consent forms should be signed and incorporated into the record.

At all times in the hospital labor and delivery area, the safety and well-being of the mother and fetus are the primary concern and responsibility of the obstetric staff. This concern, however, should not unnecessarily restrict the activity of women with uncomplicated labor and delivery or exclude people who are supportive of her. The mother should have the option to stay out of bed during the early stages of labor, to walk about the room during labor, and to rest in a comfortable chair. Concerns such as showers during labor, placement of intravenous lines, use of fetal heart rate monitoring, and restrictions on ambulation should be reviewed in departmental policies, taking into consideration physicians' preferences as well as patients' desires, comfort, and sense of participation. Likewise, the use of drugs for relief of pain during labor and delivery should depend on the needs and desires of the woman. The development of a birth plan that has been discussed previously with a woman's provider and placed in her record will promote participation in and satisfaction with her care.

The team of providers for a woman and her fetus and newborn should be in communication with each other, discussing all factors that pose a risk to her health and that of her newborn. Obstetric departmental policies should include recommendations for transmitting to the nursery those maternal and fetal historical and laboratory data that may affect the care of the newborn. Information on conditions that may influence neonatal care should also be communicated. The lack of such data, perhaps through the lack of prenatal care, should also be made known to the nursery personnel. The physician who will care for the newborn baby should be identified on the maternal chart (Appendix A).

Labor

The onset of true labor is established by observing progressive change in a woman's cervix. This may require at least two cervical examinations that are separated by an adequate time to observe change. Excitement, fear, or discomfort may influence even a well-prepared woman to arrive at the hospital labor and delivery area before true labor has begun. A policy that allows for adequate evaluation of a patient for labor and that prevents the admission of women who are not in labor to the labor and delivery unit is advisable.

False Labor at Term

Uterine contractions in the absence of cervical change is commonly called "false labor." If the results of tests of fetal status are reassuring, false labor has little predictive value for adverse perinatal outcome. Treatment for this condition should be based on individual circumstances. After observation and evaluation by appropriately trained personnel, the patient may be discharged.

Premature Rupture of Membranes

Premature rupture of membranes (PROM) is considered to be present when there is leakage of amniotic fluid at least 1 hour before the onset of labor. Preparations for labor and delivery should begin when PROM occurs, whether at or before term, because labor frequently ensues. Management of PROM is not uniform, and several different but reasonable strategies exist for the care of a patient with PROM. Each hospital's department of obstetrics and gynecology, in consultation with the department of pediatrics, should establish guidelines for the care of patients with PROM at that hospital. These guidelines should address methods of diagnosis, use of antenatal corticosteroids in preterm PROM, use of induction of labor at certain gestational ages, timing and use of antibiotics for both prophylaxis and treatment of mother and fetus, and consideration of location of the delivery in the case of anticipated preterm birth.

The diagnosis of PROM depends on history, physical examination, and laboratory confirmation. Diagnosis based on history alone is correct in more than 90% of patients. Nevertheless, all patients reporting symptoms that suggest ruptured membranes should be examined with a sterile speculum as soon as possible to confirm this diagnosis. Gross pooling of amniotic fluid in the vagina is nearly 100% diagnostic of PROM. Management is determined by the presence or absence of PROM. Supportive laboratory testing confirmation can be done by vaginal pH and fern testing.

The obstetric caregivers who perform the examination to confirm or rule out PROM should be aware of the causes of false-positive and false-negative results that occur with the use of phenaphthazine and fern testing. These causes include leakage of alkaline urine, cervical mucus, and blood. Ultrasound to determine an amniotic fluid index may help to confirm the diagnosis by documenting oligohydramnios. (See Chapter 6 for a discussion of the management of preterm PROM.)

If chorioamnionitis is diagnosed, labor should be induced with oxytocin. Tocolytic agents have been shown to be of no benefit with preterm PROM (see Chapter 6). As in any labor occurring after rupture of membranes, vaginal examinations should be limited in number and attention paid to clean technique.

Management of Labor

Ideally, any woman admitted to the labor and delivery area should know who is her designated care provider. The other members of the obstetric team should observe the patient to follow the progress of labor, record her vital signs and the fetal heart rate at regular intervals on her chart, and make an effort to ensure her understanding of the events taking place. The provider responsible for the patient's care should be kept informed of her progress and notified promptly of any abnormality. When the patient is in active labor, the provider should be readily available to provide care.

Patients in active labor should avoid oral ingestion of anything except sips of clear liquids, occasional ice chips, or preparations for moistening the mouth and lips. When significant amounts of hydration and energy substrate are needed because of a long labor, they should be given by intravenous infusion.

The progress of labor should be evaluated by periodic vaginal examinations. Attention to perineal hygiene may help reduce infection of the upper genital tract. If the membranes are ruptured, attention to clean technique is important. Sterile, water-soluble lubricants may be used to reduce discomfort during vaginal examinations. Antiseptics such as povidone-iodine and hexachlorophene have not been shown to decrease infections acquired during the intrapartum period. Furthermore, these agents may produce local irritation and are absorbed through maternal mucous membranes. Thus, lubricants containing these agents, and sprays or liquids delivering them directly to the introitus, are not recommended for use during labor.

For women who are at no increased risk of complications, evaluation of the quality of the uterine contractions and pelvic examinations should be sufficient to detect abnormalities in the progress of labor. Vital signs should be recorded at regular intervals, at least every 4 hours. This frequency may be increased, particularly as active labor progresses according to clinical signs and symptoms. Documentation of the course of a woman's labor may include, but need not be limited to, the presence of physicians or nurses, position changes, cervical status, oxygen and drug administration, blood pressure, temperature, amniotomy or spontaneous rupture of membranes, color of amniotic fluid, and Valsalva efforts.

Fetal Heart Rate Monitoring

Fetal heart rate monitoring to reflect fetal status during labor can be done by intermittent auscultation or continuous electronic means.

Guidelines should clearly delineate the procedures to be followed for using these techniques and for interpreting the observations. The intensity of fetal heart rate monitoring and the method used for fetal surveillance during labor may vary, depending on both the risk assessment at admission and the preference of the obstetric staff, which will be influenced by departmental policy and experience. If risk factors are present at admission or appear during the course of labor, there is no difference in perinatal outcome between intermittent auscultation and continuous fetal monitoring if one of the following methods for fetal heart rate monitoring is used:

• During active labor in stage I, the fetal heart rate should be determined and recorded at least every 15 minutes, preferably just after a uterine contraction, when intermittent auscultation is used. If continuous fetal heart rate monitoring is used, the heart rate tracing should be evaluated at least every 15 minutes.

• During stage II labor, the fetal heart rate should be determined and recorded at least every 5 minutes if auscultation is used. If continuous fetal heart rate monitoring is used, the tracing should be evaluated at least every 5 minutes.

If no risk factors are present at the time of the patient's admission, a standard approach to fetal surveillance is to determine and record the fetal heart rate at least every 30 minutes just after a contraction in active stage I labor and at least every 15 minutes in stage II labor.

The appropriate use of fetal monitoring includes recording and interpreting the tracings. Nonreassuring findings should be noted and communicated to the physician or nurse–midwife so that appropriate intervention can occur. When a change in the rate has been noted, it is also important to document a subsequent return to reassuring findings. Terms that describe the fetal heart rate patterns (eg, *early*, *late*, or *variable decelerations*; *accelerations*; and *beat-to-beat variability*) should be used in both chart entries and verbal communication between obstetric personnel.

Internal fetal heart rate monitoring and internal uterine pressure monitoring may be used to gain further information about fetal status and uterine contractility, respectively. Relative contraindications to internal fetal monitoring include maternal human immunodeficiency virus infection and other high-risk factors for fetal infection, including herpes simplex virus and hepatitis B virus.

A fetal scalp blood sample may be used to obtain information about fetal acid–base status during labor if the fetal heart rate pattern is nonreassuring or uninterpretable. Fetal scalp or acoustic stimulation that results in acceleration of the fetal heart rate is also reassuring if the fetal heart rate pattern is difficult to interpret.

If fetal monitoring is used, all fetal heart rate tracings should be identified with the patient's name, hospital number, and the date and time of admission. All fetal heart rate tracings should be easily retrievable from storage so that the events of labor can be studied in proper relationship to the tracings.

Induction and Augmentation of Labor

Each hospital's department of obstetrics and gynecology should develop written protocols for preparing and administering oxytocin solution. Indications for induction and augmentation of labor should be stated. The qualifications of personnel authorized to administer oxytocin for this purpose should be described. Methods for assessment of mother and fetus before and during oxytocin infusion should be specified. It is recommended that fetal heart rate monitoring be performed as delineated for high-risk patients in active labor.

Oxytocin is used to induce labor when the benefits to either the mother or the fetus outweigh those of continuing the pregnancy. The infusion should be administered by a device that permits precise control of the flow rate to ensure accurate, minute-to-minute control. Oxytocin is also used to augment labor and enhance inadequate uterine contractions in women in whom an assessment of the relationship between the maternal pelvis and fetal size is otherwise normal. Buccal or intramuscular administration of oxytocin should not be used to induce or augment labor.

Various regimens exist for the intravenous infusion of oxytocin to stimulate uterine contractions. These regimens vary in initial dose, amount of incremental dose increase, and interval between dose increases. Each hospital's department of obstetrics and gynecology should determine which regimen will be standard for that hospital so that obstetric staff in the labor and delivery area may develop guidelines for its application to individual patients. Regimens described as "low-dose" and with a less frequent increase are associated with a lower incidence of uterine hyperstimulation. Higher and more frequent dosage regimens are credited with shortening time in labor and reducing the incidence of chorioamnionitis and the number of cesarean deliveries performed for dystocia.

When oxytocin is used during labor, a physician who has privileges to perform cesarean deliveries should be readily available. The patient's record should document who is the responsible physician. A qualified member of the obstetric team should perform a vaginal examination of the patient before oxytocin infusion is initiated. Personnel who are familiar with the effects of oxytocin and who are able to identify both maternal and fetal complications should be in attendance during administration of the agent.

Cervical ripening may be beneficial if the cervix is unfavorable for induction. Acceptable interventions for preparing an unfavorable cervix for induction include mechanical dilation with laminaria placed in the cervical canal and administration of prostaglandin E_2 in doses appropriate for cervical ripening. If the fetus's estimated gestational age is near term, routine intravenous oxytocin induction is usually effective. Prostaglandin E_2 suppositories and more concentrated intravenous oxytocin regimens are both effective for terminating a pregnancy complicated by fetal death, especially at a gestational age of 28 weeks or less. Because of the risk of uterine rupture, caution should be exercised when prostaglandins are used after 28 weeks of gestation. Contraindications to the induction of labor with prostaglandins for fetal death include maternal cyanotic or ischemic cardiac disease and severe asthma.

Induction of labor by stripping the amniotic membranes is a relatively common practice. Risks associated with this procedure include infection, bleeding from an undiagnosed placenta previa or low-lying placenta, and accidental rupture of membranes. Membrane stripping may be associated with a higher frequency of spontaneous labor and with a decreased incidence of postterm gestation.

Artificial rupture of membranes is another nonpharmacologic method of labor induction that may be used, particularly when the cervix is favorable. Routine early amniotomy results in a modest reduction in the duration of labor.

When induction is essential, it is reasonable to perform amniotomy as an adjunct to oxytocin infusion, even with minimal cervical dilation, if the presenting part is well applied to the cervix and the minimal risk of cord prolapse is outweighed by the perceived benefits of rapid induction. When the situation is less urgent, it is reasonable to wait to perform an amniotomy until cervical dilatation is more advanced.

Care should be taken to palpate for an umbilical cord and avoid dislodging the fetal head. The fetal heart rate should be recorded before and immediately after the procedure.

Amnioinfusion

The transcervical infusion of sterile, balanced salt solutions during labor (amnioinfusion) is used in many hospital labor and delivery areas to ameliorate variable decelerations of the fetal heart rate tracing that are suspected to be due to umbilical cord compression. This technique has also been used to dilute thick meconium.

Analgesia and Anesthesia

Management of discomfort and pain during labor and delivery is a necessary part of good obstetric practice. Maternal request is sufficient justification for providing pain relief during labor.

Some patients tolerate the pain of labor by using techniques learned in childbirth preparation programs. The most common methods of preparation are Lamaze, Bradley, and Read. Although specific techniques vary, classes usually seek to relieve pain through the general principles of education, support, relaxation, paced breathing, focusing, and touch. The staff at the bedside should be knowledgeable about these pain-management techniques and should be supportive of the patient's decision to use them.

Unless contraindicated, pharmacologic analgesics to ameliorate the pain of contractions should be made available on request to women in labor. The choice and availability of analgesic and anesthetic techniques depend on the experience and judgment of the obstetrician and anesthesiologist, the physical condition of the patient, the circumstances of labor and delivery, and the personal preferences of the obstetrician and the patient. Parenteral opioids provide some degree of pain relief with minimal risks. High doses are potentially depressant to both mother and fetus and should be carefully monitored. Similarly, a low concentration of inhalation analgesia may be useful in the active phase of labor. Barbiturates, tranquilizers, and narcotics can be administered during prodromal and early labor to allow the patient to rest.

Of the various pharmacologic methods used for pain relief during labor and delivery, lumbar epidural block is the most flexible, effective, and least depressing to the central nervous system, allowing for an alert, participating mother. Lumbar epidural block has been associated with an increased incidence of operative abdominal and vaginal delivery. However, the administration of a dilute solution of local anesthetic (which results in less motor blockade) may minimize the increased incidence of operative delivery associated with epidural analgesia. Unless contraindications are present, women who request epidural anesthesia should be able to receive it.

Recently, some anesthesiologists have recently advocated the administration of spinal analgesia during the first stage of labor. This technique typically involves intermittent or continuous intrathecal administration of an opioid without a local anesthetic. Some physicians perform a combined spinal–epidural technique.

Paracervical block, when used for pain relief during labor, may result in fetal bradycardia. The fetal heart rate should be monitored closely before, during, and after the administration of paracervical block. Bupivacaine is contraindicated for use in paracervical block.

At the time of delivery, local infiltration of the perineum and pudendal block are safe anesthesia techniques to control the discomfort of delivery without impairing the mother's expulsive efforts. Although spinal anesthesia can provide adequate pain relief and muscle relaxation for nearly all vaginal deliveries, it typically results in profound sensory and motor blockade, which impairs maternal expulsive efforts. Thus, spinal anesthesia typically is not administered until delivery is imminent or the obstetrician has made a decision to perform an operative delivery. General anesthesia is rarely necessary for vaginal delivery and should be used only for specific indications.

For most cesarean deliveries, properly administered regional or general anesthesia is effective and has little adverse effect on the newborn. Because of the maternal risks associated with intubation and the possibility of aspiration during induction of general anesthesia, regional anesthesia may be the preferred technique and should be available in all hospitals that provide obstetric care. The advantages and disadvantages of both techniques should be discussed with the patient as completely as possible. Examples of circumstances in which rapid induction of general anesthesia may be indicated include a prolapsed umbilical cord with severe fetal bradycardia, and acute hemorrhage in a hemodynamically unstable mother.

If properly chosen and administered, analgesia or anesthesia during labor and delivery has little or no lasting effect on the physiologic status of the neonate. At present, no evidence exists that the administration of analgesia or anesthesia during childbirth per se has a significant effect on the child's later mental and neurologic development.

Because the safety of obstetric anesthesia depends primarily on the skill of the anesthesiologist, and because obstetric anesthesia must be considered emergency anesthesia, its use demands a level of competence in personnel and an availability of equipment that are similar to those required for elective surgical procedures. Regional anesthesia in obstetrics should be initiated and maintained only by providers who are approved through the institutional credentialing process to administer or supervise the administration of obstetric anesthesia. These individuals must be qualified to manage anesthetic complications. An obstetrician may administer the anesthesia if granted privileges for these procedures. However, having an anesthesiologist or anesthetist provide this care permits the obstetrician to give undivided attention to the delivery.

It is the responsibility of the director of anesthesia services to make recommendations regarding the clinical privileges of all anesthesia service personnel. If obstetric anesthesia is provided by obstetricians, the director of anesthesia services should participate with a representative of the obstetric department in the formulation of procedures designed to ensure the uniform quality of anesthesia services throughout the hospital. Specific recommendations regarding these procedures are provided in the *Accreditation Manual for Hospitals* published by the Joint Commission on Accreditation of Healthcare Organizations. The directors of departments providing anesthesia services are responsible for implementing processes to monitor and evaluate the quality and appropriateness of these services in their respective departments.

Regional anesthesia should be administered only after (1) the patient has been examined by a qualified individual and (2) the maternal and fetal status and progress of labor have been evaluated by a physician with credentials in obstetrics who concurs with the initiation of anesthesia and is readily available to supervise the labor and manage any obstetric complications that may arise. When regional anesthesia is administered during labor, the patient's vital signs should be monitored at regular intervals by a qualified member of the health care team.

The following factors place a woman at increased risk from anesthesia and should be communicated to the anesthesia care provider in advance of delivery to permit formulation of a management plan:

- Marked obesity
- Severe facial and neck edema
- Extremely short stature
- Difficulty opening her mouth
- Small mandible or protuberant teeth or both
- Arthritis of the neck
- Short neck
- Anatomic abnormalities of the face or mouth
- Large thyroid
- Asthma or other chronic pulmonary disease
- Cardiac disease
- History of problems attributable to anesthetics

- Bleeding disorders
- Severe preeclampsia/eclampsia
- Other significant medical or obstetric complications

Aspiration is a significant leading cause of anesthetic-related maternal mortality and morbidity, and the aspiration of acidic gastric contents with a pH of less than 2.5 is more harmful than the aspiration of less acidic gastric contents. Therefore, prophylactic administration of an antacid before induction of a major regional or general anesthesia is appropriate. Particulate antacids may be harmful if aspirated; a clear antacid, such as a solution of 0.3-mol/L sodium citrate or a similar preparation, may be a safer choice.

On rare occasions, it may be impossible to intubate an obstetric patient after the induction of general anesthesia. Emergency percutaneous transtracheal/cricothyroid ventilation may be lifesaving in this circumstance, and the necessary equipment for performing this procedure should be immediately available whenever general anesthesia is administered.

Delivery

Vaginal Delivery

Vaginal birth is associated with less risk of operative and postoperative complications than cesarean delivery and results in shorter hospital stays. Vaginal birth requires consideration of the following:

- The probable need for additional professionals with special skills in neonatal resuscitation
- Anesthesia personnel to manage maternal anesthetic complications
- Additional obstetric attendants to the delivery
- The need to move a patient from a labor–delivery–recovery room to an operative suite

The risk assessment performed upon the patient's admission, the course of the patient's labor, the fetal presentation, any abnormalities encountered during the labor process, and the anesthetic technique in use or anticipated for delivery will all have an impact on the need for other professionals. At least one obstetric nurse, preferably the woman's designated primary nurse for the labor, should be present in the delivery room throughout the delivery. Despite the exigency of the moments immediately preceding delivery, no attempt should be made to delay birth by physical restraint or anesthetic means. Episiotomy may be used to aid in the management of delivery in some situations. The routine use of episiotomy is not necessary and leads to a delay in the patient's resumption of sexual activity.

Vaginal Birth After Cesarean Delivery

Unless vaginal delivery is contraindicated, women who have had one previous cesarean delivery with an incision in the lower uterine segment should be counseled and encouraged to attempt labor in their current pregnancy. This counseling can begin immediately after the cesarean delivery by obstetric staff attending to the woman's recovery and postpartum care. The type of uterine incision should be noted for the patient, and she should be encouraged to attempt a vaginal birth in any future pregnancy, if appropriate.

Studies of large obstetric populations show that 60–80% of patients who are candidates for vaginal birth after a low transverse uterine incision from one previous cesarean birth will have successful vaginal births. Counseling for vaginal birth after cesarean delivery should include the advantages of vaginal birth—including less risk of complications and shorter hospital stays—as well as consideration of its complications, including uterine rupture. Symptomatic uterine rupture requiring emergency intervention is infrequent (occurring in less than 1% of all attempted vaginal births after cesarean deliveries), and serious maternal and fetal consequences usually can be minimized by appropriate intrapartum surveillance. The most common sign of uterine rupture is an abrupt change in fetal heart rate pattern, including bradycardia or prolonged decelerations; therefore, plans for rapid diagnosis and appropriate intervention should be in place before a trial of labor is undertaken.

A woman who has had two or more previous cesarean deliveries with low transverse incisions can also be encouraged and permitted to attempt vaginal birth if she wishes and if there are no contraindications. Reasonable efforts should be made to document the type of previous uterine incision. If unsuccessful, a judgment must be made as to the advisability of a trial of labor. It must be recognized that in certain geographic areas the classical uterine incision continues to be used, especially for some patients who undergo cesarean delivery for extreme prematurity or malpresentation. This type of delivery is a contraindication to future vaginal birth.

No woman should be mandated to undergo a trial of labor. For an individual woman, certain social, geographic, or past obstetric circumstances may preclude a trial of labor and vaginal delivery after cesarean delivery.

Operative Vaginal Delivery

Forceps and vacuum extraction are valuable tools to effect operative vaginal delivery. The following definitions and indications relate to both techniques:

Station: The relationship of the estimated distances, in centimeters, between the leading bony portion of the fetal head and the level of the maternal ischial spines. In classifying forceps and vacuum extraction procedures, the level of engagement of the fetal head must be stated as precisely as possible. Engagement of the head occurs when the biparietal diameter has passed through the pelvic inlet. It is clinically diagnosed when the leading bony portion of the fetal head is at or below the level of the ischial spines (station 0 or more). Although the preferred method to describe station beyond the level of the ischial spines is to estimate centimeters below the spines, some continue to find it useful to refer to station in estimated thirds of the maternal pelvis below the spines. An approximate correlation of these two methods of describing station would be:

2 cm = +1/3 (mid)
4 cm = +2/3 (low)
6 cm = +3/3 (outlet)

Outlet forceps: The application of forceps when (1) the fetal scalp is visible at the introitus without separating the labia, (2) the fetal skull has reached the pelvic floor, (3) the fetal sagittal suture is in the anterior–posterior diameter or in the right or left occiput anterior or posterior position, and (4) the fetal head is at or on the perineum. According to this definition, rotation cannot exceed 45°. There is no difference in perinatal outcome when deliveries involving the use of outlet forceps are compared with similar spontaneous deliveries, and no data support the concept that rotating the head on the pelvic floor 45° or less increases morbidity.

Low forceps: The application of forceps when the leading point of the fetal skull is at station +2 or more and not on the pelvic floor. Low forceps applications have two subdivisions: (1) rotation 45° or less (eg, left or right occipitoanterior to occiput anterior, or left or right occipitoposterior to occiput posterior) and (2) rotation more than 45°.

Midforceps: The application of forceps when the fetal head is engaged but the leading point of the skull is above station +2. Under very unusual circumstances, such as the sudden onset of severe fetal or maternal compromise, application of forceps above station +2 may be attempted while simultaneously initiating preparations for a cesarean delivery in the event that the forceps maneuver is unsuccessful. Forceps should not be applied to an unengaged fetal presenting part or when the cervix is not completely dilated.

Indications for a forceps or vacuum extraction operation, including the position and station of the vertex at the time of application of the forceps or vacuum apparatus, should be identified in a detailed operative description in the patient's medical record. These indications include the following:

• Shortening the second stage of labor: Outlet forceps or vacuum extraction may be used to shorten the second stage of labor in the best interests of the mother or the fetus.

- Ending a prolonged second stage: The following time periods are approximate; when these intervals are exceeded without continuing progress, the risks and benefits of allowing labor to continue should be assessed and documented:
  — Nulliparous patients—more than 3 hours with a regional anesthetic or more than 2 hours without a regional anesthetic
  — Parous patients—more than 2 hours with a regional anesthetic or more than 1 hour without a regional anesthetic
- Nonreassuring fetal heart rate
- Maternal indications (eg, cardiac disease, exhaustion)

The following conditions are required for forceps or vacuum extraction operations:

- A person experienced in performing these procedures or supervising the procedure
- Assessment of maternal pelvis–fetal size relationship
- Adequate anesthesia
- Willingness to abandon attempted operative vaginal delivery
- Ability to perform emergency cesarean delivery

Cesarean Delivery

All hospitals offering labor and delivery services should be equipped to perform emergency cesarean delivery. The required personnel, including nurses, anesthetists, neonatal resuscitation team members, and obstetric attendants, should be in the hospital or readily available. Any hospital providing an obstetric service should have the capability of responding to an obstetric emergency. No data correlate the timing of intervention with outcome, and there is little likelihood that any will be obtained. However, consensus has been that hospitals should have the capability of beginning a cesarean delivery within 30 minutes of the decision to operate. Not all indications for a cesarean delivery will require a 30-minute response time. Examples of those mandating the need for expeditious delivery include hemorrhage from placenta previa, abruptio placentae, prolapse of the umbilical cord, and uterine rupture. Sterile materials and supplies needed for emergency cesarean delivery should be kept sealed but properly arranged so that the instrument table can be made ready at once for an obstetric emergency. In-house obstetric and anesthesia coverage should be available in subspecialty units. The anesthesia staff responsible for covering the labor and delivery unit should be informed in advance when a complicated delivery is anticipated and when a patient with risk factors requiring a high-acuity level of care is admitted. Elective repeat cesarean delivery does not establish a high-risk situation for the neonate. However, a qualified person who is skilled in neonatal resuscitation should be in the operative delivery room, with all equipment needed for neonatal resuscitation, to care for the neonate. The duties of the surgical and anesthetic teams may prevent them from performing immediate neonatal care of the newborn.

In women requiring cesarean delivery, fetal surveillance should continue until abdominal sterile preparation is begun. If internal fetal heart rate monitoring is in use, it should be continued until the abdominal sterile preparation is complete.

Prior to elective repeat cesarean delivery, the maturity of the fetus should be established. For patients with an indication for an elective repeat cesarean delivery, fetal maturity may be assumed if one of the following criteria is met:

- Fetal heart tones have been documented for 20 weeks by nonelectronic fetoscope or for 30 weeks by Doppler ultrasound.

- Thirty-six weeks have elapsed since positive results were obtained from a serum or urine human chorionic gonadotropin pregnancy test performed by a reliable laboratory.

- An ultrasound measurement of the crown–rump length obtained at 6–11 weeks of gestation supports a current gestational age of 39 weeks or more.

- Clinical history and physical and ultrasound examinations performed at 12–20 weeks of gestation support a current gestational age of 39 weeks or more.

These criteria are not intended to preclude the use of menstrual dating. If any one criterion confirms gestational age assessment in a patient who has normal menstrual cycles and no immediate antecedent use of oral contraceptives, it is appropriate to schedule delivery at

39 weeks or later on the basis of menstrual dates. Another option is to await the onset of spontaneous labor.

Support Persons in the Delivery Room

Childbirth is a momentous family experience. Obstetric caregivers should willingly provide opportunities for those accompanying and supporting the woman giving birth to participate in the process. These support persons must be informed about requirements for safety and must be willing to follow the directions of the obstetric staff concerning behavior in the delivery room. They should also understand the normal events and procedures in the labor and delivery area. They must conform to the dress code required of personnel in attendance in a delivery room. Both the obstetrician and the patient should consent to the presence of fathers or other support persons in the delivery room. Support persons should realize that their major function is to provide psychologic support to the mother during labor and delivery.

The judgment of the obstetric staff, the individual obstetrician, the anesthesiologist, and the pediatric support personnel, as well as the policies of the hospital, determine whether support persons may be present at a cesarean birth. A written policy developed by all involved hospital staff is recommended.

Immediate Postpartum Maternal Care

Monitoring of maternal status is dictated in part by the events of the delivery process and the complications identified. Blood pressure and pulse should be monitored at least every 15 minutes and more frequently if complications are encountered. Temperature should be taken at least every 4 hours.

Postanesthesia care must be provided as outlined and assigned by prearrangement with the anesthetists responsible for administering obstetric anesthesia. Nursing staff assigned to the delivery and immediate recovery of a woman should have no other obligations. Discharge from the delivery room, which may involve recovery from an anesthetic, should be at the discretion of the physician or certified nurse–midwife or the anesthesiologist in charge.

Neonatal Resuscitation

Both routine assessment and care of the baby at the time of delivery and the possible provision of extensive resuscitation should be provided in accordance with the American Heart Association/American Academy of Pediatrics Neonatal Resuscitation Program. Hospital medical staff concerned with care and resuscitation of the newborn, including obstetricians, anesthetists, and pediatricians, should determine the qualifications needed for performance of neonatal resuscitation, including completion of the American Heart Association/ American Academy of Pediatrics Neonatal Resuscitation program. At least one person who is skilled in initiating resuscitation should be present at every delivery. A second individual to assist in resuscitation should also be readily available.

Recognition and immediate resuscitation of a distressed neonate requires an organized plan of action and the immediate availability of qualified personnel and equipment as described in the American Academy of Pediatrics and the American Heart Association *Textbook of Neonatal Resuscitation.* Responsibility for identification and resuscitation of a distressed neonate should be assigned to a qualified individual, who may be a physician or an appropriately trained nurse–midwife, labor and delivery nurse, nurse–anesthetist, nursery nurse, or respiratory therapist. The provision of services and equipment for resuscitation should be planned jointly by the directors of the departments of obstetrics, anesthesia, and pediatrics, with the approval of the medical staff. A physician should be designated to assume primary responsibility for initiating, supervising, and reviewing the plan for management of depressed neonates in the delivery room. The following factors should be considered in this plan:

- A list of maternal and fetal complications that require the presence in the delivery room of someone specifically qualified in all aspects of newborn resuscitation should be developed.
- Individuals qualified to perform neonatal resuscitation should demonstrate the following capabilities:
  — Skills in rapid and accurate evaluation of the newborn condition, including Apgar scoring.

— Knowledge of the pathogenesis and causes of a low Apgar score (eg, hypoxia, drugs, hypovolemia, trauma, anomalies, infections, and prematurity), as well as specific indications for resuscitation.

— Skills in airway management (eg, laryngoscopy, endotracheal intubation, suctioning of the airway), artificial ventilation, cardiac massage, emergency administration of drugs and fluids, and maintenance of thermal stability. The ability to recognize and decompress tension pneumothorax by needle aspiration is also a desirable skill.

• Procedures should be developed to ensure the readiness of equipment and personnel and to provide for intermittent review and evaluation of the effectiveness of the system.

• Contingency plans should be established for multiple births and other unusual circumstances.

• A physician for the neonate need not be present at a delivery, provided that no complications are anticipated and another skilled individual is present to care for the neonate.

• The resuscitation steps should be documented in the records.

Apgar Score

Apgar scores are useful for describing the status of the infant at birth and his or her subsequent adaptation to the extrauterine environment. Apgar scores (Table 5–1) should be obtained at 1 minute and 5 minutes after birth and for an extended period until the Apgar score is 7 or greater.

When necessary, resuscitation should be initiated before the 1-minute Apgar score is obtained. The Apgar score should be assigned by someone not directly involved in resuscitating the neonate. Low scores (<3), especially those associated with a delay in the return of tone, are useful in identifying the neonate who is significantly depressed; the change between the 1-minute score and the 5-minute score is useful in assessing the efficacy of resuscitation.

If a low Apgar score is anticipated or assigned, rapid assessment of the neonate's condition is necessary to delineate a plan of care. Um-

Table 5–1. Criteria for Assigning an Apgar Score

Sign	Apgar Score		
	0	1	2
Heart rate	Absent	<100 beats per minute	≥100 beats per minute
Respirations	Absent	Weak cry; hypoventilation	Good, strong cry
Muscle tone	Limp	Some flexion	Active motion
Reflex irritability	No response	Grimace	Cry or active withdrawal
Color	Blue or pale	Body, pink; extremities, blue	Completely pink

bilical cord blood gas and pH analyses may help to distinguish metabolic acidemia secondary to hypoxia from other causes of low Apgar scores in the depressed neonate.

Maintenance of Body Temperature

Immediately following delivery, the neonate should be put in a warm place and dried completely. Drying the neonate with prewarmed towels immediately after birth reduces evaporative heat loss. It is recommended that a radiant warmer with a servocontrol mechanism be placed in the resuscitation area, because such devices allow easy access to the neonate during resuscitation procedures.

Suctioning

The neonate's mouth may be suctioned gently to remove excess mucus or blood. Although clear mucus is suctioned from the mouth routinely in most centers, there is no evidence to support the value of this practice. Vigorous suctioning of the posterior pharynx should be avoided, as this may produce significant bradycardia.

If there is meconium in the amniotic fluid, the mouth and hypopharynx should be thoroughly suctioned with a mechanical device before delivery of the shoulders in a cephalic presentation and immediately after delivery of the head in a breech presentation. In the presence of thick or particulate meconium, the larynx should be visualized and any meconium present removed. If meconium is present and the infant is depressed, the clinician should intubate the trachea and suction to remove meconium or other aspirated material from beneath the glottis. If the infant is vigorous, the indication for vocal cord visualization and tracheal aspiration of meconium is less clear. It has been suggested that for the vigorous and spontaneously breathing infant who may have aspirated the meconium, less indication exists for aggressive removal. Furthermore, injury to the vocal cords is more likely to occur in attempting to intubate a vigorous infant. When using a mechanical suction apparatus, the suction pressure should be set so that when the suction tubing is occluded the negative pressure does not exceed 100 mm Hg.

Ventilation

The normal neonate breathes within seconds of delivery and has established regular respiration within 1 minute of delivery. A flaccid neonate who is not breathing spontaneously and whose heart rate is less than 100 beats per minute requires immediate positive pressure ventilation. A bag and mask can often provide effective ventilation (Fig. 5–1), but it may be difficult to use this method in premature neonates with noncompliant lungs. If the neonate's heart rate does not rise promptly to more than 60–80 beats per minute, endotracheal intubation is required.

Before applying positive pressure ventilation, it is important to ensure that the airway has been cleared. The head should be placed in a sniffing position, with care to avoid hyperextension of the neck. The middle or fourth finger should be placed behind the posterior ramus of the mandible, thrusting the mandible forward; no fingers (or any part of the mask) should rest on the soft tissues of the neck. Initial lung inflation may require 30–40 cm H_2O, and 15–20 cm H_2O is often adequate for succeeding breaths, which should be provided at a rate of 40–60 per minute. With rare exceptions, depressed neonates respond promptly to adequate ventilation, and this is the only resuscitation maneuver required.

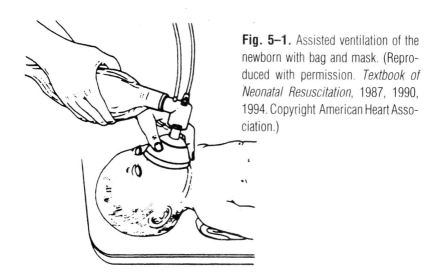

Fig. 5–1. Assisted ventilation of the newborn with bag and mask. (Reproduced with permission. *Textbook of Neonatal Resuscitation,* 1987, 1990, 1994. Copyright American Heart Association.)

Symmetric movement of the apices of the chest; equal breath sounds (heard in the axillae); and improvement in heart rate, color, and muscle tone indicate satisfactory ventilation. The response of the heart rate is the most useful and readily measurable criterion of adequate resuscitation. If the response to ventilation is not prompt, the seal between the face and the mask or the position of the endotracheal tube should be checked. If chest movement and breath sounds appear satisfactory in an intubated neonate, yet the neonate is not responding, the position of the endotracheal tube should be checked by direct visualization of the larynx with a laryngoscope.

External Cardiac Massage

If the heart rate does not rise promptly to more than 60–80 beats per minute after effective ventilation with oxygen, external cardiac massage should be instituted while ventilation is continued. Two techniques are illustrated in Figure 5–2. Chest compressions should be carried out at a rate of 90 compressions and 30 ventilations per minute (ratio of 3:1) to a depth of ½–¾ inch. If there is no response in the heart

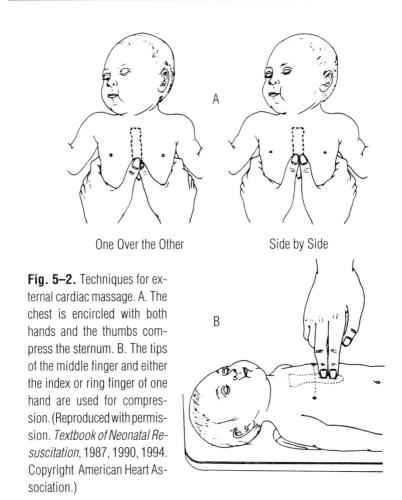

One Over the Other   Side by Side

Fig. 5–2. Techniques for external cardiac massage. A. The chest is encircled with both hands and the thumbs compress the sternum. B. The tips of the middle finger and either the index or ring finger of one hand are used for compression. (Reproduced with permission. *Textbook of Neonatal Resuscitation*, 1987, 1990, 1994. Copyright American Heart Association.)

rate, appropriate drug therapy (and volume expansion, if indicated) should be instituted.

Drugs and Volume Expansion

The use of drugs for resuscitation of the neonate is rarely necessary in the delivery room. When drugs are needed, they should not be administered until ventilation and circulation have been established. The emergency route of administration is the umbilical vein. The infusion of epinephrine into the trachea via an endotracheal tube may also be an effective route of administration.

Acidosis. Severely depressed neonates may have a combined metabolic and respiratory acidosis. The treatment of acidosis is treatment of the cause. Thus, respiratory acidosis, which is the result of hypoventilation, is treated by providing positive pressure ventilation. Metabolic acidosis is the result of hypoxemia or hypoperfusion, and the correction of these factors should correct the acidosis.

Significant acidemia is detrimental to myocardial function in the hypoxic heart. Sodium bicarbonate may be useful in a prolonged resuscitation to help correct a documented metabolic acidosis, but its use is discouraged in brief arrests or episodes of bradycardia. In the absence of adequate ventilation, sodium bicarbonate will not improve blood pH significantly. One molar sodium (8.4%) bicarbonate should not be used. One-half molar sodium (4.2%) bicarbonate or lesser concentrations are acceptable.

Bradycardia. Epinephrine hydrochloride may be indicated for bradycardia that persists after adequate ventilation and cardiac massage.

Hypovolemia. It is important to recognize that most severely depressed neonates are not hypovolemic and that there may be potential hazards (eg, intracranial hemorrhage) to rapid volume expansion. Conditions associated with hypovolemia include significant hemorrhage from the fetoplacental unit (eg, vasa praevia, fetomaternal bleeding) and compression of the umbilical cord.

If significant hypovolemia is suspected, it should be treated with repeated infusions of volume expanders (10 ml/kg). The neonate's response should be assessed after each infusion. Therapy is stopped when tissue perfusion is adequate.

Narcotic-Induced Respiratory Depression. If respiratory depression is the result of narcotics administered to the mother prior to delivery, naloxone hydrochloride, 0.1 mg/kg, may be administered to the neonate in conjunction with assisted ventilation.

Transfer of Responsibility for Resuscitation

Hospital policy should address who will be responsible for assessment and initiation of resuscitation of the baby as required. This policy should indicate circumstances in which a pediatrician (or designated newborn resuscitation personnel) may be called to attend the delivery or to take over resuscitation in an emergency. The process of transfer of responsibility for this care should also be specified.

Neonates are assessed for their individual needs to determine the best facility for care. They may be admitted to the admission and observation area, the intermediate care area, or the intensive care area in the same hospital, or they may be transferred to a hospital that provides specialty or subspecialty care (see Chapter 3).

The delivering physician or nurse–midwife is responsible for ascertaining that the newborn's adaptations to extrauterine life are proceeding normally and for ensuring immediate postdelivery care of the newborn. Such care may be provided by other health care personnel or transferred to another physician, who will assume responsibility for the ongoing care of the neonate. The routine care of a healthy newborn may be transferred to a family physician or pediatrician. The care of a newborn with additional needs should be transferred to a physician with appropriate training in neonatal care, as indicated by hospital policy. This policy should delineate the communication that should precede acceptance of this responsibility and the method by which the care of the baby will be transferred.

Assessment of Infants in the Delivery Room

An initial evaluation of the baby's condition should be performed in the delivery room to determine the level of care required. After appropriate care in the resuscitation area, babies who are small, sick, or at risk of becoming sick should be transferred to an intermediate or intensive care area in the same hospital or may be transferred to a hospital that provides specialty or subspecialty care. If the baby's condition is stable, breastfeeding can be initiated in the delivery room.

Because umbilical arterial blood best reflects the fetal condition immediately before delivery, umbilical-artery pH and blood gas measurements may be helpful in ruling out acidemia when a low Apgar score has been assigned. Umbilical venous blood better reflects uteroplacental circulation than it does fetal condition, but if fetal metabolic acidemia is truly present, a venous sample should also indicate its presence. This sample is also helpful when samples of the umbilical artery or chorionic surface artery are unobtainable.

Umbilical arterial blood with a pH of less than 7.20 is traditionally accepted as a sign of newborn acidemia, but this value is arbitrarily high. The precise cord blood pH value that defines chemically significant acidemia is not known; however, umbilical-artery blood pH values of less than 7.00 (with a metabolic component and a base deficit of >10 mEq/L) realistically represent clinically significant acidosis.

Neither Apgar score nor pH value alone can define or classify the degree of perinatal asphyxia in a newborn. Many factors other than perinatal asphyxia can result in low 1- and 5-minute Apgar scores. Thus it is suggested that the terms *fetal distress* and *birth asphyxia* be discarded as imprecise. The term *asphyxia* should be reserved to describe a neonate with all of the following conditions:

- Profound metabolic or mixed acidemia (pH <7.0) on an umbilical-cord artery blood sample, if obtained
- Apgar score of 0–3 for longer than 5 minutes
- Neonatal neurologic manifestations (eg, seizures, coma, or hypotonia)
- Multisystem organ dysfunction (eg, cardiovascular, gastrointestinal, hematologic, pulmonary, or renal system)

Meconium staining of the amniotic fluid, nonreassuring fetal heart rate patterns, low 1-minute Apgar scores, and prolonged labor, in the absence of signs of encephalopathy and seizures, have no predictive value for long-term neurologic injury or cerebral palsy.

Identification

While the newborn is still in the delivery room, identical bands that indicate the mother's admission number, the neonate's sex, the date and time of birth, and other information specified in hospital policy should be secured to the mother and the infant. Delivery room and nursery personnel should exercise meticulous care in the preparation and placement of the neonate's identification bands. The nurse in the delivery room should be responsible for preparing and securely fastening these identification bands on the neonate. Footprinting and fingerprinting alone are not adequate methods of patient identification. The birth records and identification bands should be checked before the neonate leaves the delivery room. When the neonate is taken to the nursery, both the delivery room nurse and the admitting nurse should check the neonate's identification bands and birth records, verify the sex of the neonate, and sign the neonate's record. The admitting nurse should fill out the bassinet card and attach it to the bassinet. When the neonate is shown to the mother, she should be asked to verify the information on the identification bands and the sex of the neonate.

If the condition of the baby does not allow placement of identification bands (eg, extreme prematurity), they should accompany the baby and should be placed on the incubator or warmer to be attached as soon as is practical.

With multiple births, the umbilical cords should be identified according to hospital policy (eg, use of different clamps) so that cord blood specimens may be correctly labeled. All cord blood samples must be labeled correctly with an indication that these are samples of the baby's cord blood and not that of the mother.

Ongoing Care

Resuscitation in the delivery room does not always end with the establishment of normal breathing, heart rate, and color. If the baby requires ongoing support, a continuing plan for management by personnel who are experienced in the care of such babies must be established. All babies who require more than 30 seconds of assisted ventilation or who require epinephrine, volume expanders, or chest compressions should be cared for in an area that can provide careful observation and clinical monitoring to meet the continuing needs of the baby.

Immediate plans for the baby should be discussed with the mother (and father or other support person) before the baby leaves the delivery room. Whenever possible, they should have the opportunity to see and touch the baby before he or she is transferred to a nursery.

The physician or other responsible person delivering the baby should also be advised of the status and plans for the baby. Communication regarding the potential transfer of care of the baby must be initiated before the baby leaves the delivery room, especially when specialized ongoing care is required.

Bibliography

American Academy of Pediatrics, American College of Obstetricians and Gynecologists. Use and abuse of the Apgar score. Pediatrics 1996;98:141–142

American College of Obstetricians and Gynecologists. Dystocia and the augmentation of labor. Technical Bulletin 218. Washington, DC: ACOG, 1995

American College of Obstetricians and Gynecologists. Fetal distress and birth asphyxia. ACOG Committee Opinion 137. Washington, DC: ACOG, 1994

American College of Obstetricians and Gynecologists. Induction of labor. ACOG Technical Bulletin 217. Washington, DC: 1995

American College of Obstetricians and Gynecologists. Operative vaginal delivery. ACOG Technical Bulletin 196. Washington, DC: ACOG, 1994

American College of Obstetricians and Gynecologists. Umbilical artery blood acid–base analysis. Technical Bulletin 216. Washington, DC: ACOG, 1995

American College of Obstetricians and Gynecologists. Utility of umbilical cord blood acid–base assessment. ACOG Committee Opinion 138. Washington, DC: ACOG, 1994

American College of Obstetricians and Gynecologists. Vaginal delivery after previous cesarean birth. ACOG Practice Patterns 1. Washington, DC: ACOG, 1995

American College of Obstetricians and Gynecologists and American Academy of Pediatrics. Use and abuse of the Apgar score. ACOG Committee Opinion 174. Washington, DC: ACOG, 1996

Bloom RS, Cropley C, eds. Textbook of neonatal resuscitation. American Academy of Pediatrics/American Heart Association NRP Steering Committee. Dallas, Texas: American Heart Association, 1994

Wright LL, Merenstein GB, Hirtz D, eds. Report of the Workshop on Acute Perinatal Asphyxia in Term Infants. NIH publication no. 96-3823. Washington, DC: National Institute of Child Health and Human Development, 1996

Chapter 6

Obstetric Complications

Certain complications of pregnancy, labor, or delivery may require more intensive surveillance, monitoring, and special care of the obstetric patient. Often complications can arise without warning. In some cases, early detection and timely intervention can improve outcome. When there is a high risk of complications, it may be advisable to make arrangements for such care in advance.

Management of Preterm Birth

Preterm birth is defined as delivery before 37 weeks of gestation. It pertains to approximately 8% of all births in the United States and as many as 15% of births from socioeconomically underprivileged populations.

Of all preterm births, 25–50% result from preterm labor, 33% from preterm premature rupture of the membranes (PROM), and 25% from maternal medical or obstetric complications. Ideally, preterm birth should occur in a hospital setting with personnel and equipment appropriate for the stage of gestation. Very low-birthweight infants (weighing <1,500 g) should be delivered in a subspecialty facility whenever possible. Although no definitive method of preventing preterm birth has yet been discovered, corticosteroids are effective in enhancing fetal maturity when a woman is at risk of preterm birth.

Preterm Labor

Strategies for reducing the incidence of preterm birth in the United States have focused on enhanced provider and patient education about the risks for preterm labor, as well as programs to detect uterine activity prior to term. These approaches are used to ensure that women in preterm labor are evaluated during labor and, when possible, treated at the earliest possible time to prevent preterm birth. Care of the patient who develops preterm labor is directed toward optimizing the outcome for the preterm newborn.

Diagnosis

The timely diagnosis of preterm labor remains problematic. The suggested criteria for diagnosis include the following:

- Gestation of 20 weeks or greater but less than 37 weeks
- Persistent uterine contractions (4 every 20 minutes or 8 every 60 minutes)

  and
  — Documented cervical change

  or
  — Cervical effacement of 80% or greater

  or
  — Cervical dilatation of greater than 1 cm

Patients with suspected preterm labor should be examined and observed for 1–2 hours and should have their activity restricted in order to confirm whether uterine activity is significant and whether the cervix has changed since the most recent examination. After observation, the cervical examination should be repeated, preferably by the same examiner, to help determine whether cervical dilatation or effacement is taking place. Because preterm labor is often associated with urinary tract infections, an examination of urine with a microscope and urine culture may be helpful. Based on the results, antibiotic treatment can be instituted. Ultrasound examination might be considered to confirm gestational age and to assess the presence of any congenital anomalies.

Women diagnosed as having false labor may be discharged once true labor has been excluded. Depending on gestational age and clinical condition, consideration should be given to initiating interventions such as tocolysis, corticosteroid therapy, and chemoprophylaxis for group B streptococcus (GBS) infection when preterm labor is diagnosed (see "Group B Streptococcus," Chapter 9).

Occult Infection

Because infections have been implicated as both a cause and a consequence of ruptured membranes, the diagnosis of infection is an important component of the evaluation of preterm labor. This diagnosis may be difficult to establish, however, because clinical signs of infection may be absent at the time of initial evaluation. A variety of organisms, including GBS, *Neisseria gonorrhoeae*, *Listeria monocytogenes*, *Mycoplasma* species, *Bacteroides* species, and *Ureaplasma* species have been identified in amniotic fluid. Although the threshold at which colonization is significant enough to result in preterm labor has not yet been defined and the exact proportion of preterm labor that is attributable to infection is unknown, the incidence of infection is highest with ruptured membranes. In the presence of infection, the time from the onset of preterm labor to delivery is shorter and preterm PROM is more likely.

Intraamniotic Infection

Preterm labor may be the first sign of intraamniotic infection in the absence of rupture of the membranes. Organisms may be recovered from the chorioamnion in as many as 60% of women in preterm labor with intact membranes and from the amniotic fluid in 10–15% of women who are not in labor and have intact membranes. Women with poor nutrition or of a low socioeconomic background may be at higher risk for this complication. Intraamniotic infection also may follow amniocentesis or cervical cerclage.

All patients in preterm labor should be evaluated for evidence of chorioamnionitis. Maternal temperature and white blood cell count should be documented and the uterus palpated for tenderness. Maternal or fetal tachycardia could indicate chorioamnionitis. Amniocentesis may be appropriate to detect the presence of occult chorioamnionitis. When chorioamnionitis is diagnosed during pregnancy, broad-spectrum antibiotic therapy should be initiated and delivery effected. Vaginal delivery should be anticipated, and cesarean delivery should be reserved for standard obstetric indications. The choice of antibiotics should take into consideration the polymicrobial nature of most uterine infections, which reflect endogenous vaginal flora. Antibiotics should be given intravenously to prevent serious complications of infection in the mother and to prevent or treat transplacental infection of the fetus.

Tocolysis

Although tocolytic agents have been used for the past two decades, it is not readily apparent that their use has decreased the rate of preterm birth or associated perinatal mortality. In some patients, however, tocolytic agents are successful in delaying birth for at least 48 hours. This delay may provide a window of opportunity for transporting the patient to a regional subspecialty obstetric center and administering antenatal corticosteroid therapy.

Many clinicians attempt to arrest idiopathic preterm labor by using tocolytic agents at less than 34 weeks of gestation; the use of these agents is generally not recommended after 34 weeks of gestation. Attempts at tocolysis are rarely effective when cervical dilatation has reached 4 cm or more, especially if the cervix is well effaced. The potential risks and benefits of tocolytic therapy must be weighed against the risk of preterm delivery. Conditions that limit the chance of success of tocolysis include incompetent cervix, ruptured membranes, and advanced labor (cervix dilated ≥4 cm and well effaced).

When preterm labor is suspected, a decision must be made regarding the appropriateness of tocolytic therapy and the choice of agent. Antenatal corticosteroid therapy should be given at less than 34 weeks of gestation to enhance fetal maturation. The medical history should be reviewed and a physical examination repeated to determine whether there are any contraindications to such therapy. Relative and absolute contraindications to tocolysis that are based on clinical circumstances (particularly gestational age) should take into account the risks of continuing the pregnancy versus those of delivery. Following are contraindications for tocolytic use:

General contraindications

- Acute fetal distress (except when used for intrauterine resuscitation)
- Chorioamnionitis
- Eclampsia or severe preeclampsia
- Fetal demise (singleton)
- Fetal maturity
- Maternal hemodynamic instability

Contraindications for specific tocolytic agents

- Beta-mimetic agents
  — Maternal cardiac rhythm disturbance or other cardiac disease
  — Poorly controlled diabetes, thyrotoxicosis, or hypertension

- Magnesium sulfate
  — Hypocalcemia
  — Myasthenia gravis
  — Renal failure

- Indomethacin
  — Asthma
  — Coronary artery disease
  — Gastrointestinal bleeding (current or past)
  — Oligohydramnios
  — Renal failure
  — Suspected fetal cardiac or renal anomaly

- Nifedipine: maternal liver disease

Currently, the two most accepted classes of tocolytic therapy are beta-sympathomimetic agents and intravenous magnesium sulfate. Less widely used are calcium channel blockers, such as nifedipine, and prostaglandin synthetase inhibitors, such as indomethacin. Ritodrine hydrochloride remains the only drug approved by the U.S. Food and Drug Administration for the treatment of preterm labor. Terbutaline sulfate has actions and side effects similar to those of ritodrine. Although labeled for the treatment of asthma, terbutaline is extensively used off-label for preterm labor because of its relative advantages in cost and routes of administration. Magnesium sulfate is similar in efficacy to the beta-sympathomimetics and has a more favorable risk–benefit profile.

Preterm Premature Rupture of Membranes

Preterm PROM is a major risk factor for obstetric complications because of its association with perinatal infection, preterm delivery, and resultant complications. Preterm PROM is responsible for 25–50% of all preterm deliveries, depending on racial and socioeconomic considerations.

The following information may be helpful in planning the management of patients with preterm PROM:

- Gestational age
- Presence or absence of chorioamnionitis
- Rectal and vaginal cultures for GBS
- Consideration of amniocentesis for Gram stain and culture of amniotic fluid
- Presence or absence of labor
- Possibility of a compromised fetus

The status of the fetus should be assessed by fetal heart rate monitoring, with particular attention to variable decelerations that are consistent with umbilical cord compression. Determining whether the woman is in labor may be difficult because digital examination of the cervix should be avoided until active labor occurs or until the decision has been made to induce labor.

When preterm PROM occurs, expectant management with close observation is usually attempted. If fetal pulmonary maturity can be confirmed by assessment of amniotic fluid, delivery is usually chosen, especially if the gestational age is known to be greater than or equal to 34 weeks. Many caregivers will proceed with delivery if preterm PROM has occurred at or beyond 34 weeks, based on the belief that the risks of complications from infection outweigh the risks of premature delivery at this point. A hospital's departments of obstetrics and gynecology and pediatrics should develop guidelines for the management of preterm PROM, recognizing the need to individualize patient care. If expectant management is chosen in a woman with preterm PROM, bed rest is indicated. Repeat evaluations should be performed to detect chorioamnionitis and fetal compromise resulting from umbilical cord compression.

The prophylactic use of antibiotics can prolong gestation in women with preterm PROM and may result in a decrease in neonatal morbidity but no effect on neonatal mortality. A culture for GBS is not needed if prophylactic antibiotics are used.

The use of corticosteroids to accelerate fetal pulmonary maturity requires further data to support a definitive recommendation in patients undergoing expectant management for preterm PROM. Tocolytic agents have been shown to have no benefit in patients with preterm PROM. Discharge from the hospital is an option in some circumstances.

When preterm PROM occurs before a viable gestational age, the likelihood of delivering a healthy infant with conservative management is low. Such management may produce very premature infants, resulting in significant short- and long-term morbidity. Some patients may elect induction of labor with no expectation of neonatal survival or resuscitation. If the mother elects to continue the pregnancy, management at home may be considered. It is strongly suggested that women who have preterm PROM at a previable gestational age be counseled by both an obstetrician and a pediatrician. A woman should participate fully in the decision regarding her pregnancy, and adequate time should be allowed for her to make an informed decision. In the presence of chorioamnionitis, delivery is indicated.

For women with preterm PROM at a gestational age of presumed viability, amniocentesis may be considered to exclude or confirm the presence of subclinical amnionitis. The utility of the procedure for this indication is controversial, however, because of the high rate of false-negative and false-positive diagnoses. In the absence of convincing evidence showing the efficacy of amniocentesis in improving outcome, its routine use is not considered appropriate.

Antenatal Corticosteroid Administration

Following a 1994 Consensus Conference, the National Institutes of Health concluded that the use of antenatal corticosteroid therapy to induce fetal maturation is effective in reducing respiratory distress syndrome, intraventricular hemorrhage, and mortality in preterm infants. These benefits accrue at less than 34 weeks of gestation and are not limited by sex or race. Optimal benefits begin 24 hours after the initiation of therapy and last 7 days, although treatment of less than 24 hours may also improve outcome. Furthermore, antenatal corticosteroid therapy may complement the benefit of postnatal surfactant therapy. More data are needed regarding the risk and benefits of antenatal corticosteroid therapy in the presence of preterm PROM, as well as the benefits and efficacy of weekly repeat doses. Treatment should consist of either two doses of 12 mg of betamethasone given intramuscularly 24 hours apart, or 6 mg of dexamethasone given intramuscularly 12 hours apart for a total of four doses.

Data from trials involving the follow-up of children for as long as 12 years indicate that antenatal corticosteroid therapy does not adversely affect physical growth or psychomotor development. Therefore, with few exceptions, antenatal corticosteroid therapy is indicated for women with anticipated preterm delivery at less than 34 weeks of gestation. Its implementation will result in a substantial decrease in neonatal morbidity and mortality as well as a reduction in health care costs. The use of antenatal corticosteroids for fetal maturation is a rare example of an intervention technology that yields substantial cost savings in addition to improving health.

Births at the Threshold of Viability

The anticipated birth of an infant at the threshold of viability presents a variety of complex medical, social, and ethical concerns. It is important to counsel the parents anticipating such a birth regarding the expectations for infant outcome and the risks and benefits of various approaches to care. Ideally, obstetric and neonatal health care providers will confer before counseling the parents. If time allows, additional input from other important sources, such as clergy and social workers, can be offered to the parents. It is recommended that counseling in anticipation of extreme prematurity include the following information:

- An overview of the potential problems and their treatment and complications

- A range of the most current possible survival rates, allowing for some error in the best estimate of gestational age and estimated fetal weight (see "Introduction," Figs. I–1 and I–2)

- The possibility of long-term disabilities, including blindness, cerebral palsy, mental retardation, and requirements for special education

- The absence of data documenting improved neonatal outcome from obstetric management (eg, cesarean delivery)

- The possibility that expectations for the newborn may change after birth, based on a more accurate assessment of the gestational age and condition of the newborn

In some instances, counseling could result in parents choosing a nonintervention approach, such as remaining in a community hospital or electing vaginal rather than cesarean birth. Because the benefits of various obstetric management approaches have not yet been established, families should be supported in such decisions. When a decision is made not to resuscitate or to discontinue resuscitation because of nonviability, the family should be treated with dignity and compassion.

Preeclampsia

Preeclampsia is a disorder of unknown cause that is characterized by hypertension, proteinuria, and edema occurring after 20 weeks of pregnancy. Preeclampsia complicates approximately 8% of pregnancies and is a major cause of maternal and perinatal morbidity and mortality. Treatment of preeclampsia should be directed primarily toward ensuring the safety of the mother, followed closely by the delivery of a healthy, mature infant. When preeclampsia is diagnosed during the intrapartum period, initial management should include assessing the condition of both the mother and the fetus and administering prophylaxis for maternal seizures. Although the most effective treatment is delivery, other considerations also affect management:

- Severity of preeclampsia
- Gestational age
- Maternal condition
- Fetal condition
- Presence of labor
- Availability of hospital staff and resources
- Capability of hospital staff

Mild preeclampsia prior to term can often be managed with in-hospital observation. The disease process is regarded as mild unless one or more of the following criteria are present:

- Blood pressure of greater than or equal to 160 mm Hg systolic or greater than or equal to 110 mm Hg diastolic on two occasions at least 6 hours apart with the patient at bed rest
- Proteinuria of greater than or equal to 5 g in a 24-hour urine collection or 3+ or greater on two random urine samples collected at least 4 hours apart
- Oliguria of less than 500 ml in 24 hours
- Cerebral or visual disturbances
- Pulmonary edema or cyanosis
- Epigastric or right upper quadrant pain
- Impaired liver function
- Thrombocytopenia
- Fetal growth restriction

The persistence of severe preeclampsia usually warrants delivery of the infant, irrespective of gestational age or fetal maturity. Fetuses of preeclamptic women are at increased risk of a nonreassuring heart rate during labor. Once labor is established, the route of delivery is determined by obstetric factors. Oxytocin augmentation of labor can be used if needed.

Seizure Prophylaxis

Magnesium sulfate USP ($MgSO_4$–$7H_2O$) is the drug of choice for the prevention or treatment of eclamptic convulsions. Therapy with $MgSO_4$ should be initiated intravenously with a loading dose followed by a continuous infusion. In most situations, clinical assessment of respirations, deep tendon reflexes, and urine output is adequate to monitor for maternal magnesium toxicity without the need to determine actual maternal serum magnesium levels. If toxic serum levels or side effects are encountered, $MgSO_4$ infusion must be discontinued, and calcium gluconate may be administered to reverse these effects.

Antihypertensive Therapy

Severe hypertension with a diastolic blood pressure of 110 mm Hg or greater increases the maternal risks of cerebrovascular accidents and congestive heart failure. Reducing diastolic blood pressure to 90–100 mm Hg is recommended.

Hydralazine is the most widely used agent for the treatment of acute hypertension in pregnancy, has almost universal efficacy, and is extremely safe. Labetalol is equally effective, although it has a wide range of individual dosing requirements. The calcium antagonist nifedipine, when administered orally (not sublingually) to postpartum patients with severe preeclampsia, offers good blood-pressure control and cardiorenal protection. Caution should be exercised to avoid the possibility of sudden hypotension if a calcium channel blocker (such as nifedipine) is used in conjunction with $MgSO_4$ infusion.

Fluid Balance

Patients with severe preeclampsia are at increased risk of fluid overload and pulmonary edema. Fluid intake and urine output should be assessed hourly before delivery. Total intravenous intake should rarely exceed 100–125 ml/h. Because intrapartum oliguria is common (especially with oxytocin usage), its presence should not be treated with repetitive "bolus" crystalloid infusions. Following delivery (especially cesarean birth), oliguria is most commonly caused by hypovolemia. The initial management of postdelivery oliguria is directed at volume replacement with an infusion of 500 ml of crystalloid over 20 minutes. If oliguria persists after delivery and the woman is anemic, the need for a packed red blood cell transfusion should be considered. Repetitive bolus infusions of crystalloid solution in such patients without red blood cell replacement increase the risk of pulmonary edema and acute renal failure. In rare instances, oliguria that persists despite conservative measures is an indication for invasive hemodynamic monitoring to guide fluid, electrolyte, and blood replacement more accurately.

Trauma During Pregnancy

Trauma and other forms of violence are the leading causes of death in women of reproductive age and one of the leading causes of nonobstetric maternal death. Physical trauma is estimated to complicate 1 of every 12 pregnancies. Obstetricians are uniquely qualified to play a vital role in the management of trauma during pregnancy. They understand the effects of altered maternal physiology and anatomy on the management of trauma and its effects on the fetus. The obstetrician's role in ensuring both maternal and fetal well-being is paramount in the management of pregnant trauma victims. Whether acting as a consultant or as a primary physician when seeing a pregnant trauma victim, the obstetrician should provide maternal–fetal care that is timely and systematic to ensure maternal medical stabilization and fetal evaluation.

Evaluation

Pregnancy should not restrict the use of any of the usual diagnostic, pharmacologic, or resuscitative procedures or maneuvers provided to trauma victims. The more seriously injured the mother, the more important it is to follow a methodical evaluation that ensures her complete assessment and stabilization. Serious or life-threatening maternal injuries could be overlooked if maternal evaluation is not thorough during stabilization. The finding of nonreasurring fetal status by heart rate monitoring or ultrasound may alert the clinician to more severe maternal injuries than were initially appreciated. To prevent supine hypotension syndrome, deflection of the uterus off the inferior vena cava and abdominal aorta can be obtained by placing the patient in the lateral decubitus position. This position should be maintained throughout evaluation.

Following stabilization, a more detailed secondary survey of the patient, including a thorough ultrasound evaluation of the pregnancy, should be performed. Sonography in this setting can be useful to determine estimated gestational age, placental localization, fetal cardiac function or demise, amniotic fluid volume, and the presence of intraabdominal fluid.

Once the woman's condition has been stabilized, continuous fetal monitoring is recommended when the fetus's gestational age approaches viability. Monitoring and further evaluation are warranted if uterine contractions, a nonreassuring fetal heart rate pattern, vaginal bleeding, significant uterine tenderness or irritability, serious maternal injury, or rupture of the amniotic membranes is present. Monitoring periods of 2–6 hours are usually adequate if there are no uterine contractions, uterine tenderness, or bleeding. Abruptio placentae usually becomes apparent shortly after injury.

Use of open peritoneal lavage to diagnose intraperitoneal hemorrhage has been shown to be safe, sensitive, and specific during pregnancy, particularly in association with abdominal signs and symptoms of intraperitoneal bleeding, altered sensorium, major thoracic injury, unexplained shock, and multiple major orthopedic injuries. This procedure is unnecessary if clinically obvious intraperitoneal bleeding is present or if ultrasound findings are highly suggestive of free blood in the peritoneal cavity.

Treatment

In general, aggressive exploratory laparotomy is advocated for gunshot wounds and other penetrating trauma to the abdomen during pregnancy. Laparotomy alone is not an indication to perform cesarean delivery. The fetus usually tolerates surgery and anesthesia well if adequate oxygenation and uterine perfusion are maintained. The uterus should be carefully inspected for injury at the time of laparotomy.

Administration of 300 µg of D (Rho[D]) immune globulin within 72 hours of injury should protect nearly all (90%) D-negative trauma victims with substantial abdominal trauma and possible D isoimmunization. The Kleihauer–Betke test or a similar quantitative assay of fetal–maternal hemorrhage may be used to detect a fetomaternal transfusion of 30 ml or greater, which may require additional D immune globulin.

Following evaluation and hospital discharge, the patient should be instructed to seek care if she develops vaginal bleeding, leakage of fluid, decreased fetal movement, or severe abdominal pain. Measures to prevent the recurrence of trauma should also be discussed (eg, use of safety belts, leaving a situation involving domestic violence).

Postmortem cesarean delivery after more than 10–15 minutes of maternal death is unlikely to result in neonatal survival. If a fetus does survive, there may be a high risk of adverse neurodevelopmental sequelae. After 5 minutes of unsuccessful maternal cardiac resuscitation, perimortem cesarean delivery can be undertaken to facilitate resuscitative efforts and avoid fetal compromise or death.

Maternal Hemorrhage

Hemorrhage remains one of the leading causes of maternal mortality. Excessive maternal blood loss is the most common cause of hypotension in obstetric patients. Facilities that provide labor and delivery services should be prepared to manage maternal hemorrhage. Written policies should clearly define the steps necessary to treat obstetric hemorrhage, and services should be readily available for use in the labor and delivery area. Proper preparation to manage maternal hemorrhage can be lifesaving.

An attempt should be made to identify patients with known risk factors for postpartum uterine atony. These risk factors include an overdistended uterus, precipitous or prolonged labor, fetal macrosomia, high parity, and chorioamnionitis. Policies to ensure the need for rapid availability of blood products for transfusion in the event of hemorrhage must be balanced with the need to conserve valuable blood bank reserves.

Hemorrhagic Shock

Obstetric hemorrhage can be of a volume large enough to precipitate a state of generalized circulatory failure, resulting in decreased tissue perfusion that progresses to hypoxia, acidosis, and irreversible tissue damage. The goal of therapy should be timely intervention to first identify and remedy the cause of hemorrhage in conjunction with reversing the effects leading to shock. Most cases of shock arising from obstetric hemorrhage result from hypovolemia secondary to excessive blood loss. Hemodynamic assessment with a central venous pressure or Swan–Ganz catheter is rarely needed for patients with acute hemorrhagic shock. The central venous pressure and Swan–Ganz catheter may be helpful for managing volume replacement therapy in obstetric patients with sepsis. Written policies should be developed to define when to use these catheters in the labor and delivery area and to assign responsibilities for their placement and for interpretation of the data.

Postpartum Hemorrhage

Factors associated with obstetric hemorrhage include uterine atony (the most common cause of postpartum hemorrhage), uterine inversion, obstetric lacerations, and retained placental fragments resulting from placentation abnormalities such as placenta accreta and succenturiate placental lobe. Most postpartum hemorrhage occurs immediately or soon after delivery. Maternal postpartum observation should be tailored to the need for timely identification of signs of excessive blood loss, including hypotension and tachycardia. Maternal blood pressure and pulse should be assessed and recorded immediately after delivery and repeated every 15 minutes for the first hour. These evaluations may be undertaken more frequently if warranted by the patient's condition or findings. The amount of vaginal bleeding should be evaluated often, and the uterine fundus should be identified and massaged and its size and degree of contraction noted. A dilute solution of oxytocin (20 U/L) routinely administered intravenously after placental delivery reduces the incidence of postpartum hemorrhage resulting from uterine atony.

If abnormal or excessive vaginal bleeding occurs after delivery, and if symptoms of perineal or pelvic pain are present, the provider must perform a thorough examination, including careful palpation of the uterus and inspection and palpation of the perineum, vagina, cervix, and vulva for lacerations or hematoma formation. When postpartum hemorrhage is diagnosed, therapy is instituted promptly to ameliorate or prevent the hemodynamic sequela of excessive loss of blood volume. Large-bore intravenous access is secured; Foley catheterization of the bladder should be instituted to monitor urinary output; and volume should be replaced by infusion of Ringer's lactate, normal saline, or packed red blood cells (see the guidelines set forth in the section "Transfusion" in this chapter) in an amount that will maintain a urinary output of 30 ml/h or greater. Labor and delivery areas should have 15-α-methyl-prostaglandin $F_{2\alpha}$ and ergot alkaloids readily available for further treatment of uterine atony.

Appropriate maneuvers, including medical therapy, may fail to control postpartum hemorrhage. The responsible physician and obstetric support staff must be prepared to initiate surgical management when it is deemed necessary. Uterine packing, radiographic embolization, or surgical ligation of the appropriate pelvic vessels or hypogastric arteries occasionally may be appropriate. Puerperal hysterectomy may be indicated, depending on the woman's parity and desire for childbearing; the extent and cause of the hemorrhage; and especially, the judgment, experience, and skill of the surgeon. At the time that postpartum hemorrhage is diagnosed, responsible obstetric staff members, operating room personnel, and anesthesiologists, as deemed appropriate by the physician, should be alerted to the potential for emergency surgery.

Transfusion

Transfusion therapy is used to prevent or treat hemorrhagic shock and its consequences. Blood loss estimated to be 1,500 ml or greater represents approximately 25% of a pregnant woman's total estimated blood volume (6,000 ml). In some clinical circumstances, a pregnant patient might benefit from transfusion of red blood cells before the blood loss has reached such levels. The circulating blood volume must be maintained in the pregnant patient, and therapy should be directed at the prevention of inadequate cardiac output and resultant decreased tissue perfusion.

Some women have a religious objection to the receipt of any blood product. Written policies to guide the management of these patients during treatment are advisable. Hydroxyethyl starch is a synthetic colloid that could be an acceptable alternative for these patients.

Before Delivery

The goal of red blood cell transfusion therapy is to avoid irreversible tissue damage due to hypoperfusion from inadequate circulating blood volume. In the obstetric patient, the need for adequate blood volume is made more pressing by the presence of the fetus.

Before delivery, red blood cell transfusion may be indicated in a woman with active or arrested hemorrhage, taking into consideration her hemodynamic status and clinical conditions such as the following:

- Appreciable bleeding continues.
- A major surgical procedure is under way.
- Signs or symptoms of hypovolemia (eg, shock) are present.
- Oliguria and vasoconstriction persist.

The end point of red blood cell transfusion therapy varies with the clinical situation. A hematocrit of 30% or greater has been generally recommended as a goal of therapy in a pregnant patient who is actively bleeding or who is at continued risk for significant obstetric hemorrhage, such as in the presence of placenta previa. In a clinically stable patient who has responded appropriately to therapy, however, the decision to transfuse should be based on individual circumstances.

After Delivery

If active bleeding has ceased after delivery, transfusion can be withheld despite laboratory determinations of significant anemia in patients with normal tissue perfusion, including a normal urine output of 30 ml/h or greater and no appreciable postural hypotension or tachycardia. The patient's compensatory mechanisms of increased erythropoiesis and plasma volume expansion, along with iron supplementation, will correct the red blood cell deficit.

When obstetric hemorrhage is diagnosed, packed red blood cells should be typed and cross-matched (prior typed and screened red blood cells are equally safe), and the hospital's blood bank personnel should be notified of the potential for massive transfusion. Until the blood loss is controlled by medical or surgical therapy, it is advisable to ensure the ready availability of packed red blood cell units for use if rapid transfusion is required. Obstetric blood loss of greater than 1,500 ml, or of lesser amounts due to placental causes, may result in inadequate coagulation in otherwise healthy patients. Component therapy, including fresh-frozen plasma and cryoprecipitate, should be available if needed for temporary correction of deficits in clotting factors. If massive transfusion is required, monitoring for coagulation deficiency will direct the need for blood products to replace coagulation factors. Cryoprecipitate will correct a fibrinogen deficiency, whereas fresh-frozen plasma will increase the level of all clotting factors.

The adequacy of transfusion therapy should be monitored by evaluation of the patient for signs and symptoms of shock, including measurements of pulse, blood pressure, tissue perfusion, and oxygenation. The hematocrit should be measured sequentially, and urinary output should be measured and recorded.

Endometritis

Postpartum endometritis occurs in 1–3% of vaginal deliveries and in 10–50% of cesarean deliveries. Risk factors for endometritis include cesarean delivery, prolonged rupture of membranes, prolonged labor with multiple vaginal examinations, intrapartum fever, and disadvantaged socioeconomic status.

Prophylaxis Against Postcesarean Endometritis

A short course of prophylactic antibiotics significantly lowers the risk of endometritis after nonelective cesarean delivery (ie, cesarean delivery after rupture of membranes or labor of any duration). Intravenous administration of an antibiotic immediately after cord clamping has been demonstrated to be as effective as administration before the procedure is initiated. For procedures lasting less than 2 hours, a single dose is as effective as a longer course of therapy. If excessive intraoperative blood loss occurs, a second dose may be indicated. A first-generation cephalosporin is as effective as broad-spectrum agents and is less expensive. Broad-spectrum antibiotics should be reserved for therapy rather than prophylaxis.

Management

Endometritis is usually diagnosed within a few days after delivery. Infection is often caused by several organisms, including aerobic streptococci (group B alpha-hemolytic streptococci and the enterococci), gram-negative aerobes (especially *Escherichia coli*), gram-negative anaerobic rods (especially *Bacteroides bivius*), and anaerobic cocci (*Peptococcus* species and *Peptostreptococcus* species). Clinically, endometritis is characterized by fever, uterine tenderness, malaise, tachycardia, abdominal pain, or foul-smelling lochia. Of these, fever is the most characteristic and may be the only sign early in the course of infection.

A woman with postpartum fever should be evaluated by pertinent history, physical examination, blood count, and urine culture. Blood cultures rarely influence therapeutic decisions but could be indicated if septicemia is suspected. Cervical, vaginal, or endometrial cultures need not be routinely performed because these results might not indicate the infecting organism.

Principles for managing postpartum endometritis are as follows:

- Parenteral, broad-spectrum antibiotic treatment should be initiated according to a proven regimen and continued until the patient is afebrile. A combination of clindamycin and gentamicin, with the addition of ampicillin in refractory cases, is recommended for cost-effective therapy.
- Response is usually prompt. If fever persists, a search for alternative etiologies, including pelvic abscess, wound infection, septic

pelvic thrombophlebitis, inadequate antibiotic coverage, and retained placental tissue, should be performed.

- Because postpartum endometritis may have neonatal implications, information about the mother's condition should be provided to the neonate's care providers.

Bibliography

American Academy of Pediatrics, American College of Obstetricians and Gynecologists. Perinatal care at the threshold of viability. Committee Opinion 163. Washington, DC: ACOG, 1995; and Pediatrics 1995;96:974-976

American College of Obstetricians and Gynecologists. Antenatal corticosteroid therapy for fetal maturation. Committee Opinion 147. Washington, DC: ACOG, 1994

American College of Obstetricians and Gynecologists. Hypertension in pregnancy. ACOG Technical Bulletin 218. Washington, DC: ACOG, 1996

American College of Obstetricians and Gynecologists. Preterm labor. Technical Bulletin 206. Washington, DC: ACOG, 1995

American College of Obstetricians and Gynecologists. Trauma during pregnancy. Technical Bulletin 161. Washington, DC: ACOG, 1991

National Institutes of Health. Effect of corticosteroids for fetal maturation on perinatal outcomes. NIH publication no. 95-3784. NIH consensus statement 1994;12:1–24

Chapter 7

Postpartum and Follow-Up Care

Postpartum hospitalization has two purposes: (1) to identify maternal and neonatal complications, and (2) to provide professional assistance during the time when the mother is likely to need support and care. The continuum of perinatal care that began in the antepartum period should be reinforced during hospitalization to ensure that care extends beyond discharge. A multidisciplinary, collaborative approach is often used to promote this continuity and to ensure that care is comprehensive.

Postpartum care begins immediately after delivery, either in the birthing room or in a designated recovery area where the family unit can begin the process of bonding and the mother can be observed for postpartum complications. Stabilization of the neonate usually occurs within the first 6 hours after birth, during which time the condition of the neonate is closely monitored. A healthy neonate need not be separated from the mother for this stabilization period if the facilities and personnel needed for observation are located in the mother's recovery or postpartum area. Adequate nursing personnel should be available to observe and evaluate the neonate. The father or other supporting persons can remain with the new mother during the immediate postpartum period. Parents should be encouraged to interact with the neonate unless such interaction is precluded by maternal or neonatal considerations. This is an excellent time to introduce breastfeeding. Besides its nutritional benefits, breastfeeding is important for mother–infant bonding and for control of uterine bleeding. Interaction with the neonate can also be encouraged for a woman who has undergone cesarean delivery. Analgesia should be available to facilitate this process.

Maternal Care

Immediate Postpartum Care

When regional or general anesthesia has been used for either vaginal or cesarean delivery, the mother should be observed in an appropriately equipped labor–delivery–recovery room, or in an appropriately staffed and equipped postanesthesia care unit or equivalent area, until she has recovered from the anesthetic. After cesarean delivery, standards for postanesthesia care should not differ from those applied to nonobstetric surgical patients receiving major anesthesia. Policy should ensure that a physician is available in the facility, or at least is nearby, to manage anesthetic complications and provide cardiopulmonary resuscitation for patients in the postanesthesia care unit. The patient should be discharged from the recovery area only at the discretion of, and after communication between, the attending physician or a certified nurse–midwife, anesthesiologist, or certified registered nurse–anesthetist in charge. Vital signs and additional signs or events should be monitored and recorded as they occur.

In evaluating the feasibility and safety or advisability of immediate postpartum sterilization, consideration must be given to the advent of maternal or neonatal problems and other demands on obstetric and anesthesia staff. If postpartum tubal ligation is planned, the delivery has been uncomplicated, and the anesthetic can be continued safely, there is no contraindication to proceeding directly to the sterilization procedure. Preoperative care and evaluation thus become part of delivery room care, especially if the delivery has taken place in a room designed and equipped for abdominal surgery. The obstetrician and anesthesiologist/anesthetist should exercise medical judgment regarding the risks, benefits, and safety of the procedure.

Subsequent Postpartum Care

The medical and nursing staff should cooperatively establish specific postpartum policies and procedures. In the postpartum period, staff should help the mother in learning how to care for herself and her baby and should identify potential problems related to her general health.

The physician should note postpartum orders on the patient's chart. If routine postpartum orders are used, they should be printed or written on the chart, reviewed and modified as necessary for the particular patient, and signed by the physician before the patient is transferred to the postpartum unit. When a birthing labor–delivery–recovery room is used, the same standards of care should apply.

Bed Rest, Ambulation, and Diet

The new mother must be allowed to sleep, regain her strength, and recover from the effects of any analgesic or anesthetic agents that she may have received during labor. In the absence of complications, she may have a regular diet as soon as she wishes. Because early ambulation has been shown to decrease the incidence of subsequent thrombophlebitis, the mother should be encouraged to walk as soon as she feels able to do so. She should not attempt to get out of bed for the first time without assistance. She may shower as soon as she wishes. It may be necessary to administer fluids intravenously for hydration. If the patient has an intravenous line in place, her fluid and hematologic status should be evaluated before it is removed.

Care of the Vulva

The patient should be taught to cleanse the vulva from anterior vulva to perineum and anus rather than in the reverse direction. Application of an ice bag to the perineum during the first 24 hours after delivery may help reduce edema, pain, and swelling that have resulted from pressure of the neonate's head. Orally administered analgesics are often required and are usually sufficient for relief of discomfort from episiotomy. Pain that is not relieved by such medication suggests hematoma formation and mandates a careful examination of the vulva, vagina, and rectum. Beginning 24 hours after delivery, moist heat in the form of a warm sitz bath may reduce local discomfort and promote healing.

Care of the Bladder

Women should be encouraged to void as soon as possible after delivery. Often women have difficulty voiding immediately after delivery, possibly because of trauma to the bladder during labor and delivery, regional anesthesia, or vulvar–perineal pain and swelling. In addition, the diuresis that often follows delivery can distend the bladder before the patient is aware of a sensation of a full bladder. To ensure adequate emptying of the bladder, the patient should be checked frequently during the first 24 hours after delivery, with particular attention to displacement of the uterine fundus and any indication of the presence of a fluid-filled bladder above the symphysis. Although every effort should be made to help the patient void spontaneously, single catheterization may be necessary. If the patient continues to find voiding difficult, use of a single indwelling catheter is preferable to repeated catheterization.

Care of the Breasts

The mother's decision about breastfeeding determines the appropriate care of the breasts. Breast care for a woman who chooses to breastfeed is outlined in Chapter 11. The woman who chooses not to breastfeed should be reassured that milk production will abate over the first few days after delivery if she does not breastfeed. During the stage of engorgement, the breasts may become painful and should be supported with a well-fitting brassiere. Ice packs and analgesics can help relieve discomfort during this period. Medications for lactation cessation are discouraged. Women who do not wish to breastfeed should be encouraged to avoid nipple stimulation and should be cautioned against continued manual expression of milk.

Temperature Elevation

The condition of all postpartum patients with an elevated temperature ($\geq$38°C [$\geq$100.4°F] on two occasions, 6 hours apart) should be evaluated (see Chapter 6). The nursery should be notified if the mother develops a fever at any time during the postpartum period, especially after the first 24 hours. The neonate need not be separated from the mother for infection control.

Postpartum Analgesia

After vaginal delivery, analgesic medication may be necessary to relieve perineal and episiotomy pain and facilitate maternal mobility. This is best addressed by administering the drug on an as-needed basis according to postpartum orders. Most mothers experience considerable pain in the first 24 hours after cesarean birth. Although at one time pain was most often treated by intramuscular injections of narcotics, newer techniques, such as spinal or epidural opiates and patient-controlled analgesia, provide better pain relief and greater patient satisfaction. Regardless of the route of administration, opioids can potentially cause respiratory depression and decrease intestinal motility. Thus, adequate supervision and monitoring should be ensured for all postpartum patients receiving these drugs.

Immunization: D Immune Globulin and Rubella

An unsensitized, D-negative woman who delivers a D-positive or D^u-positive neonate should receive 300 µg of D (Rho[D]) immune globulin postpartum, ideally within 72 hours, even when D immune globulin has been administered in the antepartum period. This dose may be inadequate in circumstances in which there is a potential for fetal-to-maternal hemorrhage, such as abruptio placentae, placenta previa, intrauterine manipulation, and manual removal of the placenta. In these cases, laboratory analysis should be performed to detect excessive maternal-to-fetal hemorrhage and thus determine the proper dose. If indicated, additional D immune globulin should be given.

A patient who is identified as susceptible to rubella virus infection should receive the rubella vaccine in the postpartum period. Rubella vaccine can be administered before discharge, even if the patient is breastfeeding. Patients should be informed of the possibility of transient arthralgia and low-grade fever after rubella immunization.

Neonatal Care

For a healthy neonate born after an uncomplicated pregnancy, an individualized care plan should be established that includes appropriate observation for the stabilization–transition period—the first 6–12 hours—and the remainder of the hospital stay. Health care providers should carefully evaluate and document the baby's status and care and communicate this information when transferring care to other providers or health care agencies.

Pediatric Information

Care of the baby after birth is aided by effective communication to the pediatrician of information about the mother and fetus. With an uncomplicated pregnancy, labor, and delivery, information on the record accompanying the baby will suffice. The obstetric staff should record the following information, which should also be available on a chart that accompanies the baby during any transfer of responsibility for care:

- The mother's name, medical record number, blood type, serology result, rubella status, hepatitis B virus test result, and history of substance use
- Other maternal test results, if obtained, that are relevant to neonatal care, such as human immunodeficiency virus (HIV) test results and colonization with group B streptococcus (in some states, it is necessary to obtain the mother's written authorization prior to disclosing her HIV status to health care providers who are not part of her health care team, such as her baby's pediatrician)
- Intrapartum maternal antibiotic therapy
- Maternal illness potentially affecting the pregnancy, evidence of chorioamnionitis, and maternal use of any medications (including tocolytics and glucocorticoids)
- Complications of pregnancy associated with abnormal fetal growth, fetal anomalies, or abnormal results from tests of fetal well-being and the corresponding interpretation
- Information regarding the delivery (eg, method and time in labor), complications of labor (eg, nonreassuring fetal heart rate),

duration of rupture of amniotic membranes, and presence or absence of meconium in amniotic fluid

The obstetric staff should communicate problems before and after delivery in a timely manner to the physician who will be caring for the baby. For some high-risk pregnancies, a neonatal consultation during antepartum care can help in obstetric management and assist the parents in understanding what to expect for their baby. This is of particular importance when fetal abnormalities are significant or a very preterm baby is expected.

Assessment of the Newborn

Intrauterine Growth Status

The neonate's gestational age can be estimated from the mother's menstrual history or the results of ultrasound examination prior to 20 weeks of gestation (see Chapter 4) and from the pediatrician's assessment of gestational age (Fig. 7–1). The gestational age should be assigned by the pediatrician after all data, both pediatric and obstetric, have been assessed. Any marked discrepancy between the presumed duration of pregnancy by obstetric assessment and the physical and neurologic findings in the neonate should be documented on the chart.

Data from each baby should be plotted on a birth weight–gestational age chart that is appropriate for the population of babies in that geographic area. Determination of gestational age and its relationship to weight can be used to identify neonates at risk for postnatal complications. For example, neonates who are either large or small for their gestational ages are at relatively increased risk for hypoglycemia and polycythemia, and appropriate tests (eg, serum glucose screen or hematocrit determination) are indicated.

Risk Assessment

No later than 2 hours after birth, nursery admitting personnel should evaluate the neonate's status and assess risks. Clinical data that are deemed necessary but are initially unavailable should be either obtained or requested at this time. Risks can be assessed through the history and physical examination as documented on the antepartum

Neuromuscular maturity

	-1	0	1	2	3	4	5
Posture							
Square window (wrist)	<90°	90°	60°	45°	30°	0°	
Arm recoil		180°	140–180°	110–140°	90–110°	<90°	
Popliteal angle	180°	160°	140°	120°	100°	90°	<90°
Scarf sign							
Heel to ear							

Physical maturity

Skin	Sticky, friable, transparent	Gelatinous, red, translucent	Smooth, pink, visible veins	Superficial peeling &/or rash, few veins	Cracking, pale areas, rare veins	Parchment, deep cracking, no vessels	Leathery, cracked, wrinkled
Lanugo	None	Sparse	Abundant	Thinning	Bald areas	Mostly bald	
Plantar surface	Heel–toe 40–50 mm:-1 <40 mm:-2	<50 mm, no crease	Faint red marks	Anterior transverse crease only	Creases on ant. 2/3	Creases over entire sole	
Breast	Imperceptible	Barely perceptible	Flat areola– no bud	Stripped areola, 1–2 mm bud	Raised areola, 3–4 mm bud	Full areola, 5–10 mm bud	
Eye/ear	Lids fused loosely (-1), tightly (-2)	Lids open, pinna flat, stays folded	Slightly curved pinna; soft; slow recoil	Well-curved pinna, soft but ready recoil	Formed & firm, instant recoil	Thick cartilage, ear stiff	
Genitals male	Scrotum flat, smooth	Scrotum empty, faint rugae	Testes in upper canal, rare rugae	Testes descending, few rugae	Testes down, good rugae	Testes pendulous, deep rugae	
Genitals female	Clitoris prominent, labia flat	Prominent clitoris, small labia minora	Prominent clitoris, enlarging minora	Majora & minora equally prominent	Majora large, minora small	Majora cover clitoris & minora	

Maturity rating

Score	Weeks
-10	20
-5	22
0	24
5	26
10	28
15	30
20	32
25	34
30	36
35	38
40	40
45	42
50	44

Fig. 7–1. The expanded new Ballard Score includes extremely premature infants and has been refined to improve accuracy in more mature infants. (Ballard JL, Khoury JC, Wedig K, Wang L, Eilers-Walsman BL, Lipp R. New Ballard Score, expanded to include extremely premature infants. J Pediatr 1991;119:417–423)

and intrapartum records. If the baby's physician (or other health care provider) is not present at the delivery, he or she should be notified of the admission and of the status of the baby within a time frame established by institutional policy.

The neonate's physician or health care provider, as defined by institutional policy, should examine the apparently normal neonate no later than 24 hours after birth and within 24 hours before discharge from the hospital. This may be accomplished with one physical examination. The results should be recorded on the neonate's chart and discussed with the parents.

Immediate Care

Following an initial evaluation of the neonate's condition, a care plan should be established, and the neonate should be carefully observed during the subsequent stabilization–transition period (the first 6–12 hours after birth). Temperature, heart and respiratory rates, skin color, adequacy of peripheral circulation, type of respiration, level of consciousness, tone, and activity should be monitored and recorded at least once every 30 minutes until the neonate's condition has remained stable for 2 hours.

After these observations have been made, the neonate with no identified problems may be placed in the newborn nursery or in the mother's room for continued surveillance and care until discharge. Feeding can be initiated as soon as possible after delivery. If the neonate remains with the mother, the physician or nurse should assess and document the neonate's condition according to the routine of the transitional nursery. The neonate should be observed for any of the following signs of illness:

- Temperature instability
- Change in activity, including refusal of feedings
- Unusual skin color
- Abnormal cardiac or respiratory rate and rhythm
- Delayed or abnormal stools or voiding
- Abdominal distension, bilious vomiting, and excessive lethargy and sleeping

The normal full-term neonate passes meconium within the first 24 hours after birth. If a full-term neonate has not passed meconium by 48 hours after birth, the lower gastrointestinal tract may be obstructed. Urine is normally passed within the first 12 hours after birth. Failure to void within the first 24 hours may indicate genitourinary obstruction or abnormality.

After appropriate care in the resuscitation area, neonates who are born sick, small, or at high risk of becoming sick (as determined by history or physical examination) should be transferred to an intermediate or intensive care area. Subsequently, observations should be made and recorded at an interval consistent with the acuity of the newborn's illness.

Eye Care

Prophylaxis against gonococcal ophthalmia neonatorum is mandatory for all neonates, including those born by cesarean delivery. A variety of topical agents appear to be equally efficacious. Acceptable prophylactic regimens are application of two drops of 1% silver nitrate in single-dose containers and a 1–2-cm ribbon of sterile ophthalmic ointment containing tetracycline (1%) or erythromycin (0.5%) in single-use tubes. Care should be taken to ensure that the agent reaches all parts of the conjunctival sac. The eyes should not be irrigated with saline or distilled water after instillation of any of these agents; however, after 1 minute, excess solution or ointment can be wiped away with sterile cotton. Instillation may be delayed up to 1 hour after birth.

Vitamin K

To prevent vitamin K-dependent hemorrhagic disease of the newborn, every neonate should receive a single parenteral 0.5–1.0-mg dose of natural vitamin K$_1$ oxide (phytonadione) within 1 hour of birth. Oral administration of vitamin K has not been shown to be as efficacious as parenteral administration. Furthermore, no commercial oral vitamin K preparations are approved for use in the United States.

Subsequent Care

The condition of the neonate should be evaluated upon admission to the nursery. This evaluation should include a review of the neonate's identification, the mother's health prior to pregnancy and during the prenatal and intrapartum periods, the neonate's condition at birth, and the neonate's ability to adapt to extrauterine life.

Nursery guidelines should delineate those conditions (eg, low birth weight, small for gestational age) that require specific actions by nurses or immediate notification of the physician. Clinical conditions such as maternal substance use, maternal fever or infection, or low Apgar scores at 5 minutes or more are associated with increased risk for neonatal illness and should prompt immediate notification of the physician. The obstetrician should be notified of the baby's status in a timely manner, particularly if problems or complications arise.

Weighing

Each neonate should be weighed daily. The neonate must be kept warm during weighing. The scale pan should be covered with clean paper before each neonate is weighed. The accuracy of the nursery scales should be checked once a month.

Clothing

Most neonates require only a cotton shirt or gown without buttons in addition to a soft diaper. They may be clothed only in a diaper during hot weather if the nursery is not air conditioned. A supply of soft, clean, cotton clothing, bed pads, sheets, and blankets should be kept at the bedside. Nontoxic dyes should be used to mark clothing, blankets, or other items used in the care of newborns.

Skin Care

Skin care, including bathing, may be important for the health and appearance of the individual neonate and for infection control within the nursery. The first bath should be postponed until the neonate's thermal stability is ensured. The medical and nursing services of each hospital should develop guidelines regarding the time of the first bath, circumstances and method of skin cleansing, and the roles of personnel and parents.

Effects on the neonate's skin should be considered in selecting skin care techniques. Some agents are absorbed and may be toxic; others change skin flora and may increase the risk of infection. Whole-body bathing of the neonate may not be necessary. Localized skin care or techniques that minimize exposure to water may reduce the neonate's heat loss. Sterile cotton sponges (not gauze) soaked with warm water may be used to remove blood and meconium from the neonate's face, head, and body. Alternatively, the baby can be cleansed with a mild, nonmedicated soap and then rinsed with water. Careful drying of the neonate's skin and removal of blood after birth may minimize the risk of infection with potentially contaminating microorganisms, such as hepatitis B virus, herpes simplex virus, and HIV. If the neonate's skin is not grossly soiled, it may not require much cleansing.

For the remainder of the neonate's stay in the hospital nursery, the buttocks and perianal regions should be cleansed with fresh water and cotton, or with a mild soap and water, at diaper changes. The gelatinous skin of extremely immature neonates should be cleaned with sterile water and only when necessary. Ideally, agents used on the newborn's skin should be dispensed in single-use containers, or each neonate should have a personal dispenser.

Various antiseptic compounds for skin care have been studied to determine their safety and effectiveness in preventing colonization and infection in neonates. Hexachlorophene, although relatively effective against gram-positive bacteria, particularly *Staphylococcus au-*

reus, should not be used routinely for bathing neonates because of its potential for neurotoxic effects in neonates. Although iodophors are good antiseptics, they have not been proved to be both safe and effective for routine skin care. Chlorhexidine gluconate, a compound that is poorly absorbed through intact skin, is useful for bathing or for localized skin care. No single method of cord care has proved to be superior in preventing colonization and disease. Current methods include the local application of antimicrobial agents, such as bacitracin, or of triple-dye agents. The skin absorption and toxicity of triple-dye agents in newborns have not been carefully studied. Alcohol is probably not effective in preventing cord colonization and omphalitis.

Circumcision

Newborn circumcision is an elective procedure to be performed at the request of the parents on baby boys who are physiologically and clinically stable. The exact incidence of complications after circumcision is not known, but data indicate that the rate is low and that the most common complications are local infection and bleeding. A possible benefit of circumcision may be a reduced incidence of urinary tract infection.

Although circumcision is a painful procedure, the preferred methods for anesthesia or analgesia have not been determined. Many techniques have been used, with various degrees of success, to lessen the infant's stress response. Swaddling, sucrose by mouth, and acetaminophen administration may reduce the stress response. Dorsal penile blocks have exhibited efficacy, but rare complications can occur. More studies are needed to assess the potential short-term and long-term side effects and absorption rates of these agents. Although lidocaine has been shown to be effective when used to block the dorsal penile nerves, concern remains about the long-term effects of lidocaine infiltration on the nervous or vascular tissues of the penis and the risk of elevated blood levels of lidocaine. Use of topical anesthetic cream has not been shown to be effective.

The uncircumcised penis is easy to keep clean. The foreskin usually does not fully retract for several years and should not be forced. Gentle washing of the genital area while bathing is sufficient for normal hygiene. Later, when the foreskin is fully retractable, boys should be taught the importance of washing underneath the foreskin on a regular basis.

Preventive Care

Hepatitis Immunization

Immunization against hepatitis B virus is often initiated in the nursery. Each hospital should establish procedures to assess the neonate's status regarding hepatitis exposure and timely, appropriate intervention and immunization (see Chapter 9).

Universal Neonatal Screening

Newborn screening is a preventive public health procedure that should be available to all neonates. Although all states have newborn screening programs, some neonates with disorders included in the newborn screening battery will be missed, even when properly screened. This may be due to individual or biologic variations, very early discharge, or administrative or laboratory error.

An adequate neonatal screening program involves laboratory tests, education, administration, follow-up, management, and evaluation components. Systematic follow-up and management should be part of the comprehensive newborn screening program. A comprehensive screening program includes the following components:

- Education of parents and practitioners about newborn screening and about their participation in the activity
- Reliable acquisition and transportation of adequate specimens
- Reliable and prompt performance of screening tests
- Prompt retrieval and follow-up of individuals with abnormal test results
- Accurate diagnosis of individuals with confirmed positive test results
- Education, genetic counseling, and psychosocial support for families with affected neonates

Every nursery should establish routines to provide total participation of all newborns in the screening program in accordance with state law. Premature neonates, neonates receiving parenteral feeding, or neonates being treated for illness should have a specimen of blood serum obtained for screening at or near 7 days of age if a specimen has not been obtained before that time, regardless of feeding status. An adequate specimen should be provided to the laboratory for analysis. Cord blood is not adequate for detection of phenylketonuria or other disorders in which metabolite accumulation occurs after birth and after the initiation of feeding. If a neonate requires transfusion or dialysis prior to the routine time for acquisition of the newborn screening specimen, appropriate modifications should be made in the screening procedure to allow accurate diagnosis. If the initial specimen is obtained before 24 hours of age, then a second specimen should be obtained at 1–2 weeks of age to decrease the probability that phenylketonuria and other disorders with metabolite accumulation will be missed as a consequence of testing on the first day of life.

The responsibility for transmitting the screening test results to the physician should rest with the authority or agency that performed the test. Screening status should be entered into the patient's record. The pediatrician should recognize the need for careful documentation of newborn screening results on each baby entering the practice for the purpose of comprehensive care.

In the absence of risk factors and symptoms, screening for hypertension or hypotension by blood pressure measurements, for hyperglycemia or hypoglycemia by blood glucose screening, and for polycythemia or anemia by hematocrit determination are not warranted. Screening for blood glucose and hematocrit abnormalities is appropriate for high-risk babies, such as those born to diabetic mothers and in cases of intrauterine growth restriction and twin-to-twin transfusion.

Hearing Screening

The prevalence of newborn and infant hearing loss is estimated at 1.5–6.0 per 1,000 live births. Detection of hearing loss as early as possible, preferably before 3 months of age, facilitates early intervention and the possibility of improved functional outcome.

Programs should be in place to provide assessment services to neonates identified to be at risk for hearing problems. Neonates should be screened for hearing loss if the following risk factors are present:

- Family history of hereditary childhood sensorineural hearing loss
- In utero infection, such as cytomegalovirus, rubella, syphilis, herpes, or toxoplasmosis
- Craniofacial anomalies, including infants with morphologic abnormalities of the pinnae and ear canals
- Birth weight less than 1,500 g
- Hyperbilirubinemia at a serum level requiring exchange transfusion
- Ototoxic medications, including, but not limited to, aminoglycosides used in multiple courses or in combination with loop diuretics
- Bacterial meningitis
- Apgar score of 0–4 at 1 minute or 0–6 at 5 minutes after birth
- Mechanical ventilation lasting 5 days or longer
- Stigmata or other findings associated with a syndrome known to include a sensorineural or conductive hearing loss

When hearing loss is identified in an infant, evaluation and early intervention services should be provided. The multidisciplinary evaluation and assessment of an infant identified with hearing loss should be performed by a team of professionals working in conjunction with the parent or caregiver.

Visiting

The father or supporting person may remain with the mother throughout the intrapartum and postpartum periods. Whenever possible, parents of neonates in continuing care, intermediate care, or intensive care areas should be allowed unrestricted visits. Provisions should be made for feeding (particularly breastfeeding), handling, and holding these neonates. Flexible and liberal visiting policies for families are encouraged.

Some institutions offer sibling classes to prepare other children in a family for the event of childbirth. Contact with the mother and newborn in the hospital helps prepare siblings for the new family member and is reassuring for younger children. The presence of siblings may be appropriate in labor, at delivery, or in the postpartum period, as local policy permits. The children must be accompanied by an adult to help them understand what is occurring and to remove them if circumstances demand.

Physical contact of siblings with neonates is a topic of current concern because of the possible transmission of viral infectious diseases. If siblings are allowed to have direct contact with the newborn, the visit may take place in the mother's private room or, if the mother is not in a private room, in a special sibling visitation area. Thorough hand-washing should be required. Parents should share the responsibility of preventing the exposure of their newborn to a sibling with a contagious illness. Contact of the newborn with children other than siblings should be avoided (see also Chapter 10).

An institution that allows sibling visitation should have clearly defined, written policies and procedures that are based on currently available information. Basic guidelines for sibling visits, which may serve as the basis for policy formulation, are as follows:

- Sibling visits should be encouraged in both the healthy-baby nursery and the newborn intensive care nursery.

- Before the visit, a nurse or physician should interview the parents at a site outside the unit to assess the current health of each sibling visitor. No child with fever or symptoms of an acute illness, such as upper respiratory infection or gastroenteritis, should be allowed to visit. Siblings who have been recently exposed to a known communicable disease (eg, chickenpox) should not be allowed to visit.

- Children should be prepared in advance for their visit.

- All visitors should be adequately observed and monitored by the medical and nursing staff.

- The visiting sibling should visit only his or her sibling.
- Children should carefully wash their hands before patient contact.
- Throughout the visit, sibling activity should be supervised by parents or a responsible adult.

Because available data on the risks and benefits of sibling visitation are limited, continued evaluation and reporting are needed. Evaluation should include both psychologic and infectious-disease factors. Institutions that have not introduced sibling visitation should consider the opportunity to use controlled trials to study the effects of these programs. Institutions offering controlled sibling visitation in neonatal intensive care units have noted no adverse effects, but more study is needed before a general recommendation can be made.

Discharge

The hospital stay of the mother and neonate should be long enough to allow identification of problems and to ensure that the mother is sufficiently recovered and prepared to care for herself and her baby at home. Many neonatal cardiopulmonary problems that are related to the transition from the intrauterine to the extrauterine environment usually become apparent during the first 12 hours after birth. Other neonatal problems, such as jaundice, ductal-dependent cardiac lesions, and gastrointestinal obstruction, may require a longer period of observation by skilled and experienced personnel. Likewise, significant maternal complications, such as endometritis, may not become apparent during the first day after delivery. The length of stay should therefore be based on the unique characteristics of each mother–infant dyad, including the health of the mother, the health and stability of the baby, the ability and confidence of the mother to care for herself and her baby, the adequacy of support systems at home, and access to appropriate follow-up care. All efforts should be made to keep mothers and babies together and to ensure simultaneous discharge.

The timing of discharge from the hospital should be the decision of the physicians caring for the mother and the baby. The decision of when to discharge should be made in consultation with the family and should not be based on arbitrary policies established by third-party payers.

A shortened hospital stay (<48 hours after delivery) for healthy term infants can be accomplished but is not appropriate for every mother and neonate. Each mother–baby dyad should be evaluated individually to determine the optimal time of discharge. Local institution of discharge guidelines is best accomplished through the collaborative efforts of all concerned parties. Institutions should develop guidelines through their professional staff in collaboration with appropriate community agencies, including third-party payers, to establish hospital stay programs for healthy term infants and their mothers. State and local public health agencies should also be involved in the oversight of existing hospital stay programs for quality assurance and monitoring.

Maternal Considerations

When no complications are present, the postpartum hospital stay ranges from 48 hours for vaginal delivery to 96 hours for cesarean birth, excluding the day of delivery. When the physician and the mother want a shortened hospital stay, certain minimal criteria should be met:

- The mother is afebrile, with pulse and respirations of normal rate and quality.
- Her blood pressure is within the normal range.
- The amount and color of lochia are appropriate for the duration of recovery.
- The uterine fundus is firm.
- Urinary output is adequate.
- Any surgical repair or wound has minimal edema and no evidence of infection and appears to be healing without complication.
- The mother is able to ambulate with ease.
- There are no abnormal physical or emotional findings.
- The mother is able to eat and drink without difficulty.

- Arrangements have been made for postpartum follow-up care.
- The mother has been instructed in caring for herself and the baby at home, is aware of deviations from normal, and is prepared to recognize and respond to danger signs and symptoms.
- The mother demonstrates readiness to care for herself and her baby.
- Pertinent laboratory results are available, including a postpartum measurement of hemoglobin or hematocrit.
- ABO blood group and D type are known, and, if indicated, the appropriate amount of D immune globulin has been administered.
- The mother has received instructions on postpartum activity and exercises and common postpartum discomforts and relief measures.
- Family members or other support persons are available to the mother for the first few days following discharge.

The medical and nursing staff should be sensitive to potential problems associated with shortened hospital stays and should develop mechanisms to address patient questions that arise after discharge. With a shortened hospital stay, a home visit or follow-up phone conference by a health care provider such as a lactation nurse within 48 hours of discharge is encouraged.

When a pregnancy, labor, or delivery is complicated by medical or obstetric disorders, the mother's readiness for discharge may be based on the aforementioned criteria, as modified by the individual judgment of the obstetric care provider. The stability of the mother's medical condition, the need for continued inpatient observation, and treatment and risks of complications should be taken into consideration.

Neonatal Considerations

The following minimum criteria should be met before a newborn is discharged from the hospital after an uncomplicated pregnancy, labor, and delivery. It is unlikely that the fulfillment of these criteria and conditions can be met in less than 48 hours after birth:

- The antepartum, intrapartum, and postpartum courses for both mother and baby are uncomplicated.
- Delivery was vaginal.
- The baby is a single birth at 38–42 weeks of gestation, and birth weight is appropriate for gestational age according to appropriate intrauterine growth curves.
- The baby's vital signs are documented to be normal and stable for the 12 hours preceding discharge, including a respiratory rate of fewer than 60 breaths per minute, a heart rate of 100–160 beats per minute, and an axillary temperature of 36.1–37°C (97.0–98.6°F) in an open crib with appropriate clothing.
- The baby has urinated and has passed at least one stool.
- The baby has completed at least two successful feedings, and documentation has been made that the baby is able to coordinate sucking, swallowing, and breathing while feeding.
- Physical examination reveals no abnormalities that require continued hospitalization.
- There is no evidence of excessive bleeding at the circumcision site for at least 2 hours.
- There is no evidence of significant jaundice in the first 24 hours of life. (Noninvasive means of detecting jaundice may be useful.)
- The mother's knowledge, ability, and confidence to provide adequate care for her baby are documented by the fact that she has received the following training:
  — Breastfeeding or bottle-feeding—The breastfeeding mother–baby dyad should be assessed by trained staff regarding nursing position, latch-on, adequacy of swallowing, and mother's knowledge of urine and stool frequency.
  — Cord, skin, and infant genital care should be reviewed.
  — The mother should be able to recognize signs of illness and common infant problems, particularly jaundice.

— Instruction in proper infant safety (eg, proper use of a car seat and positioning for sleeping) should be provided.

• Family members or other support persons, including health care providers such as the family pediatrician or his or her designees, who are familiar with newborn care and are knowledgeable about lactation and the recognition of jaundice and dehydration are available to the mother and the baby for the first few days after discharge.

• Laboratory data are available and have been reviewed, including the following:

— Maternal syphilis and hepatitis B virus surface antigen status

— Cord or infant blood type and direct Coombs' test result, as clinically indicated

• Screening tests have been done in accordance with state regulations. If a test was done before 24 hours of milk feeding, a system for repeating the test during the follow-up visit must be in place.

• Initial hepatitis B vaccine has been administered or an appointment scheduled for its administration within the first week of life.

• A physician-directed source of continuing medical care for both the mother and the baby has been identified. For newborns discharged before 48 hours after delivery, a definitive appointment has been made for the baby to be examined within 48 hours of discharge. The follow-up visit can take place in a home or clinic setting, as long as the personnel examining the neonate are competent in newborn assessment and the results of the follow-up visit are reported to the neonate's physician or designees on the day of the visit.

• Family, environmental, and social risk factors have been assessed. When risk factors are present, the discharge should be delayed until they are resolved or a plan to safeguard the infant is in place. Such factors may include, but are not limited to, the following:

— Untreated parental substance use or positive urine toxicology results in the mother or newborn

— History of child abuse or neglect
— Mental illness in a parent who is in the home
— Lack of social support, particularly for single, first-time mothers
— No fixed home
— History of untreated domestic violence, particularly during this pregnancy
— Adolescent mother, particularly if other risk factors are present

All newborns having a shortened hospital stay should be examined by experienced health care providers within 48 hours of discharge. This follow-up visit should be considered an independent service to be reimbursed as a separate package and not as part of a global fee for labor, delivery, and routine nursery services. If it cannot be assured that this examination will take place, discharge should be deferred until a mechanism for follow-up evaluation is identified. The follow-up visit is designed to fulfill the following functions:

• Assess the newborn's general health, hydration, and degree of jaundice and identify any new problems
• Review feeding pattern and technique, including observation of breastfeeding for adequacy of position, latch-on, and swallowing
• Collect historical evidence of adequate stool and urine patterns
• Assess quality of mother–baby interaction and details of infant behavior
• Reinforce maternal or family education in neonatal care, particularly regarding feeding and sleep position
• Review results of laboratory tests performed at discharge
• Perform screening tests in accordance with state regulations and other tests that are clinically indicated
• Identify a plan for health care maintenance, including a method for obtaining emergency services, preventive care and immunizations, periodic evaluations and physical examinations, and necessary screening

High-Risk Neonates

Discharge planning for high-risk neonates should begin shortly after admission to ensure a smooth transition from the hospital to the home. The following minimum criteria should be met before discharge:

• The neonate has had a comprehensive physical examination to identify problems that may require ongoing close surveillance (eg, atypical head growth, heart murmur) and to provide data on which to base future assessments. If preterm, the neonate was tested for anemia before discharge.

• The neonate is stable physiologically and is able to maintain body temperature without cold stress when the amount of clothing worn and the room temperature are appropriate to what the neonate will experience in the home.

• The neonate is gaining weight steadily on enteral feedings.

• The neonate is able to breastfeed or bottle-feed adequately. If the neonate's clinical condition precludes adequate nipple feeding, the parents or other care providers are competent in alternative feeding techniques.

• The neonate is free of apnea or can be monitored appropriately at home.

• The mother's knowledge, ability, and confidence to provide adequate care for her baby are documented by the fact that she has been assessed by trained staff in the following areas:

— Preparation, dosing accuracy, and proper storage and administration of medications (eg, diuretics and bronchodilators for infants with chronic lung disease)

— Use of oxygen therapy or monitoring equipment (eg, apnea monitor), including the ability to set up and monitor oxygen delivery system or monitoring equipment

— Ability to provide appropriate nutrition to the infant, including adequate frequency and volume of feeding and the ability to mix calorically dense formulas

— Recognition of signs of illness and acute deterioration (eg, wheezing in infants with chronic lung disease)

— Basic neonatal cardiopulmonary resuscitation
— Proper infant safety, including car seat adaptations for infants weighing less than 2,000 g and recommended sleeping positions for premature infants

• Appropriate immunizations have been given (see Chapter 9).

• Hearing screening has been accomplished or an appointment for hearing evaluation has been scheduled.

• Ophthalmologic assessment of neonates born at less than 27 weeks of gestational age or weighing 1,250 g or less at birth (as determined by hospital policy) has been performed, and a follow-up appointment has been scheduled.

• A physician-directed source of continuing medical care, including periodic assessment of infant development, has been identified.

• Family, environmental, and social risk factors have been assessed and, if present, have been resolved, or a plan to safeguard the infant is in place. These factors may include, but are not limited to, the following:

— Untreated parental substance use or positive urine toxicology results in the mother or newborn
— History of child abuse or neglect
— Mental illness in a parent who is in the home
— Lack of social support
— No fixed home
— History of untreated domestic violence, particularly during this pregnancy
— Infrequent visitation or phone inquiry during the baby's hospital stay

Education and Psychosocial Factors

The reduction in the average length of a patient's hospital stay has compromised the opportunity for parent education. Hospital resources that have traditionally been extended to parents can no longer be accommodated within the shortened hospital stay. Physicians should be willing to accept, understand, and respond to parent inquiries that arise throughout the perinatal period and should make every effort to ensure that educational aspects of care are provided before and after hospitalization.

Closed-circuit television films that have been previewed and approved by the obstetric and pediatric staff, printed materials, and counseling by hospital personnel (eg, postpartum and nursery nurses, registered dietitians/nutritionists, and physical therapists) have been helpful to parents. Other beneficial activities are group or individual educational sessions held regularly during the postpartum period to teach and discuss patient self-care, including exercises and self-examination of the breasts; parent–neonate relationships; care of the neonate, including bathing and feeding; and child growth and development. Family-planning techniques appropriate to the patient's needs and desires should be explained in detail.

The newborn undergoes rapid changes in physiology that should be explained to the parents. The neonate's cardiovascular, pulmonary, renal, and neurologic maturation should be observed by the parents with the guidance of qualified personnel. Parents should be familiar with normal and abnormal changes in wake–sleep patterns, temperature, respiration, voiding, stooling, and the appearance of the skin, including jaundice. They should also observe and become familiar with the behavior, temperament, and neurologic capabilities of the newborn. Awareness of infant cardiopulmonary resuscitation techniques may also be helpful.

During the postpartum hospital stay, health care personnel can provide the mother with professional assistance when she is most likely to be uncomfortable and can help her to anticipate how she may feel once she is home. The new mother may be unsure of the normal physical changes that occur after delivery and of her ability to care for the newborn. The mother should be evaluated when she is with her neonate to identify any problems she is having so that appropriate instructions with education can be provided before and after discharge. Prenatal instructions given to prepare the family for the neonate's care at home should also be reinforced.

Both in-hospital and community agencies are often available to assist the family. Information on public and private groups that provide services to families with newborns, and the circumstances under which these organizations may be asked for such assistance, should be available in the hospital. Sources may include the following:

- The in-hospital social service department, as an integral part of the interdisciplinary effort to coordinate hospital and discharge activities, to obtain public or private assistance, and to render psychosocial support
- Members of the home care services, for home visits to assess the parents' child-rearing skills, the home environment, the mother's emotional stability, and the neonate's status and development (under the physician's direction, these nurses may administer drugs or provide other types of therapy)
- Groups that lend support and provide education on special activities (eg, breastfeeding)

Sleep Position

Sudden infant death syndrome (SIDS) is the leading cause of infant mortality after 1 month and before 1 year of age in the United States. Recent investigations on the hazards of prone sleeping and reviews of the epidemiology of SIDS with attention to sleep position have resulted in the recommendation that healthy neonates not be placed in the prone position for sleeping. Although supine positioning (lying wholly on the back) carries the lowest risk of SIDS and is preferred, side positioning is a reasonable alternative. For neonates with gastroesophageal reflux, obstructive sleep apnea, or certain congenital malformations, the physician should recommend specific sleep positioning.

Declines in deaths due to SIDS have been documented in countries where parents have changed from placing babies in prone positions to back positions for sleeping. No adverse effects of supine positioning have become apparent. Although prospectively collected data may clarify the issues, the supine position appears to be a prudent recommendation for placing the healthy neonate for sleeping.

Postpartum Considerations

Before discharge, the mother should receive information about normal postpartum events, including the following:

- Changes in lochia pattern expected in the first few weeks

- Range of activities that she may reasonably undertake
- Care of the breasts, perineum, and bladder
- Dietary needs, particularly if she is breastfeeding
- Recommended amount of exercise
- Emotional responses
- Signs of complications (eg, temperature elevation, chills, leg pains, episiotomy or wound drainage, increased vaginal bleeding)

The length of convalescence that the patient can expect, based on the type of delivery, should also be discussed. For women who have had cesarean delivery, additional precautions may be appropriate, such as wound care and temporary abstinence from lifting objects heavier than the baby and from driving motor vehicles. It is helpful to reinforce oral discussions with written information.

The earliest time at which coitus may be resumed safely after childbirth is unknown. Resumption of coitus should be discussed with the couple. Risks of hemorrhage and infection are minimal approximately 2 weeks postpartum. By this time the uterus has involuted markedly and the endometrium and cervix have begun to reepithelialize. Thereafter, coitus can be resumed, depending on the patient's desire and comfort and on resolution of contraceptive issues.

Sexual difficulties that are common in the early months after childbirth should be discussed. Healing at the episiotomy site can cause the woman some discomfort during intercourse within the first year following delivery. In the lactating woman, the vagina is often atrophic and dry. Lubrication during sexual excitement may be unsatisfactory. Furthermore, the demands of the neonate's care alter the couple's ability to find time for physical intimacy.

Methods of contraception should be fully reviewed and implemented. Nonnursing mothers may begin using a contraceptive soon after delivery if they wish to avoid becoming pregnant. Combined oral contraceptives may be prescribed, or levonorgestrel implants or depot medroxyprogesterone acetate can be initiated before discharge. Nonnursing mothers may receive depot medroxyprogesterone acetate within 5 days after delivery. Nursing mothers should delay such an injection until lactation is established.

Nursing mothers may begin using oral contraceptives as soon as their milk supply is established. Progesterone-only contraceptives do not appear to have adverse effects on lactation. An intrauterine device that contains copper is also an option that does not interfere with breast milk. However, intrauterine devices are generally not inserted until 4–6 weeks postpartum. A diaphragm or a cervical cap cannot be fitted adequately during the immediate postpartum period and should be delayed until the 4–6-week examination.

Patients for whom the use of oral contraceptives is contraindicated or who prefer other methods of contraception, such as foam or condoms, should be offered instruction in their use. Spermicides and barrier methods have no effect on breastfeeding. Lubricated condoms may offset vaginal dryness secondary to breastfeeding. Fertility awareness methods, such as the rhythm method, are difficult to practice accurately before the resumption of menses and therefore are not recommended.

At the time of discharge, the family should be given the name of the person to contact if questions or problems arise for either the mother or the neonate. Arrangements should be made for a follow-up examination and specific instructions conveyed to the mother, including when contact is advisable.

In general, the following points should be reviewed with the mother or, preferably, with both parents; specific information to be conveyed is discussed within this section.

• Condition of the neonate

• Immediate needs of the neonate (eg, feeding methods and environmental supports)

• Feeding techniques; skin care, including cord care; temperature assessment and measurement with a thermometer; and assessment of neonatal well-being and recognition of illness

• Roles of the obstetrician, pediatrician, and other members of the health care team concerned with the continuous medical care of the mother and neonate

• Availability of support systems, including psychosocial support

• Instructions to follow in the event of a complication or emergency

• Importance of maintaining newborn immunization, beginning with an initial dose of hepatitis B virus vaccine

Follow-Up Care

The physical and psychosocial status of the mother and neonate should be subject to ongoing assessment after discharge. The new mother needs personalized care during the postpartum period to hasten the development of a healthy mother–infant relationship and a sense of maternal confidence. Support and reassurance should be provided as the mother masters neonatal-care tasks and adapts to her maternal role. Involving the father and encouraging him to participate in the neonate's care not only can provide additional support to the mother but can also enhance the father–infant relationship.

The postpartum period is a time of developmental adjustment for the whole family. Family members now have new roles and relationships, and an effort should be made to assess the progress of the family's adaptation. If a family member—mother, father, or sibling—finds it difficult to assume the new role, the health care team should arrange for sensitive, supportive assistance. This is particularly important for adolescent mothers, for whom it may be necessary to mobilize multiple resources within the community.

Maternal Considerations

Approximately 4–6 weeks after delivery, the mother should visit her physician for a postpartum review and examination. This interval may be modified according to the needs of the patient with medical, obstetric, or intercurrent complications. A visit within 7–14 days of delivery may be advisable after a cesarean delivery or a complicated gestation.

The review at the first postpartum visit should include obtaining an interval history and performing a physical examination to evaluate the patient's current status and her adaptation to the newborn. Specific inquiries regarding breastfeeding should be made. The examination should include an evaluation of weight, blood pressure, breasts, and abdomen, as well as a pelvic examination. Episiotomy repair and uterine involution should be evaluated and a Pap test done, if needed. Methods of birth control should be reviewed or initiated.

Many women experience some degree of emotional lability in the postpartum period. If this persists or develops into clinically significant depression, intervention may be needed. The emotional status of a woman whose pregnancy had an abnormal outcome should also be reviewed. Counseling should address specific issues regarding her future health and pregnancies. For example, it may be advantageous to discuss vaginal birth after a cesarean delivery or the implications of diabetes, intrauterine growth restriction, prematurity, hypertension, fetal anomalies, or other conditions that may recur in any future pregnancies. Laboratory data should be obtained as indicated. This is a good time to review immunizations, including rubella vaccination for women who are susceptible and did not receive the vaccine immediately postpartum, and to discuss any special problems. The patient should be encouraged to return for subsequent periodic examinations.

The postpartum visit is an excellent time to begin preconception counseling for patients who may wish to have future pregnancies. This counseling includes risk assessment to facilitate the planning, spacing, and timing of the next pregnancy; health promotion measures; and timely intervention to reduce medical and psychosocial risks. Such intervention may include treatment of infections, counseling regarding behaviors such as those related to HIV transmission, nutrition counseling, supplementation, and appropriate referrals for follow-up care. Although physiologic considerations indicate that a woman can return to a normal work schedule 4–6 weeks after delivery, attention should also be given to maternal–infant bonding.

Neonatal Considerations

The frequency of follow-up visits for normal neonates varies with patient, locale, and community practices. The interval should be consistent with the American Academy of Pediatrics' guidelines on preventive health care. Regular follow-up visits and good records of development should be maintained.

The intervals of follow-up visits required by high-risk neonates should be determined by the needs of the individual infant and family. It may be necessary to examine some of these infants weekly or bi-monthly at first. Neurologic, developmental, behavioral, and sensory status should be assessed more than once during the first year in high-risk infants to ensure early identification of problems and referral for remedial care. A perinatal follow-up program with an appropriate staff of multidisciplinary personnel is useful in providing these assessments.

Physicians and other professionals who provide follow-up care to mothers and infants should be aware of and look for the physical, social, and psychologic factors associated with child abuse, including the following:

- Prematurity
- Neonatal illness with long periods of hospitalization, especially in neonatal intensive care units
- Single parenthood
- Adolescent motherhood
- Closely spaced pregnancies
- Infrequent family visits to hospitalized infants
- Substance use

Children born prematurely have been shown to have a greater incidence of irritability, hyperkinesis, and increased dependency. Prolonged hospitalization inevitably disrupts family relationships, particularly the parent–child relationship. Infants and parents with such a history or with other factors associated with child abuse require closer follow-up than does the average family. The interaction of the parents, especially the mother, with the infant should be evaluated periodically. The infant or child who fails to thrive may be a victim of neglect, if not outright abuse, and a causal relationship between neglect and failure to thrive should always be suspected. In every state, providers of health care to children are legally obligated to report suspected child abuse.

Assessment

Growth parameters of the infant should be assessed, including continued monitoring of the adequacy of weight gain, linear growth, and head growth. Growth should be plotted on standardized growth curves. Review of nutritional intake and calculation of caloric intake are helpful in case management.

Physical examination should assess neuromotor, cardiac, pulmonary, and gastrointestinal status, as well as any hernias, anomalies, or orthopedic deformities. Parents of infants who were cared for in the neonatal intensive care unit are often concerned about minor scars secondary to procedures performed in the unit, and they benefit from reassurance.

Medication dosage should be reevaluated, doses increased with weight gain and age, and blood levels monitored when indicated. Immunization status should be reviewed. Follow-up audiologic and visual assessments should be obtained when indicated.

In the primary physician's office, neurologic assessment should include an appraisal of muscle tone, reflexes, and visual and auditory responses. In addition, a standard developmental screening tool, such as the Denver Developmental Screening Test, should be used. When neurologic findings are suspicious or when developmental delays are suggested, infants should be referred for more in-depth assessment, either to a neonatal follow-up program or to equivalent facilities or programs capable of providing detailed neurodevelopmental assessments.

Early Intervention

Intervention programs for neurodevelopmental disabilities offer therapeutic guidelines for families, parent support groups, respite care programs, and innovative therapy modalities. Although no definitive data confirm the beneficial effects of infant stimulation programs, indications are that early intervention may improve the social adaptation of infants with neurodevelopmental disabilities, as well as that of their families.

Technology-Dependent Neonates

In recent years, with improvements in survival rates of low-birth-weight neonates, an increasing number of babies, including those with bronchopulmonary dysplasia and those with persistent apnea, require cardiopulmonary monitoring for a considerable period at home. Many children with chronic lung disease require equipment to deliver oxygen at home, cardiopulmonary monitoring when appropriate, and assessment of oxygen status by pulse oximetry. The appropriate management of these neonates will require the coordinated team efforts of the tertiary-care physicians, primary care physicians, discharge planning personnel, social workers, visiting nurses, and providers of home care products. In many medical communities, tertiary-care personnel take responsibility for coordinating the management and follow-up of these children.

Adoption

Health care for babies who are to be adopted should focus on the needs of the child, the adoptive family, and the birth parents. These babies may have acute and long-term medical, psychologic, and developmental problems because of their genetic, emotional, cultural, psychosocial, or medical backgrounds. The pediatrician should perform a careful medical assessment of the child and should counsel the adopting family appropriately. Just as a birth family cannot be certain that its biologic child will be healthy, an adoptive family cannot be guaranteed that a child will not have future health problems. Most adopted children, even those from high-risk backgrounds, are healthy. Those with certain disorders and special problems, however, can also be successfully adopted. Risks should be defined and carefully explained to the family so that problems can be anticipated and addressed expediently.

The pediatrician's role is not to judge the advisability of a proposed adoption, but to apprise the prospective parents and any involved agency clearly and honestly of any special health needs detected at examination or anticipated in the future. Pediatricians evaluating a newborn for adoption should obtain an extensive history from the birth parents and enter these data into the formal medical record. There may never again be a comparable opportunity to obtain this information. If the pediatrician is unable to interview the parents personally, an adoption agency social worker who is trained to do a skilled genetic and medical interview should obtain a complete prenatal and postpartum history. The prenatal history should include information on the birth parents' lifestyle that may affect the fetus at birth or later in development. Physicians and adoption agency social workers should be trained to obtain lifestyle information in a manner that is sensitive to psychologic and cultural issues. Such information includes parental use of alcohol or other drugs and history of sexual practices that increase the risk of sexually transmissible infections in both birth parents. The increased risk of genetically inherited disorders by neonates of incestuous matings may require special consultations. After reviewing whatever history is available, the pediatrician should examine the adopted child carefully and perform metabolic, genetic, and other assessments as indicated.

Physicians must be careful with semantics when dealing with the adoptive family. This is an "adoptive family," not only an "adopted child." The term *parents* applies to the parents in the adoptive family; the *birth parents* are those who conceived the child. *Real* or *natural parent(s)* are confusing terms that should be eliminated because they may reflect negatively on adoptive families and imply a temporary or less-than-genuine relationship between adoptive families and their children.

The physician should be aware of state laws on adoption procedures. Hospital nurseries should have policies regarding the handling of adoptions in accordance with these laws.

Bibliography

American Academy of Pediatrics, Committee on Children with Disabilities. Guidelines for home care of infants, children, and adolescents with chronic disease. Pediatrics 1995;96:161–164

American Academy of Pediatrics, Committee on Fetus and Newborn. Hospital stay for healthy term newborns. Pediatrics 1995;96:788–790

American Academy of Pediatrics, Committee on Fetus and Newborn. The initiation or withdrawal of treatment for high-risk newborns. Pediatrics 1995;96:362–363

American Academy of Pediatrics, Committee on Genetics. Newborn screening fact sheets. Pediatrics 1996;98:473–501

American Academy of Pediatrics, Joint Committee on Infant Hearing. Joint Committee on Infant Hearing 1994 position statement. Pediatrics 1995; 95:152–156

American Academy of Pediatrics, Task Force on Circumcision. Care of the uncircumcised penis. Elk Grove Village, Illinois: AAP, 1996

American Academy of Pediatrics, Task Force on Circumcision. Report of the Task Force on Circumcision. Pediatrics 1989;84:388–391 (erratum in Pediatrics 1989;84:761)

American Academy of Pediatrics, Task Force on Infant Positioning and SIDS. Positioning and sudden infant death syndrome (SIDS): update. Pediatrics 1996;98:1216-1218

American Academy of Pediatrics, Vitamin K Ad Hoc Task Force. Controversies concerning vitamin K and the newborn. Pediatrics 1993;91:1001–1003

American Academy of Pediatrics, American College of Obstetricians and Gynecologists. Perinatal care at the threshold of viability. Committee Opinion 163. Washington, DC: ACOG, 1995

American Academy of Pediatrics, American College of Obstetricians and Gynecologists. Use and abuse of the Apgar score. Pediatrics 1996;98:141–142

Ballard JL, Khoury JC, Wedig K, Wang L, Eilers-Walsman BL, Lipp R. New Ballard Score, expanded to include extremely premature infants. J Pediatr 1991;119:417–423

Chapter 8

Neonatal Special Concerns

Some neonatal conditions and treatments are of special concern because of advances in knowledge, controversies surrounding these issues, or their importance to the family. Whenever possible, therapies should be based on the best evidence available, preferably from well-designed, randomized, controlled trials.

Hyperbilirubinemia

Although bilirubin may be toxic to the central nervous system and may cause neurologic impairment, the factors that determine the toxicity of bilirubin to the brain cells of neonates are many, complex, and incompletely understood. Factors include those that affect serum albumin concentration and the binding of bilirubin to albumin, the penetration of bilirubin into the brain, and the vulnerability of brain cells to the toxic effects of bilirubin. In addition, the interrelationships between serum bilirubin concentrations and kernicterus (a condition characterized by yellow discoloration of the brain and specific yellow staining of the nuclear areas) and bilirubin encephalopathy (brain damage due to bilirubin) are not clear. The incidence of mild neurologic impairment caused by bilirubin is not known, nor is it known at what bilirubin concentration or under what circumstances the risk of brain damage exceeds that of treatment. In addition to uncertainty about the cause and effect of the disorder, differences in patient populations, geographic locations, and practice settings contribute to variations in the management of hyperbilirubinemia.

Bilirubin Toxicity

A direct association between severe, unconjugated hyperbilirubinemia, kernicterus, and bilirubin encephalopathy has been demonstrated in neonates with erythroblastosis fetalis. In the past, survivors often manifested serious sequelae, particularly the athetoid form of cerebral palsy, hearing loss, paralysis of upward gaze, and dentoalveolar dysplasia. In most studies of otherwise healthy term infants without hemolysis, total serum bilirubin levels of less than 25 mg/dl (428 μmol/L) have not been associated with either cognitive or serious neurologic abnormalities.

Studies of low-birth-weight neonates have failed to identify a specific serum bilirubin concentration as a risk factor for kernicterus. As a result of reported autopsy findings of yellow-stained cerebral tissues in premature neonates whose bilirubin concentrations never exceeded 10 mg/dl (171 μmol/L), published guidelines for the management of jaundice in such neonates have suggested early phototherapy and exchange transfusion at bilirubin concentrations of as low as 10 mg/dl (171 μmol/L). Several studies of low-birth-weight neonates, however, have failed to confirm a relationship between serum bilirubin concentrations and later neurodevelopmental handicap, particularly if serum bilirubin concentrations did not exceed 20 mg/dl (342 μmol/L).

Management of Jaundice

Data from numerous studies of bilirubin toxicity are so complex that it is difficult to derive a single rational approach to jaundiced neonates. One principle is well accepted: If the infant's clinical course suggests that the jaundice is not physiologic, the cause should be investigated. Jaundice that persists beyond 3 weeks requires further investigation, including a measurement of total and direct serum levels.

Term Infants with Hemolytic Disease

Clinical observation of term neonates with hemolytic disease has confirmed that the occurrence of clinical kernicterus is highly unlikely if serum unconjugated bilirubin concentrations are less than 20 mg/dl (342 μmol/L). The physician may elect to perform an exchange transfusion before the serum bilirubin concentration reaches 20 mg/dl (342 μmol/L) if several determinations of bilirubin levels indicate that the concentration is likely to reach that point. Women who are likely to deliver neonates with edema hydrops fetalis should be cared for in perinatal centers that are capable of the full range of obstetric and neonatal intensive care.

Term Infants Without Hemolytic Disease

There are no properly designed studies, or even observational data, on low-birth-weight or term neonates without hemolytic disease on which to base clinical guidelines for the treatment of neonates with serum bilirubin concentrations of less than 20 mg/dl (342 μmol/L). A review of available follow-up data for apparently healthy term infants whose serum bilirubin concentrations were as high as 25 mg/dl (428 μmol/L) showed no apparent ill effects from these concentrations. On the basis of these observations, the American Academy of Pediatrics developed guidelines for managing healthy term infants (defined as those born at ≥37 weeks of gestation) who have hyperbilirubinemia but no signs of illness or apparent hemolytic disease (Table 8–1).

Table 8–1. Management of Hyperbilirubinemia in the Healthy Term Newborn

	Total Serum Bilirubin Levels (mg/dl)			
Age (hours)	Consider Phototherapy*	Phototherapy	Exchange Transfusion If Intensive Phototherapy Fails	Exchange Transfusion and Intensive Phototherapy
< 24	Term infants who are clinically jaundiced at < 24 hours are not considered "healthy" and require evaluation			
25–48	≥12	≥15	≥20	≥25
49–72	≥15	≥18	≥25	≥30
≥73	≥17	≥20	≥25	≥30

* Phototherapy at these levels is a clinical option; that is, the intervention is available and may be used on the basis of individual clinical judgment.

Modified from the American Academy of Pediatrics, Provisional Committee for Quality Improvement and Subcommittee on Hyperbilirubinemia. Practice parameter: management of hyperbilirubinemia in the healthy term neonate. Pediatrics 1994;94:558–565.

Low-Birth-Weight Infants

Some pediatricians recommend initiating phototherapy early and performing exchange transfusions in selected low-birth-weight neonates who have serum bilirubin concentrations of as low as 10 mg/dl (171 μmol/L). However, this approach cannot guarantee the prevention of kernicterus. Some pediatricians allow serum bilirubin to reach 15–20 mg/dl (257–342 μmol/L) before considering exchange transfusion. Both of these approaches are reasonable.

Breastfed Infants

Composite data from several studies reveal that breastfed neonates have a higher incidence of elevated serum bilirubin concentrations than do bottle-fed neonates. The finding of an association between breastfeeding and increased serum concentrations of bilirubin does not imply a causal relationship.

Some evidence indicates that frequent breastfeeding (8–10 times per 24 hours) may reduce the incidence of hyperbilirubinemia. Supplementing nursing with water or dextrose–water will not lower serum bilirubin levels in jaundiced, healthy, breastfeeding infants. When an indirect serum bilirubin concentration is elevated by some pathologic cause, there is no reason to discontinue breastfeeding.

In the 1–2% of breastfed neonates who develop the syndrome of breast milk jaundice, an elevated serum concentration of unconjugated bilirubin may persist for several weeks. Although no cases of overt bilirubin encephalopathy related to breast milk jaundice have been reported, there is no reason to believe that significant elevations of serum bilirubin in breastfed neonates are less threatening than are similar elevations in bottle-fed neonates. If the bilirubin concentration in a breastfed neonate is rising and seems likely to reach 25 mg/dl (428 μmol/L), nursing may be interrupted for 48 hours.

Mothers who must temporarily cease nursing should be given positive and enthusiastic support. They should be encouraged to maintain lactation by using a breast pump or manual expression during the period of interrupted nursing. They should also be reassured that the nutritional value of their milk is not compromised by the use of these methods.

Hydration

There is no evidence that excess fluid administered to the infant lowers serum bilirubin concentration. Some infants who are admitted to the hospital with high bilirubin levels may also be mildly dehydrated and may need supplemental fluid intake to correct dehydration. In the absence of dehydration, routine supplementation (with dextrose–water) of infants receiving phototherapy is not indicated.

Phototherapy

Phototherapy is effective in reducing serum bilirubin concentrations in neonates with nonhemolytic jaundice. Phototherapy is less effective in neonates with ABO and CDE (Rh) hemolytic disease, reducing, but not eliminating, the need for exchange transfusions in these infants. Exchange transfusion is the treatment of choice when the bilirubin concentration appears to pose an imminent threat to the health of the neonate.

There is no standardized method for delivering phototherapy. However, detailed recommendations on phototherapy can be found in the hyperbilirubinemia practice parameters of the American Academy of Pediatrics. Commonly used phototherapy units contain daylight, cool white, blue, or "special blue" fluorescent tubes. Other units use tungsten–halogen lamps in different configurations, either freestanding or as part of a radiant-warming device. Fiberoptic systems have been developed that deliver high-intensity light to a fiberoptic blanket.

The efficacy of phototherapy is influenced by the energy output of the phototherapy light, the spectrum of light, and the amount of surface area of the infant exposed to the light source. In most instances, it is acceptable to interrupt phototherapy during feeding or brief parental visits. If the serum bilirubin level continues to rise despite the use of conventional phototherapy, or if the bilirubin levels approach the range at which exchange transfusion might be indicated (Table 8–1), intensive phototherapy should be used. This level can be achieved by increasing the surface area exposed to the lights.

Although phototherapy has many biologic effects, it has no known lasting toxic effects in the human neonate. Because experiments in animals have documented retinal damage from phototherapy, the infant's eyes should be covered with opaque patches when they are exposed to phototherapy light. These patches can become displaced and obstruct the nares, so appropriate supervision is necessary.

Some infants with uncomplicated nonhemolytic jaundice may be treated with phototherapy at home. Guidelines should be developed by each institution to define criteria for infants who are eligible for home phototherapy. Home care requires appropriate follow-up and supervision by a health care professional with access to serum bilirubin determinations as clinically indicated. With proper instruction of the parents or guardians, phototherapy can be provided by using a free-standing device or a fiberoptic blanket. If serum bilirubin levels do not decline in response to conventional phototherapy, admission to the hospital may be indicated for more intensive phototherapy or exchange transfusion and for possible evaluation of the underlying cause.

Clinical Considerations in the Use of Oxygen

The hazards associated with the indiscriminate administration of supplemental oxygen to premature infants have been recognized for many years. Studies conducted in the 1950s indicated that excessive and prolonged oxygen therapy is associated with retinopathy of prematurity, formerly called *retrolental fibroplasia.* The ensuing indiscriminate restriction of ambient oxygen therapy resulted in a marked decrease in retinopathy of prematurity at the cost of a marked increase in mortality and morbidity. Current practice includes the prudent use of supplemental oxygen, guarding against its potential risks.

When supplemental oxygen therapy is considered, the potential risks, in terms of both hypoxia and hyperoxia, should be weighed. Clinical judgment of physical signs alone as a guide to the amount of supplemental oxygen needed is acceptable for short periods. However, some newborns require prolonged use of supplemental oxygen, a clinical judgment that must be supported by a method to monitor oxygen tension or oxygen saturation.

Administration and Monitoring

In an emergency, high concentrations of supplemental oxygen may be administered by a face mask or endotracheal tube. When an infant requires oxygen therapy beyond the emergency period, the delivery of oxygen should be carefully monitored and controlled. The ambient oxygen should be warmed, humidified, and delivered via a system capable of regulating the concentration. Oxygen can be delivered via an endotracheal tube, oxygen hood, nasal prong, or incubator. Oxygen analyzers should be calibrated in accordance with manufacturers' recommendations. Orders for oxygen therapy should be written in terms of desired ambient concentration and should indicate the intervals at which the concentration (or flow rate, when nasal prongs are used) is routinely checked. There should be an institutional policy for documenting oxygen therapy and monitoring.

Periodic measurement of arterial oxygen tension (Pao_2) in samples from an umbilical or peripheral artery catheter is the most reliable method of measuring the level of oxygen therapy. If an indwelling arterial catheter is not in place, radial artery puncture can be used, but repeated sampling from these sites is not always possible. When arterial blood sampling is not possible, arterialized capillary sampling is an acceptable alternative. This measurement produces fairly reliable estimates of arterial pH and arterial carbon dioxide ($Paco_2$) but underestimates Pao_2.

An important development in the care of infants who require oxygen therapy has been the ability to monitor oxygenation continuously with noninvasive techniques. The transcutaneous oxygen analyzer provides an indirect measurement of Pao_2, and the pulse oximeter measures oxyhemoglobin saturation. Because neither technique measures Pao_2 directly, they should be used as adjuncts to, rather than substitutes for, arterial blood gas sampling, especially in infants with moderate to severe respiratory distress.

In infants whose condition is unstable, noninvasive measurements should be correlated with Pao_2 at least every 8–12 hours. More frequent analyses of arterial blood gas may be indicated for the assessment of pH and Pco_2. In infants whose condition is stable, correlation with arterial blood gas samples may be performed less frequently.

The use of either transcutaneous oxygen measurement or pulse oximetry may shorten the time required to determine optimum inspired oxygen concentration and ventilator settings in the acute care setting. Both measurements are particularly useful in monitoring oxygen therapy in infants who are recovering from respiratory distress or who require long-term supplemental oxygen. Because transcutaneous oxygen measurements underestimate oxygenation in older infants with chronic lung disease, pulse oximetry may be a more suitable method for monitoring oxygen therapy in these infants.

In consideration of the current, but incomplete, understanding of the effects of oxygen administration, the following recommendations are offered:

- Supplemental oxygen should not be used without a specific indication, such as cyanosis, low Pao_2, or low oxygen saturation.

- The use of supplemental oxygen other than for resuscitation should be monitored by regular assessments of Pao_2. Infants less than 36 weeks of gestational age who require oxygen therapy should be transferred immediately to a facility able to monitor Pao_2. More mature newborn infants may be administered oxygen for a few hours without such monitoring before a decision is made regarding their transfer. For infants who require oxygen therapy for acute care, measurements of blood pressure, blood pH, and $Paco_2$ should accompany measurements of Pao_2. In addition, a record of blood gas, details of the oxygen delivery system (eg, ventilator, settings, CPAP [continuous postitive airway pressure]), and ambient oxygen concentrations (or liter of flow per minute, if nasal prongs are used) should be maintained.

- When supplemental oxygen is administered to a premature infant, attempts should be made to maintain Pao_2 at 50–80 mm Hg. Oxygen tensions in this range should be adequate for tissue needs, given normal hemoglobin concentrations and blood flow. Even with careful monitoring, however, Pao_2 may fluctuate outside this range, particularly in infants with cardiopulmonary disease. It is sometimes prudent to maintain Pao_2 above 100 mm Hg, especially if attempts to decrease the inspired oxygen concentration dramatically reduce Pao_2 to hypoxemic levels. The increased risk of retinopathy of prematurity may be unavoidable during such periods. In this situation, the medical record should reflect the physician's observations, concerns, and decisions relating to oxygen administration, as well as any discussion with the parents about these decisions and their associated risks and benefits.

- Hourly measurement and recording of the concentration of oxygen delivered to the infant is recommended. The oxygen analyzer should be recalibrated every 8 hours with the use of room air and 100% oxygen.

- Except in emergencies, air–oxygen mixtures should be warmed and humidified before they are administered to newborn infants.

- An individual with experience in neonatal ophthalmology and indirect ophthalmoscopy should examine the retinas of all preterm infants (ie, those delivered at <28 weeks of gestational age or weighing ≤1,500 g at birth). The examination should be performed at 4–6 weeks of chronologic age or at 31–33 weeks postconceptional age (gestational age at birth plus chronologic age), as determined by the infant's attending pediatrician or neonatologist. Follow-up examinations are best determined by the findings of the first examination, using the International Classification of Retinopathy of Prematurity. Infants with threshold disease should be considered candidates for ablative therapy of at least one eye within 72 hours of diagnosis. A written hospital policy for this issue is useful.

Retinopathy of Prematurity

Myriad factors other than hyperoxia may contribute to the pathogenesis of retinopathy of prematurity. Vitamin E deficiency; ambient light; clinical conditions, including acidosis, shock, sepsis, apnea, anemia, and patent ductus arteriosus; and prolonged ventilatory support (especially when accompanied by episodes of hypoxia and hypercapnia) have been associated with retinopathy of prematurity.

To date, a direct relationship between Pao_2 and retinopathy of prematurity has not been established. Retinopathy of prematurity has occurred in premature infants who have never received supplemental oxygen therapy and in infants with cyanotic congenital heart disease in whom Pao_2 levels never exceeded 50 mm Hg. Conversely, retinopathy of prematurity has not developed in some premature infants after prolonged periods of hyperoxia. Finally, continuous close monitoring of transcutaneous oxygen tension has not resulted in a decrease in the incidence of retinopathy of prematurity.

On the basis of published data, the following statements regarding retinopathy of prematurity and oxygen use are warranted:

- Retinopathy of prematurity is not preventable in some infants, especially extremely low-birth-weight infants.

- Many factors other than hyperoxia are important in the pathogenesis of retinopathy of prematurity.

- Transient hyperoxia alone cannot be considered sufficient to cause retinopathy of prematurity.

- No existing standard of care for supplemental oxygen therapy can completely prevent complications or side effects.

Drug Exposure

Neonatal Implications

An increasing number of infants are being admitted to special-care nurseries for complications caused by intrauterine exposure to alcohol and other drugs. Drug exposure often is unrecognized, and the infants are discharged from the nursery to homes where they are at increased risk for a complex of medical and social problems, including abuse and neglect. Symptoms of neonatal opiate withdrawal are often present soon after birth but may not reach a peak until 3–4 days or as late as 10–14 days after birth. Evidence of withdrawal from narcotics can persist in a subacute form for 4–6 months after birth.

Common features of neonatal abstinence syndrome mimic those of an adult's withdrawal from narcotics. Significant signs and symptoms for the neonate include a high-pitched cry, sweating, tremulousness, excoriation of the extremities, and gastrointestinal disturbances. Withdrawal from nonnarcotic substances does not appear to result in as severe a syndrome of abstinence as does withdrawal from narcotics. Increased research is needed to define the degree of permanent residual effects in these infants.

Illicit drugs reach the fetal circulation by crossing the placenta and the newborn through breast milk. They can cause direct toxic effects on the fetus, as well as fetal and maternal dependency. An opiate-exposed fetus may experience withdrawal in utero when drugs are withdrawn from a dependent mother or after delivery, when the mother's use no longer directly affects her newborn. Although, in general, substance-using mothers do not breastfeed their babies, nursing mothers should be counseled about the hazards of substance use.

Cocaine abuse during pregnancy should be considered a major perinatal risk. Cocaine-exposed infants may have an increased incidence of premature birth, impaired fetal growth, and neonatal seizures. A specific cocaine withdrawal syndrome in the neonate has not been defined, but there may be signs of irritability and tremulousness, lethargy, or an inability to respond appropriately to stimulation.

Pediatric Implications

Long-term effects on learning and school performance of children exposed to illicit drugs in utero have not been well documented. Physicians should discuss with all professionals and agencies involved how multifaceted problems resulting from drug exposure in utero might best be addressed in their communities. Environmental factors also place drug-exposed children at high risk for abuse, neglect, and developmental delay. Infants and children of substance-using parents or guardians are at increased risk for physical, sexual, and emotional abuse. Pediatricians should therefore work with their state social service agencies and state legislatures to extend the assistance now available through child protective services. Until that is accomplishe pediatricians should consider recruiting the assistance of the l child protective services agency to provide multidisciplinary ment and support for the affected mother, child, and fa general, a coordinated multidisciplinary approach in the dev of a plan without criminal sanctions has the best chanc children and families.

Respiratory Distress Syndrome

Respiratory distress syndrome is associated with prematurity-related surfactant deficiency. Multiple randomized, controlled clinical trials indicate the benefits of surfactant replacement therapy, including reduction in the severity of respiratory distress syndrome, improvement in survival rate, and fewer pulmonary complications.

Surfactant Replacement Therapy

The prospect of the universal availability of surfactant replacement therapy raises concerns about its potential misuse. One concern is that very low-birth-weight infants with multisystem disorders may be treated with surfactant and may stay in nurseries without adequate facilities and personnel to care for them. This is a critical issue because these high-risk, low-birth-weight infants may have multisystem morbidities that are not beneficially affected by surfactant. Caring for these infants in nurseries that do not have the full range of required capabilities may adversely affect overall outcome. Thus, the availability of surfactant therapy should not alter the referral criteria for high-risk maternal and neonatal transfers, specifically early-gestational-age and low-birth-weight infants.

Following are recommendations for administration of surfactant therapy:

- Surfactant replacement therapy should be directed by physicians who are trained in the respiratory management of low-birth-weight infants and have knowledge and experience in mechanical tion.

spiratory therapy personnel who are experienced f low-birth-weight infants, including the use n, should be available on site when surtered.

or managing and monitoring low-g that needed for mechanical venti-on site when surfactant therapy is

- Radiology and laboratory support to manage a broad range of needs of very low-birth-weight infants should be available.

- An institutionally approved protocol for administering surfactant therapy should be a mandatory component of a quality-assessment program.

- If an emergency situation arises and if indications are present in an institution in which any of the recommended staff and equipment are not present, surfactant therapy may be given, but only by a physician who is skilled in endotracheal intubation. Infants should be transferred from such institutions as soon as feasible to a center with appropriate facilities and trained staff to care for multisystem morbidity in low-birth-weight infants.

Postnatal Corticosteroid Therapy

Antenatal use of corticosteroids has been shown to be effective in reducing the incidence of respiratory distress syndrome, intraventricular hemorrhage, patent ductus arteriosus, and death in low-birth-weight infants. Although corticosteroid therapy for the prevention and treatment of chronic lung disease is prescribed by many physicians, its efficacy is controversial.

Transfusion and Erythropoietin

Transfusion of erythrocytes to newborn infants, especially very low-birth-weight (birth weight <1,500 g), preterm infants, is common. As many as 70–80% of very low-birth-weight infants require at least one transfusion. Although indications for erythrocyte transfusion to newborn infants should be based on objective clinical criteria and not on a single determination of hemoglobin or hematocrit levels, indications for red blood cell transfusion have not been clearly defined by controlled clinical trials. Guidelines for erythrocyte transfusion to newborn infants, maintenance of oxygen-carrying capacity, and symptomatic anemia should be developed for each neonatal service.

During the past several years, clinical trials in very low-birth-weight infants have been performed to evaluate recombinant human erythropoietin in the treatment of anemia of prematurity. The efficacy of this treatment, however, is still inconclusive. Although future management strategies might aim to prevent additional donor exposure by initiating recombinant human erythropoietin, treatment of very low-birth-weight infants with this modality should remain investigational for the present.

The volume of blood removed for testing correlates with the amount transfused. Thus, physician behavior with respect to blood sampling and transfusion practices should be reviewed and modified.

Surgical Procedures in the Neonatal Intensive Care Unit

Infants in the neonatal intensive care unit often require surgical procedures during hospitalization. These procedures range from venous access procedures to laparotomy for necrotizing enterocolitis or thoracotomy for ligation of a patent ductus arteriosus. The transport of an acutely ill neonate to the operating room may be associated with a number of risks, including hypothermia, changes in blood pressure, and dislodging of an intravenous catheter or endotracheal tube. For this reason, in many centers selected surgical procedures are performed in the setting of the neonatal intensive care unit. Studies of central venous catheter insertion, extracorporeal membrane oxygenation cannulation or decannulation, patent ductus arteriosus ligation, laparotomy, and other procedures have suggested that this approach can be safe and effective and may result in improved outcome.

With the exception of relatively minor procedures, surgery must be performed in an area of the neonatal intensive care unit that is separate from other infants, is equipped with adequate lighting and working space, and permits ongoing monitoring and anesthetic management. Personnel should wear appropriate operating room attire, and strict sterile technique must be used. Hospital policy governing these procedures should be developed in conjunction with the institutional operating room committee to ensure that appropriate guidelines are met.

Analgesia

Pain consists of the perception of painful stimuli (nociception) and the psychologic response to them (anxiety). Recent studies measuring a variety of physiologic factors, including oxygen saturation, beta-endorphin, glucose and cortisol concentrations, and epinephrine levels, confirm that infants of all gestational ages have a nociceptive response to pain stimuli. Studies performed in adults reveal that, although nociceptive responses to painful stimuli are similar, individual perception of the severity of pain and its psychologic significance varies widely. Observations of infant behavior suggest that anxiety is also a component of the infantile pain response, but its character, intensity, and duration remain undeterminable. Therefore, the true significance of anxiety in the newborn remains unknown.

Pain management for the newborn should be based on considerations similar to those used for the management of pain in adults. Several recent surveys of physicians in the United States and Canada confirm a general acceptance of this principle. For major surgical procedures, general anesthesia by inhalation of anesthetic gases, intravenous administration of narcotic agents, or regional techniques can be safe and effective. The use of paralytic agents without analgesia during surgery cannot be condoned. Physicians who are specially trained in the administration of neonatal anesthesia should provide anesthesia for preterm infants and other ill infants for whom such agents may have an adverse effect.

Postoperative pain management in the newborn has frequently been overlooked. The use of analgesic agents is important in the immediate postoperative period and should be continued as required. The infant may be carefully observed for physical signs of pain until biochemical markers become more available.

Although consensus has been reached on the use of anesthesia for major procedures, the use of anesthesia and analgesia for certain common procedures remains controversial. The need to provide the newborn with anxiolysis, an essential aspect of adult care, is also uncertain.

Skin Punctures

Repeated skin punctures to obtain blood and other fluid samples have been shown to elicit a pain response in the neonate. The need for and frequency of testing should be a major concern of management, and efforts should be made to minimize the number of skin punctures. Although the use of topical anesthetic creams appears to attenuate the physiologic response to skin punctures, clinicians are concerned about the transdermal absorption of these agents. Because this risk is increased in premature infants, care must be taken to avoid excessive application and duration of exposure. The routine use of topical anesthetic cream for amelioration of the pain of skin punctures cannot be recommended at this time.

Sedation for Prolonged Endotracheal Intubation

Case reports from adults treated with prolonged endotracheal intubation reveal this to be an uncomfortable and anxiety-provoking procedure. Because anxiety appears to be the major affective component, it is difficult to extrapolate the significance of these reports to the neonate. Medications that have been employed as anxiolytic agents in the neonate include morphine, fentanyl, midazolam, lorazepam, and chloral hydrate. Most of these agents have profound pharmacologic effects in addition to analgesia and anxiolysis.

Use of analgesic and anxiolytic agents in newborns for amelioration of the discomfort associated with prolonged endotracheal intubation should be undertaken only after careful consideration of the observed response to pain and anxiety, as demonstrated by the individual neonate, and the side effects of the commonly used agents. These agents appear to be safe when used judiciously in the intraoperative and postoperative period, but no such reassurance can be made when their use extends over several days or weeks.

Fentanyl induces significant habituation early in treatment. In addition, increasing clearance rates result in the need for ever-larger doses to maintain the desired level of analgesia. Although these side effects may be insignificant for short-term postoperative use, their importance increases with duration of use. Fentanyl, midazolam, and lorazepam, both separately and in combination, have been reported to cause troubling and long-lasting neurologic abnormalities in neonates.

Immunization

All neonatal intensive care nurseries should implement a policy for the immunization of preterm infants. Preterm infants, including those of low birth weight, should be immunized at the usual chronologic age of 2 months, in most cases. Vaccine doses should not be reduced for preterm infants. If an infant is still in the hospital at 2 months of age, the immunization schedule, including the administration of whole-cell or acellular diphtheria–tetanus–pertussis vaccine, *Haemophilus influenzae* conjugate, and hepatitis B and poliovirus vaccines, should be initiated. To avoid nosocomial transmission of poliovirus in the nursery, oral poliovirus vaccine should not be used.

The dose and schedule for hepatitis B virus vaccination is determined according to the gestational age of the infant and the hepatitis B surface antigen status of the mother (see Chapter 9). Preterm infants who develop chronic respiratory disease should be given influenza immunization annually in the fall, beginning at 6 months of age.

Perinatal Loss and Fetal Death

Loss of a pregnancy or death of an infant touches many aspects of a family's life. The intense emotions of grieving can be confusing and overwhelming. Every effort should be made to determine the cause of the loss and to understand the family's grief response.

Fetal death accounts for almost 50% of cases of perinatal mortality; in 50% of those cases, the cause of fetal death is unknown. A fetal death occurring before 20 weeks of gestation in which the conceptus is retained in utero is called *missed abortion*. This condition may be managed gynecologically, although admission to the labor and delivery area may be appropriate in some situations involving a missed abortion at 16–20 weeks of gestation. Management of this condition should be the subject of a written protocol, developed by a hospital's department of obstetrics and gynecology in conjunction with nursing staff responsible for the care of pregnant women throughout the hospital.

Management

Fetal death is often suspected when fetal movement is absent or fetal heart tones cannot be heard after having been present earlier. Confirmation of this diagnosis with ultrasound should not be delayed.

Coagulopathy will be seen in about one fourth of women who retain a dead fetus for longer than 4 weeks. Hypofibrinogenemia is the most common change found by laboratory testing. The platelet count, prothrombin time, and partial thromboplastin time may also be affected. The coagulopathy should be corrected with fresh-frozen plasma or cryoprecipitate, followed by prompt delivery.

If delivery is to be performed because of coagulopathy or intrauterine infection, cervical status should be assessed. (For additional information on cervical ripening, see Chapter 5.) If hemorrhage occurs during termination of pregnancy for fetal death in the presence of coagulopathy, treatment should be instituted with aggressive use of appropriate blood products to correct coagulation defects.

Grieving and Mourning

The most important complication of fetal death relates to the psychologic and emotional consequences for the mother. Care should be taken to explain the findings and the medical situation to her. Time for initial grieving should be allowed. It may be beneficial to postpone a discussion of planned delivery of the dead fetus with the patient for a short time.

Investigations into grief and mourning have suggested that parents should be encouraged to be involved in all aspects of the medical management of fetal death in order to promote a more realistic identification with and subsequent resolution of the grieving process. A sense of attachment between mother and fetus has already formed— fetal heart tones have probably been heard, fetal movement has been felt, and possibly the fetus has been viewed by ultrasound. The loss felt by those who experience fetal death is intense. All obstetric caregivers should be aware of the stages of the grief process—shock, searching, disorientation, and reorganization—and should strive to support a woman and her partner during the process. There may be considerable overlap between and recurrence of the so-called stages of grief, which can lead to diverse somatic complaints and manifestations. A member of the obstetric care team with special training in grieving processes may be designated to maintain contact with the mother at regular intervals postpartum and after discharge from the hospital.

Every mother and her partner should be encouraged to make as many choices as possible about medical care, including the timing of delivery, the presence of visitors during labor and delivery, and the use of analgesia and anesthesia. Use of sedative and analgesic medications should serve to relieve pain and discomfort but should not interfere with grieving, although this may be requested by the woman herself. As soon as they are able, after being informed of an established fetal death, the mother and her partner should consider their needs and desires for a private room, viewing and holding their baby, naming the baby, photographs and remembrances, baptism, and burial arrangements.

An autopsy should be requested with sensitivity and tactful timing. Emphasis on the relief that may be derived from knowing the cause of death, or from learning of the absence of malformations, may aid in the discussion of autopsy. The limitations of autopsy should be delineated for the couple as well.

Assessment

When a fetal or neonatal death occurs, an effort should be made to determine the cause of the death. This process is helpful for several reasons:

- It helps the family to understand the medical reason for the death.
- It provides a basis for counseling, especially in the areas of family planning, genetic counseling, and obstetric and neonatal management of any future pregnancies.
- It provides a correct diagnosis for the perinatal data base and the statistical reporting of congenital defects and important perinatal events.

Components of the evaluation include the following:

- Complete medical and prenatal history, including this pregnancy and previous pregnancies and information as to previous pregnancy loss and neonatal deaths. Any family history of birth defects or genetic diseases should be noted.

- Autopsy, including both gross and microscopic evaluation of the stillborn or neonate and evaluation of the cord, membranes, and placenta. Consent for an autopsy is most likely to be given when the parents are approached by the physician who managed the pregnancy or the newborn's care.

- Photographs—both total-body and close-up pictures should be taken with appropriate centimeter markers of dysmorphic features.

- Full-body X-ray with posteroanterior and lateral views. Additional X-rays, especially in cases with limb or other structural abnormalities, may be needed.

- Cytogenetic studies should be considered, especially in the presence of congenital anomalies or dysmorphic features; a family history of chromosomal abnormalities; or previous multiple perinatal deaths, spontaneous abortions, or unexplained fetal deaths. Specimens may be obtained from blood or appropriate tissue.

- Special tests such as serology (for a variety of infectious diseases) or frozen sections of liver (for inborn errors of metabolism) may be helpful in special cases.

After such an evaluation has been performed, the family should meet with the physician who is coordinating the investigation. This physician may be the obstetrician, pediatrician, neonatologist, maternal–fetal specialist, geneticist, dysmorphologist, and, in some instances, surgical specialist. Clinical-pathologic correlation is best done by a team comprising obstetricians, neonatologists, pathologists, and geneticists. Families should be given adequate time to have their questions answered after the postmortem evaluation is performed and to return for additional medical counseling, if needed. Copies of the final autopsy report should be made available to both the parents and the referring physicians.

The causes of fetal death should be identified as accurately as possible. Systematic review of fetal and infant mortality will help to distinguish possibly preventable causes from unpreventable causes, as well as clustering of events that may indicate environmental effects. Perinatal statistics should be computed using only deaths of fetuses and infants weighing 500 g or more at delivery or in accordance with state reporting requirements.

Obstetric units should adopt a method for recording each perinatal event by specific birth weight (rather than ranges); actual hours or days of life, in the case of live births; and gestational age of the fetus or infant as determined by crown–rump length or first-trimester ultrasound. These data can then be aggregated into categories that are appropriate and useful. In this way, different reporting requirements can be met without additional data collection, but statistical analysis can be based on valid comparisons of consistent data. Standard definitions (see Appendix E) should be used.

In-Hospital Support and Counseling

Bereavement counseling has an important impact in family members' ability to adjust to their loss and to continue with their lives. Counseling should be tailored to the specific circumstances surrounding the death; should be sensitive to specific ethical, cultural, religious, and family considerations; and should be provided by specific staff within the hospital.

The time in the hospital after the baby has died is the parents' only opportunity to create a memory of the child. Specific management procedures can help parents cope with their grief:

- Offer the parents an opportunity to see, hold, and spend time with the baby.

- Obtain pictures and remembrances (eg, identification tags, footprints, a lock of hair, birth and death certificates, height and weight records, a receiving blanket for the baby). Even if the parents say initially that they do not want these mementos, they frequently ask for them days, weeks, or months later.

- Encourage the family to name the baby, for it is easier to connect memories to a child if parents can refer to him or her by name.

- Provide information about options for burial, cremation, funerals, or memorial services. Encourage both parents to take an active part in making these arrangements.

- Visit the parents daily while the mother is in the hospital, listen to them sympathetically, and give them information as it becomes available. Physicians should be aware that the staff's potential reactions—a sense of guilt, failure, and uncertainty—may cause them to avoid the parents, thereby impeding discussion of the deceased infant with the family.

- Ensure that the parents have access to support from their families, clergy, and friends. Anticipate with parents the difficulties they may have in sharing information about the loss with other children, family, and friends. Provide information and suggestions on how they might handle difficult situations or times.

- Provide reliable preliminary information from the appropriate medical professionals concerning the cause and circumstances of death.

- Explain the grieving process so that the parents understand the usual reactions. Parents frequently demonstrate reactions of acute grief, such as somatic disturbances, a preoccupation with the newborn's appearance or probable future appearance, guilt, hostility, and loss of ability to function. Mourning should be allowed and encouraged to proceed.

- Encourage the parents to communicate their thoughts and feelings openly with one another. Help them understand and accept the differences in how each of them grieves.

- Provide written materials for the parents to read in the hospital and after discharge. The period after a fetal or neonatal death always has an element of confusion because of the continuing grief, the tasks of informing relatives and friends, and the need to make final arrangements. Although there can be no substitute for a multidisciplinary group of professionals carefully organized to provide support, written materials can provide concrete information about specific procedures, such as autopsy and funeral arrangements, as well as guidance on long-term issues, such as grief, marriage, explanations for young children, and consideration of another pregnancy. These materials can be designed by the individual hospital or obtained through various associations.

Finally, because families may come from a distance and thus may not be well acquainted with the attending physicians, it is especially important that tertiary-care referral centers designate a member of the team to be an advocate for the family during the hospital stay and after discharge. The designated individual is also responsible for documenting the management and follow-up of each perinatal death. Too often families from afar are lost to follow-up, as physicians, nurses, and families avoid the sadness of bereavement.

Postdischarge Follow-Up

The responsibility for ongoing bereavement counseling depends on the specific circumstances of the death and on the family's relationship to the physician. Bereavement counseling is best provided with a multidisciplinary approach. In the case of fetal death, counseling is coordinated by the obstetrician, whereas in the case of neonatal death, it is coordinated by the neonatologist or pediatrician. The family should receive bereavement counseling that includes the following:

- Schedule the first session 4–6 weeks after the death.
- Assess the grieving process.
- Obtain additional genetic services if needed.
- Begin review of preliminary autopsy data.
- Answer specific questions.
- Set up future follow-up visits.
- Refer patients for genetic counseling, if appropriate.
- Provide education and reassurance regarding the normal grieving process.
- Refer family members to bereavement support groups or bereavement counselors.

Bibliography

American Academy of Pediatrics. Peter G, ed. 1997 Red book: report of the Committee on Infectious Diseases. 24th ed. Elk Grove Village, Illinois: AAP, 1997

American Academy of Pediatrics, Committee on Substance Abuse. Drug-exposed infants. Pediatrics 1995;96:364–367

American Academy of Pediatrics, Provisional Committee on Quality Improvement and Subcommittee on Hyperbilirubinemia in the Healthy Term Newborn. Practice parameter: management of hyperbilirubinemia in the healthy term newborn. Pediatrics 1994;94:558–565

American Association of Blood Banks, Standards Committee. Standards for blood banks and transfusion services. 17th ed. Bethesda, Maryland: AABB, 1996

American College of Obstetricians and Gynecologists. Grief related to perinatal death. ACOG Technical Bulletin 86. Washington, DC: ACOG, 1985

American College of Obstetricians and Gynecologists. Perinatal and infant mortality statistics. Committee Opinion 167. Washington, DC: ACOG, 1995

American College of Obstetricians and Gynecologists. Substance abuse in pregnancy. Technical Bulletin 195. Washington, DC: ACOG, 1994

American College of Obstetricians and Gynecologists, National Fetal and Infant Review Program. A manual for fetal and infant mortality review. Washington, DC: ACOG, 1991

Chapter 9

Perinatal Infections

Certain infections that occur in the antepartum or intrapartum period may have a significant effect on the fetus and newborn. Proper care of the mother during pregnancy and at delivery and of the newborn can reduce the frequency of or ameliorate many serious problems and can minimize the risk of subsequent transmission of infection in the nursery. Communication and cooperation among all perinatal care personnel are essential to obtain the best results. The infections discussed in this chapter have been selected on the basis of new and evolving information that affects management.

Screening for TORCH (toxoplasmosis, other viruses, rubella, cytomegalovirus [CMV], herpes simplex virus [HSV]) infections as a package is of no value in pregnancy and can lead to harmful interventions. Although the presence of antibodies does not always preclude fetal infection, the risks of clinically apparent disease or significant sequelae are very low when antibodies are present, as compared with events resulting from a primary infection.

All women who will be in the second and third trimesters of pregnancy during the influenza season should be offered influenza vaccine. Influenza vaccine is strongly recommended for women at high risk for influenza complications. Pregnant women with medical conditions that increase their risk for complications from influenza should be offered the vaccine before the influenza season, regardless of the stage of pregnancy. Administration of influenza vaccine is considered safe at any stage of pregnancy.

Viral Infections

Cytomegalovirus

Approximately 1% of all newborns are infected with CMV in utero and excrete CMV after birth. Of congenitally infected babies born to mothers with primary CMV infection, 8% are symptomatic at birth. An additional 3% may develop sensorineural hearing loss in the first few years of life.

Because there is neither a vaccine for prevention of infection nor effective therapy for acute maternal infection, routine serologic screening of either mothers or neonates is of little benefit. Testing is generally limited to women in whom specific exposure is suspected and for management of their pregnancy. Routine serologic testing of personnel in newborn nurseries is not recommended; however, testing women of childbearing potential could identify those personnel who are seropositive and thus not susceptible to infection from CMV exposure.

Although the presence of immunoglobulin M (IgM) CMV antibody is highly suggestive of primary infection, false-positive and false-negative results occur. Establishing that seroconversion has occurred is the most accurate method for documenting primary maternal infection. Isolation of the virus from either amniotic fluid or fetal blood can be used to detect fetal CMV infection. Fetal blood obtained by cordocentesis may also be tested for CMV-specific IgM, elevated hepatic enzymes (especially γ-glutaryltransferase), anemia, and thrombocytopenia.

Infection can be transmitted to neonates by transfusion of blood from seropositive donors or by ingestion of CMV-contaminated breast milk. Blood transmission has been virtually eliminated by the use of blood from CMV-negative donors, the use of frozen deglycerolized red blood cells, or by filtration to remove white blood cells. Babies born to seronegative mothers who receive milk from human milk banks are at risk of developing CMV disease. This can be minimized by limiting donor milk to CMV-negative donors or by appropriate pasteurization.

Hepatitis A Virus

Hepatitis A virus has little effect on pregnancy and rarely is transmitted perinatally. The risk of transplacental transmission to the fetus is negligible, and there is no evidence that the virus is a teratogen. The most common mode of transmission is by the fecal–oral route. Diagnosis is confirmed by the demonstration of hepatitis A virus IgM antibodies.

Hepatitis A vaccine is recommended for preexposure immunoprophylaxis, especially before travel to foreign countries in which infection is common. The safety of the vaccine's use in pregnancy has not been established, but because it is produced from inactivated virus, the risk to the developing fetus is theoretically low. Immunoglobulin is effective for both preexposure and postexposure prophylaxis and can be used during pregnancy.

In neonatal intensive care units, nosocomial outbreaks have been reported but are infrequent. Prevention of spread of the virus is based on enteric precautions, with emphasis on careful hand-washing. With appropriate hygienic precautions, breastfeeding is permissible. Although immunoglobulin has been administered to newborns in specific situations, the efficacy of this practice has not been established.

Hepatitis B Virus

Hepatitis B virus (HBV) infection accounts for approximately 35% of reported cases of viral hepatitis. Although 85–90% of older children and adults experience complete resolution following an acute infection, 6–10% will develop a chronic infection and continue to manifest HBV surface antigen (HBsAg). Transmission of HBV from mother to neonate occurs primarily during delivery. Neonates born to mothers who are antigen positive are at risk of infection. Approximately 70–90% of infected neonates become chronic carriers of HBsAg.

Maternal Infection

Because historical information about risk factors identifies fewer than half of chronic carriers, serologic testing for HBsAg is recommended as part of the routine battery of prenatal tests for pregnant women who have not been immunized or whose serologic status is unknown. Women who were not screened during pregnancy or who are at high risk for infection should be tested at the time of admission to the hospital. Women who are HBsAg negative but who have risk factors for HBV infection should be offered vaccination during pregnancy. The adult dose of HBV vaccine is 1 ml injected into the deltoid muscle; intramuscular injection in the buttocks may not be as effective and is not recommended. A series of three doses is required; the second and third doses are given 1 and 6 months after the first dose.

Hepatitis B vaccine is recommended for household contacts and sexual partners of chronic carriers of HBV (ie, those who are HBsAg positive) unless immunity has previously been demonstrated. Previously nonimmunized sexual partners of persons with acute HBV infection should receive a single dose of HBV immune globulin (HBIG) and should begin an HBV vaccine series if they are serologically negative. Serologic testing to determine susceptibility, although not usually cost-effective and not recommended routinely, is recommended in this circumstance.

Newborns Exposed to Hepatitis B Virus

Universal HBV immunization is recommended for all babies. Three intramuscular doses are required to provide effective protection (Table 9–1). For babies born to HBsAg-negative mothers, the first dose of vaccine should be administered during the newborn period or by 2 months of age, the second dose 1–2 months later, and the third dose by 6–18 months of age. Alternatively, vaccine may be administered at 2-month intervals, concurrent with other childhood vaccines, at 2, 4, and 6 months of age. The appropriate dose (Table 9–2) can be given into the deltoid muscle or into the anterolateral thigh muscle of neonates and infants.

Babies born to mothers known to be HBsAg positive should be vaccinated shortly after birth and should receive one dose of HBIG, preferably within 12 hours of birth. Prophylaxis for exposed newborns can prevent perinatal HBV infection in approximately 95% of infants when the three-dose immunization series is completed and HBIG is

Table 9–1. Recommended Schedules for Hepatitis B Virus Immunoprophylaxis of Babies to Prevent Perinatal Transmission*

Status	Dosing Schedule	Age
Babies of HBsAg-positive mothers	HBV vaccine 1	Birth (within 12 hours)
	HBIG (0.5 ml IM)	Birth (within 12 hours)
	HBV vaccine 2	1–2 months
	HBV vaccine 3	6 months
Babies of HBsAg-negative mothers	HBV vaccine 1	Birth (preferably before hospital discharge) to 2 months
	HBV vaccine 2	1–2 months after dose 1
	HBV vaccine 3	6–18 months
Babies born to mothers not screened for HBsAg before delivery	HBV vaccine 1	Birth (within 12 hours)
	HBIG	If mother is subsequently found to be HBsAg positive, give 0.5 ml IM as soon as possible (no later than 1 week after birth)
	HBV vaccine 2	1–2 months
	HBV vaccine 3	6–18 months[†]

* These recommendations may not apply to preterm infants.

[†] Babies of HBsAg-positive mothers should be vaccinated at 6 months of age.

Abbreviations: HBV = hepatitis B virus; HBsAg = HBV surface antigen; HBIG = HBV immune globulin; IM = intramuscularly.

Modified from American Academy of Pediatrics. Peter G, editor. 1997 Red book: report of the Committee on Infectious Diseases. 24th ed. Elk Grove Village, Illinois: AAP, 1997.

given within 12 hours after birth. The initial dose of HBV vaccine can be administered concurrently with HBIG but should be given at a different site. No special care of the neonate is indicated other than removal of maternal blood in order to avoid inoculation of the virus contaminating the skin. The second dose of vaccine should be administered at 1–2 months of chronologic age, regardless of the infant's

Table 9–2. Recommended Doses of Hepatitis B Virus Vaccines in Infants

Maternal Status	Vaccine Type	
	Recombivax HB	Energix-B
HBsAg-positive*	5 µg (1.0 ml)† (0.5 ml)‡	10 µg (0.5 ml)
HBsAg-negative	2.5 µg (0.5 ml)†	10 µg (0.5 ml)

* Hepatitis B immune globulin (0.5 ml) should also be given.
† Pediatric formulation.
‡ Adult formulation.
Abbreviation: HBsAg = hepatitis B virus surface antigen.
Modified from American Academy of Pediatrics. Peter G, ed. 1997 Red book: report of the Committee on Infectious Diseases. 24th ed. Elk Grove Village, Illinois: AAP, 1997.

gestational age or birth weight. The third dose should be given at 6 months of age.

At 1–3 months after completion of the immunization schedule for babies born to HBsAg-positive women, testing is indicated to ensure response or to identify babies who have become chronically infected. With appropriate immunoprophylaxis, including HBIG, breastfeeding of babies born to HBsAg-positive mothers poses no additional risk for the transmission of HBV. In developed countries, however, even a low risk for transmission of the virus by breast milk may be considered significant and sufficient reason to bottle feed.

Neonates born to mothers whose HBsAg status is unknown should receive HBV vaccine within 12 hours, in a dose appropriate for neonates born to HBsAg-positive mothers. The mother's blood should be obtained for testing upon admission. If the woman is subsequently found to be HBsAg positive, the neonate should receive HBIG as soon as possible, but within 7 days of birth, and should subsequently be vaccinated (doses 2 and 3) as recommended for infants of HBsAg-positive mothers.

For preterm infants weighing less than 2.0 kg at birth and born to HBsAg-negative women, initiation of HBV vaccination should be deferred until just before hospital discharge, providing that the infant weighs 2.0 kg or more, or until approximately 2 months of age, when other immunizations are given. For preterm infants of HBsAg-positive mothers or those of unknown status, vaccine and HBIG should be given as recommended for term infants, within 12 hours of birth.

Hepatitis C Virus

Hepatitis C virus (HCV) is the principal cause of non-A, non-B hepatitis. Until the implementation of universal screening for HCV in donors of blood products, the virus accounted for as many as 95% of cases of posttransfusion hepatitis. Transmission occurs through routes similar to those for HBV, including sexual contact, needles and syringes shared by intravenous drug users, and contact within households. However, in nearly one half of cases, the source is not identified.

Infection with HCV is diagnosed serologically by the presence of HCV antibodies. Positive test results should be confirmed by an enzyme immunoassay and a radioactive immunoblock assay. As many as 70% of patients with HCV infection develop chronic liver disease, and cirrhosis ultimately develops in 20–25%. Hence, liver enzyme and function tests should be obtained in patients who are antibody positive.

Routine serologic testing during pregnancy for HCV infection is not recommended. Testing should be reserved for those whose history suggests an increased risk of infection, such as from blood transfusion, intravenous drug use, or repeated exposure to percutaneous or mucosal blood.

Mothers who are infected with HCV should be advised that transmission of HCV by breastfeeding is possible but has not been documented. According to current guidelines of the U.S. Public Health Service, maternal HCV infection is not a contraindication to breastfeeding. The decision to do so should be based on an informed discussion between the mother and the health care provider.

Maternal–fetal (vertical) transmission of HCV occurs at a rate of only 5% (range, 0–25%). The risk of transmission, which correlates with maternal HCV RNA titer, appears to be increased for women infected with human immunodeficiency virus (HIV). The consequences of vertical transmission have not been defined.

Screening of donors of blood products for HCV antibodies and exclusion of antibody-positive donors is recommended. Immune globulin manufactured in the United States does not contain antibodies to HCV and is unlikely to prevent infection following exposure.

Herpes Simplex Virus

Treatment and Counseling During Pregnancy

All women should be questioned about a history of genital HSV infection. Patients with an active primary genital HSV lesion who deliver vaginally have a high (33–50%) risk of transmitting the infection to their neonates; if the disease is recurrent, the risk is lower (2–5%). Distinguishing between primary and recurrent HSV infection in women on the basis of clinical findings is not accurate. Most newborns infected with HSV are born to women who have asymptomatic or unrecognized infection.

The benefits of prophylactic administration of antiviral drugs such as acyclovir to pregnant women with genital HSV infection are not well established. Acyclovir may be administered intravenously to treat maternal life-threatening HSV infection (eg, disseminated infection that includes encephalitis, pneumonitis, and hepatitis). The long-term safety and efficacy of administering acyclovir systemically has not yet been established. To date, no evidence has been found of any adverse effects on the fetus.

Couples should be educated about the natural history of genital HSV infection and should be advised that, if either partner is infected, they should abstain from sexual contact while lesions are present. To minimize the risk of transmission, use of condoms is recommended for asymptomatic HSV-infected persons. Susceptible pregnant women should avoid sexual contact during the last 6–8 weeks of gestation if their partners have an active genital HSV infection.

Obstetric Management

Women with a history of genital HSV infection should be questioned about recent symptoms and should undergo a careful perineal examination when they present for delivery. Serial cervical and vaginal HSV cultures for screening asymptomatic women have not been shown to be predictive of newborn infection and therefore are not recommended. If an HSV lesion will come into contact with the baby during the birth process, cesarean delivery is recommended. Once membranes have ruptured near term, cesarean delivery should be expedited if lesions are present and vaginal delivery is not imminent. The use of scalp monitors and sampling should be avoided, if possible, in women with active genital HSV lesions. Patients with nongenital lesions may deliver vaginally if the lesion can be covered at delivery.

Contact precautions (in addition to standard precautions) should be used for women with clinically evident or serologically confirmed primary genital HSV infection or nongenital HSV infection in the labor, delivery, and postpartum care areas. For recurrent mucocutaneous lesions, standard precautions only are sufficient. Health care personnel and the woman herself should use gloves for direct contact with the infected area or with contaminated dressings, and meticulous hand-washing is essential. The labor and delivery rooms require only routine, careful cleaning and disinfection before using the rooms for another patient.

Management of Exposed Newborns

The incidence of neonatal HSV infection is very low, and congenital (intrauterine) infection is rare. Most neonatal infections are caused by HSV type 2 (HSV-2), although infection with HSV-1 can also occur. Most neonates who develop HSV infection acquire the infection during passage through the infected maternal lower genital tract, or by ascending infection to the fetus, sometimes even though membranes are apparently intact. Less common sources of neonatal infection include (1) postnatal transmission from the mother, father, hospital personnel, or other close contact, most often from a nongenital infection (eg, mouth, hands, or around the breasts); and (2) postnatal transmission in the nursery from another infected neonate, probably from the hands of personnel attending the babies.

Infection in newborns may be generalized; localized to the central nervous system; localized to the skin, eyes, or mouth; or a combination of these. Typically, clinical disease is not present at birth, but onset occurs during the first month after birth. In a large multicenter study, approximately one third of neonates with HSV infection developed localized disease with lesions of the skin, eyes, or mouth as an early manifestation. Another one third developed systemic or central nervous system disease before the mucocutaneous lesions appeared. In the remaining one third, no visible lesions were noted. Asymptomatic HSV infection occurs rarely, if at all, in newborns.

Neonates with documented perinatal exposure to HSV may be in the incubation phase of infection and should be handled expectantly. Neonates born vaginally (or by cesarean delivery if membranes have ruptured) to a mother with active HSV lesions should be physically separated from other babies and managed with contact precautions if they remain in the nursery during the incubation period; an isolation room is not essential. Alternatively, the neonate may stay with the mother in a private room after the mother has been instructed on proper preventive care to reduce postpartum transmission.

The risk of HSV infection is extremely low in neonates born to asymptomatic mothers with a history of recurrent genital herpes and in those born to symptomatic mothers by cesarean delivery before rupture of membranes. Special isolation precautions are not needed for most of these neonates. They should be observed in the nursery and followed closely after discharge. The length of in-hospital observation is empirical and is based on risk factors, local resources, and access to adequate follow-up. Parents should be instructed to report early signs of infection.

Early Diagnosis and Management of Disease in Neonates

Cultures obtained from the nasopharynx or mouth and the conjunctivae of neonates born to mothers who are known or who are strongly suspected to be infected with HSV can assist in management decisions. A positive culture obtained 24–48 hours or more after birth suggests HSV infection and is an indication for immediate institution of antiviral therapy, even in the absence of symptoms.

The early signs of HSV infection in newborns are frequently nonspecific and subtle. A neonate known to have been exposed to HSV should be observed carefully for vesicular lesions and unexplained illnesses, including respiratory distress, convulsions, and signs of sepsis. If any of these signs occur, the possibility of HSV infection, as well as of other bacterial infections, should be investigated. Skin lesions and other sites, as appropriate, should be cultured for HSV; this can be done relatively easily.

The neonate should be physically segregated and managed with contact precautions for the duration of the illness; an isolation room is desirable. Personnel having contact with skin lesions or potentially infectious secretions should use gowns and gloves. Antiviral therapy is effective in the treatment of neonatal HSV infection and should be initiated if HSV is suspected. Neonates with HSV disease should be managed in a facility that provides subspecialty care.

Although HSV infection is more likely to occur at a site of skin trauma, no data indicate that the circumcision of male neonates who may have been exposed to HSV at birth should be postponed. It may be prudent, however, to delay circumcision for about a month in babies at highest risk of disease (eg, those born vaginally to mothers with active genital lesions).

Contact of Neonates with Herpes Simplex Virus-Infected Mothers

A mother with HSV infection should be taught about her infection and about hygienic measures to prevent postpartum transmission of the infection to her neonate. Before touching her newborn, the mother should wash her hands carefully and use a clean barrier to ensure that the neonate does not come into contact with lesions or potentially infectious material. If the mother has genital HSV infection, her newborn may room with her after she has been instructed in protective measures. Breastfeeding is permissible if the mother has no vesicular herpetic lesions in the breast area and all active cutaneous lesions are covered.

A mother with herpes labialis (cold sore) or stomatitis should not kiss or nuzzle her newborn until the lesions have cleared. Careful hand-washing is important. She may wear a disposable surgical mask when she touches her newborn until the lesions have crusted and dried. Herpetic lesions on other skin sites should be covered. Direct contact of a newborn with other family members or friends who have active HSV infection should be avoided.

Human Immunodeficiency Virus

Etiology

Acquired immunodeficiency syndrome (AIDS) is caused by HIV type 1 (HIV-1) and, less commonly, HIV-2, a related virus that is extremely uncommon in the United States but is more common in West Africa. The role of cofactors, such as simultaneous infection with other infectious agents or malnutrition, in the natural history of HIV infection is not known.

Epidemiology

Human immunodeficiency virus has been isolated from blood (including lymphocytes, macrophages, and plasma), cerebrospinal fluid, pleural fluid, human milk, semen, cervical secretions, saliva, urine, and tears. However, only blood, semen, cervical secretions, and human milk have been implicated epidemiologically in the transmission of infection.

The predominant modes of HIV transmission in the United States are sexual contact (both heterosexual and homosexual), skin penetration by contaminated needles or other sharp instruments, and mother-to-infant transmission before or near the time of birth. Infection with HIV continues to spread among women of childbearing age and is occurring increasingly in rural as well as urban areas. The predominant risk behavior is unprotected sexual intercourse. The incidence of perinatal HIV infection has mirrored increases in sexually transmissible infections in women.

The risk of infection for a neonate born to an HIV-seropositive mother is estimated to be 13–39%. The exact timing of transmission from an infected mother to her baby is uncertain, but evidence suggests that transmission may occur in utero near the time of delivery or postpartum through breastfeeding. Most infections appear to occur in the perinatal period.

Management

Clear medical benefits are derived from pregnant women knowing their HIV serostatus. These benefits include early diagnosis and treatment to delay active disease in women and significant reduction in perinatal transmission through early treatment with zidovudine (ZDV). Routine testing for all pregnant women, with their consent, is recommended. When maternal serostatus is unknown, HIV testing of the newborn remains important for diagnostic and therapeutic reasons. The individual providing health care for the newborn should be informed of the mother's HIV serostatus to ensure appropriate care and testing. In some states, physicians are required to obtain the mother's written authorization before disclosing her HIV status to other health care providers who are not members of the woman's health care team, such as her baby's health care provider. For infants born to seropositive mothers, testing for HIV should be performed at least twice. Optimally, testing is done within the first few days of life, at 1 month of age, and again at 4 months of age or later, either by culture or by polymerase chain reaction. Testing in the first days of life will detect infection in 30–50% of infected infants, but a negative test does not rule out infection. Testing at 1 month of age will detect almost all infected infants. If the neonate is found to be seropositive when the maternal serostatus is unknown, the health care provider for the child should ensure that this information and its significance is relayed to the mother and, with her consent and possibly written authorization, to her health care provider.

Prenatal and intrapartum administration of ZDV to HIV-infected pregnant women has been shown to reduce the rate of HIV transmission to the newborn by 68%. In a large, multicenter study, ZDV treatment of an infected mother, beginning with oral administration at 14–34 weeks of gestation and followed by intrapartum intravenous ZDV and postnatal oral treatment of the baby for 6 weeks, reduced the transmission from 25.5% in the control group to 8.3%. No significant short-term side effects were observed from ZDV use other than mild, self-limited anemia in the babies. These infants have been followed for more than 2 years, and no untoward effects of ZDV have been observed.

A theoretical concern about the prophylactic use of ZDV remains, however, because the long-term effects are unknown. Women who take ZDV to reduce the possibility of mother-to-infant transmission theoretically may encourage resistance to ZDV, which could compromise future care. The decision to use ZDV should be made by the patient only after discussing with her doctor the benefits for and potential risks to herself and her child. The U.S. Public Health Service Task Force recommends the following ZDV regimen for HIV-infected pregnant women and their newborns:

- Eligibility (therapy should also be discussed and considered with all HIV-infected pregnant women, even those who do not meet these criteria):
  — Pregnancy at 14–34 weeks of gestation
  — No antiretroviral therapy during the current pregnancy
  — No clinical indications for antenatal antiretroviral therapy
  — CD4+ T lymphocyte count of greater than 200 cells/mm^3 at the time of entry into the study
- Maternal treatment:
  — Antepartum: Oral administration of 100 mg of ZDV five times daily, initiated at 14–34 weeks of gestation and continued throughout the pregnancy
  — Intrapartum: Intravenous administration of ZDV in a 1-hour loading dose of 2 mg/kg of body weight, followed by a continuous infusion of 1 mg/kg of body weight per hour until delivery
- Neonatal treatment: Oral administration of ZDV to the newborn (ZDV syrup at 2 mg/kg of body weight per dose every 6 hours) for the first 6 weeks of life, beginning 8–12 hours after birth

In addition, because ZDV still may be effective in reducing the transmission rate, ZDV prophylaxis should be offered to HIV-infected pregnant women whose gestation is beyond 34 weeks and to newborns whose mothers did not receive ZDV.

Human immunodeficiency virus DNA has been detected in both the cellular and cell-free fractions of human breast milk, and breast-feeding has been implicated in the transmission of HIV infection. When a safe alternative is available, HIV-infected women should be counseled not to breastfeed their babies; they should not donate to milk banks.

Using virologic diagnostic techniques such as HIV culture, polymerase chain reaction, and immune complex-dissociated p24 antigen, HIV infection can be diagnosed in 30–50% of infected infants at birth and in nearly 100% of infected neonates by 4–6 months of age. Early identification of infected babies is essential for adequate medical management. *Pneumocystis carinii* pneumonia is the most common opportunistic infection in HIV-infected children. Because *P. carinii* pneumonia in HIV-infected babies usually occurs at 3–6 months of age, *P. carinii* pneumonia prophylaxis should begin at 4–6 weeks of age in all babies born to HIV-infected women, regardless of the baby's CD4+ T lymphocyte count.

Because HIV (as well as other viral agents, such as HBV) may be present in blood, vaginal secretions, amniotic fluid, and other fluids, standard precautions should be strictly followed during all vaginal and cesarean deliveries. Gloves should be used when handling the placenta or the neonate until blood and amniotic fluid have been removed from the neonate's skin.

After delivery, HIV-infected women can receive care in the postpartum care unit, with the use of standard precautions. Few neonates with HIV infection show clinical evidence of infection in the first weeks after birth. To minimize risk to health care personnel, routine standard precautions should be used. Prompt and careful removal of blood from the neonate's skin is important. There is no need for other special precautions or for isolation of the neonate with an HIV-infected mother; rooming-in is acceptable. Gloves should be worn for contact with blood or blood-containing fluids and for procedures that entail exposure to blood. Gloves are not required for prevention of HIV transmission while changing diapers.

Human Papillomavirus

Genital warts caused by human papillomavirus (HPV) are common. Infection with certain types of HPV also appears to be related to the subsequent development of genital neoplasms. Cervical or vaginal HPV infections are usually asymptomatic. Studies using DNA diagnostic techniques detect the virus in up to 40% of sexually active young women. Pap tests are less useful for the diagnosis of subclinical cervical infection. Most genital HPV infections are sexually transmitted.

Genital HPV infections may be exacerbated during pregnancy. The papillary lesions may proliferate on the vulva and in the vagina, and lesions may become increasingly friable during pregnancy. Cryotherapy, laser therapy, and trichloroacetic acid may be used safely to treat genital HPV infection in pregnancy. Podophyllin, 5-fluorouracil, and interferon are generally not recommended during pregnancy because of concern that they may be toxic to the fetus.

The risk that a neonate whose mother has a genital HPV infection will develop subsequent laryngeal papillomatosis is very small. These lesions are thought to result from aspiration of infectious secretions during passage through the birth canal. The latent period may be several years before HPV lesions become clinically significant in children. Because the risk of respiratory papillomatosis is low, cesarean delivery is not recommended solely to protect the neonate from HPV infection. In women with extensive condylomata, however, cesarean delivery may be necessary because of poor vaginal or vulvar distensibility and the related increased likelihood of extensive vulvovaginal lacerations. Neonates born to mothers with HPV infection do not need to be managed with special precautions in the nursery.

Human Parvovirus

Erythema infectiosum is caused by parvovirus B19. When this infection occurs during pregnancy, the incidence of fetal mortality and morbidity is low. However, parvovirus B19 can infect fetal erythroid precursors and cause anemia, which can lead to hydrops and death. Most reported maternal infections that have resulted in fetal death occurred in the first half of pregnancy, and fetal death and spontaneous abortion usually have occurred 4–6 weeks after infection. Third-trimester maternal infections followed by the birth of anemic newborns have been described. Congenital anomalies due to parvovirus have not been reported, but on rare occasions the myocardium has been reported to be infected, suggesting the possibility of heart damage.

Because of widespread asymptomatic parvovirus infection in both adults and children, all women are at some risk of exposure, particularly those with school-aged children. Pregnant women who learn that they have been in contact with children who were either in the incubation period of erythema infectiosum or in aplastic crisis should be counseled about the relatively low potential risk to the fetus and should be offered the option of serologic testing. Fetal ultrasound will detect hydrops, but the frequency with which serial measurements should be performed is not known. In some cases, maternal serum alpha-fetoprotein levels may be elevated by the presence of fetal hydrops. A hydropic fetus can be treated by intrauterine transfusion when severe anemia has been documented by cordocentesis, although spontaneous resolution may occur.

In view of the high prevalence of parvovirus B19, the low risk of ill effects to the fetus, and the fact that avoidance of child care or teaching can reduce but not eliminate the risk of infection, pregnant women should not be routinely excluded from the workplace where erythema infectiosum is present. Pregnant health care workers should be aware that patients with aplastic crisis may be highly contagious and should be aware of the resulting importance of droplet precautions in caring for these patients.

Respiratory Syncytial Virus

Respiratory syncytial virus (RSV) is a common cause of respiratory infection in infancy. The disease can be very serious when a premature infant with chronic lung disease is affected. In January 1996, the U.S. Food and Drug Administration (FDA) approved licensure of intravenous RSV immune globulin (RSV-IGIV). The FDA-approved indication for RSV-IGIV use is to prevent serious RSV lower respiratory disease in infants and children less than 24 months of age with bronchopulmonary dysplasia or a history of premature birth at less than 35 weeks of gestation. Two randomized controlled trials have shown that RSV-IGIV administered monthly during RSV season resulted in a 41–65% reduction of hospitalization rates; however, RSV-IGIV is costly and the intravenous administration can be logistically demanding. RSV-IGIV should be considered for infants with bronchopulmonary dysplasia who are receiving or have received oxygen therapy in the past 6 months. Infants with a gestational age of 32 weeks or less at birth may also benefit clinically from RSV-IGIV prophylaxis. Intravenous RSV immune globulin has not been approved for use in infants with congenital heart disease, and available data indicate that, because of safety concerns, it should not be administered to children with cyanotic congenital heart disease.

Intravenous RSV immune globulin should be initiated before the onset and terminated at the end of the RSV season. There is a regional variation with regard to the time window of the RSV season. Practitioners should consult with the health department or diagnostic laboratories in their geographic area to determine the optimal schedule.

A critical aspect of RSV prevention is parent education about the importance of exposure to and transmission of the virus. Preventive measures include limiting, when feasible, exposure to contagious settings, such as child care centers. The importance of hand-washing should be emphasized in all settings, including the home, particularly during periods when contact with high-risk children who have a respiratory infection can occur.

Rubella

Prevention and Management During Pregnancy

Surveillance for susceptibility to rubella infection is essential in prenatal care. Each patient should be screened serologically at the first prenatal visit unless she is known to be immune by a previous serologic test.

Seropositive women do not need further testing, regardless of their subsequent history of exposure. If seronegative pregnant women have been exposed to rubella or develop symptoms that suggest infection, they should be retested for antibody titers to establish whether infection has occurred. Specimens should be obtained as soon as possible after exposure, again 2 weeks later, and, if necessary, 4 weeks after exposure. Serum specimens from both acute and convalescent periods should be tested on the same day in the same laboratory; a rise in titer of fourfold or greater or seroconversion indicates acute infection. Rubella-specific IgM testing or isolation of the virus from throat swabs establishes a diagnosis of acute rubella.

If rubella is diagnosed in a pregnant woman, the patient should be advised of the risks of fetal infection; the alternative of therapeutic abortion should be discussed. Structural malformation may be caused by infection during embryogenesis, but not if infection occurs after 20 weeks of gestation. If a woman chooses not to terminate her pregnancy, administration of immune globulin as soon as possible after exposure may be considered. However, no data demonstrate that immune globulin prevents fetal infection. The absence of clinical signs in a woman who has received immune globulin does not guarantee that infection has been prevented.

For rubella-susceptible women of reproductive age, vaccination is highly effective and has few side effects. For women found to be susceptible during pregnancy, offering vaccination postpartum and before discharge, if possible, is recommended. Breastfeeding is not a contradiction to receiving the rubella vaccine.

Following rubella immunization, women should be advised to avoid conception for 3 months. However, a woman who conceives within 3 months of rubella vaccination or who is inadvertently vaccinated in early pregnancy should be counseled that the teratogenic risk to the fetus is theoretic and that data do not support termination of the pregnancy. Although asymptomatic infection can occur, no case of rubella syndrome has arisen from a mother given the current rubella vaccine (human diploid vaccine RA 27/3). The Centers for Disease Control and Prevention (CDC) has discontinued its registry of women vaccinated during pregnancy. However, all suspected cases of congenital rubella syndrome, whether caused by wild-type virus or vaccine virus infection, should continue to be reported to local and state health departments.

Neonatal Management

Neonates who show signs of congenital rubella infection or who were born to women known to have had rubella during pregnancy, including neonates with few or no obvious clinical manifestations at birth, should be isolated, preferably in a private room. Care of the neonate should be provided only by personnel known to be immune to rubella. Efforts should be made to obtain viral cultures from the neonate and to document the infection. Neonates with congenital rubella should be considered contagious until 1 year of age unless nasopharyngeal and urine cultures (after 3 months of age) are repeatedly negative for rubella virus.

Varicella–Zoster Virus

Women with varicella–zoster virus (VZV) infection (chickenpox) during pregnancy are no more likely to develop varicella pneumonia than are other adults, but varicella pneumonia is more severe during pregnancy. Thus, pregnant women with VZV infection should be followed closely for pulmonary symptoms. Although no evidence indicates that maternal administration of VZV immune globulin (VZIG) after exposure reduces the rare occurrence of congenital varicella syndrome, postexposure prophylaxis with VZIG may prevent or ameliorate the illness in nonimmune pregnant women, as it does in other adults. Thus, a pregnant woman who has been exposed to VZV (through intimate or household contact) and who has no history of prior infection should be tested for immunity. If she is not immune, administration of VZIG should be considered within 96 hours of exposure. Varicella–zoster virus immune globulin is available from the American Red Cross Blood Services. Prophylactic administration of acyclovir for treatment of patients with exposure or mild disease is not of proven benefit and is not recommended.

During early pregnancy, VZV infection is infrequently associated with severe congenital malformations or fetal death. The estimated risk of embryopathy from maternal VZV infection in the first trimester of pregnancy is approximately 2%.

If the onset of clinical maternal infection occurs within 5 days before or 2 days after delivery (ie, before the development of maternal antibody, indicating that no VZV antibody has crossed the placenta), VZIG (125 U) should be administered to the neonate as soon as possible. Once VZIG is administered, the neonate can be with the mother. Administration of VZIG is not indicated for healthy, full-term infants exposed postnatally to VZV, except those born within 48 hours of maternal VZV infection. Administered to the mother within 5 days before delivery, VZIG is unlikely to reach the fetus in sufficient quantities. If the mother has herpes zoster infection (shingles), VZIG is not indicated.

Very premature neonates (born at <28 weeks of gestation) who are exposed to VZV postnatally should receive VZIG (125 U), regardless of maternal history, because of the poor transfer of antibody across the placenta early in pregnancy. Hospitalized premature babies born at 28 weeks or more of gestation who are exposed postnatally to chickenpox and whose mothers have no history of chickenpox also should receive VZIG. Hospitalized women with VZV infection must be kept under airborne and contact precautions. Hospitalized neonates born to mothers with active VZV infection should be isolated until 21 days of age (if VZIG is not given) or until 28 days of age (if VZIG is given). Hospitalized infants who are exposed postnatally should be isolated from 8 to 21 days after onset of the rash in the index case. Neonates with VZV infection should be isolated in a private room, and airborne and contact precautions should be maintained for the duration of the illness. Neonates with congenital VZV infection acquired earlier in gestation do not require special precautions or isolation.

Live-attenuated VZV vaccine, licensed in 1995, is routinely recommended for susceptible children, beginning at 12 months of age, and adolescents. Susceptible adults, particularly those in high-risk categories, also should be offered immunization. For adolescents and adults, the primary vaccination series consists of two doses administered subcutaneously 4–8 weeks apart.

Because the vaccine's possible effects on the fetus are not known, pregnant women should not be vaccinated. Women being vaccinated should be advised to avoid pregnancy for 1 month after each vaccine dose. A pregnant mother or other household member, however, is not a contraindication to vaccination of a child.

Bacterial Infections

Group B Streptococcus

Epidemiology

The proportion of pregnant women colonized with group B streptococcus (GBS) ranges from approximately 10% to 30%, but the ability to isolate the organism can be intermittent. Although antepartum rectal or genital colonization is usually asymptomatic, GBS accounts for significant peripartum infection (eg, endometritis, amnionitis, and urinary tract infections).

An estimated 7,600 episodes of GBS sepsis occur annually in newborns (a rate of 1.8 per 1,000 live births) in the United States and result in more than 300 deaths annually among infants less than 90 days of age. Invasive GBS disease in the newborn is primarily characterized by sepsis, pneumonia, and meningitis. Vertical transmission of GBS during labor or delivery may result in invasive infection in the newborn during the first week of life. Known as early-onset GBS infection, this constitutes approximately 80% of GBS disease in newborns. Late-onset GBS disease in the newborn also may occur as a result of vertical transmission or of nosocomial or community-acquired infection.

The risk of early-onset disease is increased by preterm birth (birth at <37 weeks of gestation), a prolonged interval ($\geq$18 hours) between rupture of amniotic membranes and delivery, and clinically evident amnionitis (maternal temperature of $\geq$38°C [$\geq$100.4°F]). Other factors associated with a higher risk of early-onset disease include GBS bacteriuria during pregnancy and previous delivery of an infant with GBS disease.

Prevention

The primary method of preventing GBS disease is antibiotic chemoprophylaxis. There are two equally acceptable strategies for the prevention of early-onset GBS infection in the newborn, based on (1) clinical risk factors such as those noted previously as the primary risk determinants or (2) late prenatal culture (35–37 weeks). When the risk factor strategy is used, the American Academy of Pediatrics, the American College of Obstetricians and Gynecologists, and the CDC recommend giving intrapartum antibiotics when a patient has any one of the risk factors listed in Figure 9–1. When the culture-based strategy is used, the CDC recommends offering intrapartum antibiotic prophylaxis to all women who have a positive culture, irrespective of intrapartum risk factors (Fig. 9–2). Penicillin (intravenous penicillin G, 5 mU initially and then 2.5 mU every 4 hours) is the preferred antibiotic for prophylaxis with ampicillin (intravenous ampicillin, 2 g initially and then 1 g every 4 hours until delivery) as an acceptable alternative. The number of doses of penicillin G received and the

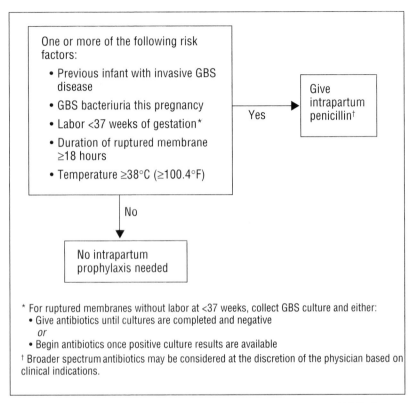

One or more of the following risk factors:

• Previous infant with invasive GBS disease
• GBS bacteriuria this pregnancy
• Labor <37 weeks of gestation*
• Duration of ruptured membrane ≥18 hours
• Temperature ≥38°C (≥100.4°F)

Yes → Give intrapartum penicillin†

No → No intrapartum prophylaxis needed

* For ruptured membranes without labor at <37 weeks, collect GBS culture and either:
• Give antibiotics until cultures are completed and negative
  or
• Begin antibiotics once positive culture results are available
† Broader spectrum antibiotics may be considered at the discretion of the physician based on clinical indications.

Fig. 9–1. Prevention strategy for early-onset group B streptococcus (GBS) disease using risk factors. (Centers for Disease Control and Prevention. Prevention of perinatal group B streptococcal disease: a public health perspective. MMWR Morb Mortal Wkly Rep 1996;45[RR-7]:1–24.)

duration of intrapartum chemoprophylaxis may be important factors in the prevention of neonatal GBS disease. With either strategy, all women who have had a previous infant with GBS disease or who have had GBS bacteriuria during the current pregnancy should be offered intrapartum chemoprophylaxis. Cultures taken before 35 weeks of gestation may have less predictive value for carrier status at delivery and thus are not recommended. Likewise, antepartum treatment for GBS carriers is not recommended.

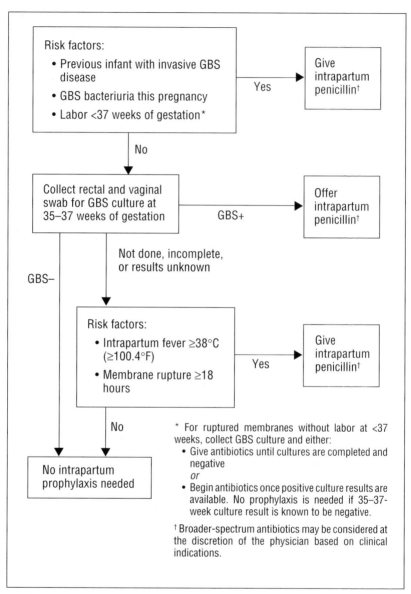

Fig. 9–2. Prevention strategy for early-onset group B streptococcus (GBS) disease using perinatal screening at 35–37 weeks. (Centers for Disease Control and Prevention. Prevention of perinatal group B streptococcal disease: a public health perspective. MMWR Morb Mortal Wkly Rep 1996;45[RR-7]:1–24.)

Obstetric providers should adopt a strategy for the prevention of early-onset GBS disease in the newborn. This strategy should be based on the intrapartum administration of antibiotic prophylaxis to women who are at increased risk of delivering an infant who will develop GBS disease. The risk may be based solely on clinical risk factors or late prenatal cultures for GBS. Women should be informed of the GBS prevention strategy used. If the strategy adopted by the provider is based solely on clinical risk factors, some women may request GBS cultures. Such requests from informed women should be honored by obtaining a culture at 35–37 weeks of gestation.

Management of Newborns

The algorithm for management of infants born to women receiving intrapartum chemoprophylaxis to prevent GBS disease is based on expert opinion (Fig. 9–3). Data to guide decision making are limited, and evaluation of alternative approaches is encouraged. The management of infants born to women receiving chemoprophylaxis is based on the following factors:

• The presence or absence of signs compatible with systemic infection at birth
• The ability to assess signs dictated by gestational age
• The number of doses of maternal chemoprophylaxis given before delivery
• The likelihood that features of early-onset GBS will occur within 48 hours of delivery

Routine administration of antibiotics for all newborns born to mothers who receive intrapartum chemoprophylaxis to prevent GBS disease is not recommended.

Neonates at Any Gestation with Signs of Systemic Infection. Regardless of whether maternal intrapartum chemoprophylaxis is given, neonates with signs of septicemia should have a complete diagnostic evaluation and initiation of empirical antimicrobial therapy, usually with ampicillin and gentamicin. Laboratory evaluation should include a complete blood count and differential, a blood culture, and, if

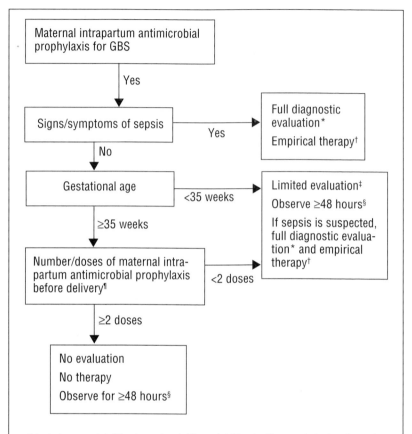

Fig. 9–3. Empirical management of a neonate born to a mother who received intrapartum antimicrobial prophylaxis for prevention of early-onset group B streptococcal (GBS) disease. (American Academy of Pediatrics, Committee on Infectious Diseases and Committee on Fetus and Newborn. Revised guidelines for prevention of early-onset group B streptococcal [GBS] infection. Pediatrics 1997;99:489–496)

respiratory symptoms are present, a chest radiograph. Although elevated total white blood cell counts and absolute neutrophil counts are usually not helpful as single indicators of septicemia, neutropenia (<1,500 total neutrophils cells per mm^3) and an elevated immature-to-total neutrophil ratio of 0.20 or greater are more often associated with systemic infection. Although other perinatal conditions can elevate immature-to-total neutrophil ratios, this measurement has a 98% negative predictive value. The value of a lumbar puncture is controversial, and the need for this procedure should be determined by the examining physician. Additional laboratory studies, such as measurement of acute-phase reactants or testing of urine for GBS antigen, may be done, but their predictive value is low, and perineal GBS contamination of urine specimens frequently produces a false-positive antigen result.

When antibiotic therapy is initiated, the duration of this empirical therapy will vary, depending on the results of the initial complete blood count, blood culture, and cerebrospinal fluid findings (if available) and the clinical course of the infant. If the laboratory evaluation and clinical course suggest that invasive infection is unlikely, therapy should be discontinued 48–72 hours after initiation.

Asymptomatic Infants of Less than 35 Weeks of Gestation. Compared with term infants, preterm neonates have a 10–15-fold increased risk for early-onset GBS sepsis. Further, as the degree of prematurity increases, clinical evaluation to ascertain the presence or absence of signs of septicemia becomes more difficult. If the results of the clinical evaluation are equivocal, the physician may choose to err on the side of implementing empirical therapy promptly.

Figure 9–3 shows a management scheme for healthy infants. Asymptomatic infants born at less than 35 weeks of gestation should be evaluated and observed in the hospital without empirical antimicrobial therapy. The evaluation could be limited to a complete blood count (with differential) and a blood culture. At least 48 hours of hospital observation (ie, no shortened hospital stay) is indicated to minimize the likelihood of early-onset GBS sepsis after discharge. If during the period of observation the clinical course suggests systemic infection, a complete diagnostic evaluation and initiation of empirical antibiotic therapy is indicated.

Asymptomatic Infants of 35 or More Weeks of Gestation. In infants with gestations of 35 weeks or more, the initial clinical evaluation of signs and symptoms should be dependable. Thus, further management would be dictated by the duration of maternal intrapartum chemoprophylaxis before delivery. High amniotic fluid concentrations of ampicillin are achieved within 3 hours after intravenous administration. Asymptomatic infants born at a gestational age of 35 weeks or more and whose mothers have received two or more doses of penicillin G prophylaxis before delivery should be observed in the hospital for at least 48 hours. More than 95% of infants with early-onset GBS disease develop symptoms within 48 hours of birth, and no instance has been reported in which maternal chemoprophylaxis has delayed the onset of early neonatal GBS sepsis.

Asymptomatic Infants and the Number of Doses of Maternal Intrapartum Chemoprophylaxis Prior to Delivery. Term infants account for about 70% of cases of early-onset GBS sepsis in neonates, but the risk for sepsis and attendant mortality are lower than that in neonates born before 37 of weeks of gestation. Asymptomatic infants of 35 or more weeks of gestation whose mothers have received two or more doses of penicillin G should account for most of those undergoing the empirical management algorithm shown in Figure 9–3. They should be managed as healthy, low-risk newborns who require neither empirical laboratory evaluation nor therapy. However, they should be observed in the hospital for at least 48 hours.

Listeriosis

The major cause of epidemic and sporadic listeriosis infections is foodborne transmission. Incriminated foods include unpasteurized milk, cheese, and other dairy products; undercooked poultry; and prepared meats, such as paté. Asymptomatic fecal and vaginal carriage can result in sporadic neonatal disease, which can cause early-onset neonatal infections from transplacental or ascending intrauterine infection or from exposure during delivery.

Maternal infection has been associated with preterm delivery and other obstetric complications. Late-onset neonatal infection results from acquisition of the organism during passage through the birth canal or possibly from environmental sources. Nosocomial transmission to newborns probably occurs as well.

Signs of listeriosis in the newborn vary widely and often are nonspecific. The clinical picture may be similar to that of GBS infection with early- and late-onset syndromes.

Listeria monocytogenes can be cultured readily, but the laboratory should be informed that this organism is suspected, because *L. monocytogenes* may be confused initially with diphtheroids, a common contaminant. Special techniques may be necessary to isolate the organism from stool and other sites with mixed flora. Gram stain of a fecal smear from an infected newborn may show the organism in profusion.

Prompt diagnosis and antibiotic treatment of maternal listeriosis may prevent fetal or perinatal infection. *Listeria monocytogenes* is highly sensitive to penicillin. Because repeated fetal infection with *L. monocytogenes* has occurred in some women, some authorities suggest that the cervix and stools of the mother of an infected neonate be cultured and the mother treated if either culture is positive. Reculturing for listeria during a subsequent pregnancy has been proposed.

Gonorrhea

Management in Pregnant Women

Gonorrhea occurs most commonly in individuals aged 15–29 years, and the highest reported incidence occurs in young men aged 20–24 years. In females, the highest rates are in adolescents aged 15–19 years. Risk factors include lower socioeconomic status, single status, early onset of sexual activity, multiple sexual partners, and substance use.

Pregnant women with risk factors or symptoms for gonorrhea should be cultured for *Neisseria gonorrhoeae* at an early prenatal visit. A repeat culture should be obtained in the third trimester for women at increased risk for gonorrhea and other sexually transmissible infections.

The treatment for gonorrhea also includes antibiotic therapy for presumptive *Chlamydia trachomatis* infection. The 1993 CDC guidelines for pregnant women recommend ceftriaxone plus erythromycin. Because of gastrointestinal toxicity, a regimen of 250 mg four times daily for 14 days is acceptable. Azithromycin in a single dose (1 g) is an acceptable alternative to erythromycin for the treatment of *C. trachomatis* infection, but well-controlled, adequate studies in pregnant women have not been performed. Animal studies suggest no adverse effect on the fetus. Spectinomycin, 2 mg intramuscularly, followed by erythromycin is indicated for infected pregnant women allergic to beta-lactam antibiotics. Tetracycline drugs are contraindicated during pregnancy because of the association of yellow-brown discoloration of the fetal deciduous teeth. A test-of-cure is not routinely recommended in persons with uncomplicated gonorrhea, provided that symptoms resolve, but is warranted in pregnant women.

Neonatal Clinical Manifestations

Routine prophylaxis administered immediately after birth usually prevents gonococcal ophthalmia. However, an occasional case of gonococcal ophthalmia or disseminated gonococcal infection can occur in neonates born to mothers with gonococcal disease. Neonates born to mothers with active gonorrhea should receive a single dose of ceftriaxone, 125 mg, intravenously or intramuscularly; for low-birth-weight neonates, the dose is 25–50 mg/kg of body weight. Cefotaxime in a single dose (100 mg/kg given intravenously or intramuscularly) is an alternative.

Neonatal involvement other than the eyes include scalp abscess, vaginitis, and systemic disease with bacteremia, arthritis, meningitis, or endocarditis. Cultures of blood, cerebrospinal fluid, and eye discharge should be obtained from neonates with clinical gonococcal disease. For those with positive cultures (ie, disseminated infection), the recommended antimicrobial therapy is ceftriaxone (25–50 mg/kg per day intravenously or intramuscularly, not to exceed 125 mg given in a single daily dose). Cefotaxime (50–100 mg/kg per day, divided into two doses given every 12 hours) is an alternative. Treatment should be given for 7 days and for 10–14 days if meningitis occurs. Infected neonates should be managed with standard precautions.

Chlamydia

Chlamydia trachomatis has been detected in the cervix of 2–13% of pregnant women and is generally found in 5% or more of women in all populations. Prevalence is highest (eg, 37%) in sexually active adolescent girls. Unrecognized infection is common. Important risk factors for chlamydial infection include unmarried status, recent change in sexual partner or multiple concurrent partners, age younger than 25 years, inner-city residence, history or presence of other sexually transmissible infections, and little or no prenatal care. Universal testing of all pregnant women for *C. trachomatis* is not recommended. Most infected women have few symptoms, but chlamydia may cause urethritis and mucopurulent (nongonococcal) cervicitis. Chlamydial infection is also associated with postpartum endometritis and infertility. Infection may be transmitted from the genital tract of infected mothers to their neonates during birth; about 50% of neonates born to infected mothers become colonized with *C. trachomatis* in the absence of prophylaxis. Purulent conjunctivitis develops a few days to several weeks after birth in 25–50% of neonates who acquire *C. trachomatis* infection, and neonatal pneumonia occurs in 5–20%.

Treatment should be administered to women who have known *C. trachomatis* infection (ie, with mucopurulent cervicitis) or whose infants are infected. Women whose sexual partners have nongonococcal urethritis or epididymitis are presumed to be infected and should also be treated. Simultaneous treatment of male partners is an important component of the therapeutic regimen. Although first-line therapy for chlamydia is oral doxycycline or azithromycin, treatment with erythromycin is recommended; doxycycline is contraindicated, and only limited data are available on the safety of azithromycin in pregnant women.

Chlamydial infections in the neonate are generally mild and responsive to antimicrobial therapy. Prophylactic cesarean delivery is not warranted. Routine instillation of topical erythromycin or tetracycline into the conjunctival sac of the neonate shortly after birth has not been proven to prevent neonatal conjunctivitis or other infections caused by chlamydia. Neonates with chlamydial conjunctivitis or chlamydial pneumonia should be treated with oral erythromycin and, if hospitalized, should be managed with drainage and secretion precautions.

Tuberculosis

Screening

Once considered rare in the United States, the incidence of tuberculosis has increased considerably in women of childbearing age. In endemic areas, the incidence of tuberculosis may approach 0.1% of pregnant women. All pregnant women who are at high risk for tuberculosis should be screened with a Mantoux skin test with purified protein derivative (PPD) when they begin receiving prenatal care. High-risk factors for tuberculosis include the following:

• HIV infection
• Close contact with persons known or suspected to have tuberculosis
• Medical risk factors known to increase risk of disease
• Birth in a country with a high prevalence of tuberculosis
• Medically underserved status
• Low socioeconomic status
• Alcohol addiction
• Intravenous drug use
• Residency in a long-term care facility (eg, correctional institutions, mental institutions, nursing homes and facilities)
• Health care professionals working in facilities where the risk of exposure to *Mycobacterium tuberculosis* is increased

In endemic urban areas, universal screening may be warranted, because essentially all patients meet risk criteria.

Management During Pregnancy

Treatment regimens for tuberculosis are based on the presence or absence of active disease, primarily determined by chest X-ray and, in the absence of active disease, the duration of PPD, or tuberculin, positivity. The risk of progression to active disease is highest in the 2 years after seroconversion to positive PPD. For this reason, the recommended medication in women known to have converted within the previous 2 years but with no evidence of active disease is isoniazid, 300 mg per day, starting after the first trimester and continuing for 9 months.

Unfortunately, the time of seroconversion is usually not known. If a chest X-ray is normal, the woman should be treated after pregnancy. For women who are HIV infected, the duration of therapy for tuberculosis is 12 months. Women less than 35 years of age with an unknown or prolonged (>2 years) duration of PPD positivity should receive isoniazid, 300 mg per day, for 6 months after delivery. For women over 35 years of age, isoniazid prophylaxis is not recommended for unknown or prolonged PPD positivity in the absence of active disease because of concerns about hepatotoxicity. All pregnant women receiving isoniazid should also take pyridoxine.

Neonatal Management

Because tuberculosis is usually transmitted by inhalation of droplet nuclei produced by an adult or adolescent with infectious primary tuberculosis, acquisition of *M. tuberculosis* by newborns generally occurs only after delivery. Infection can occur before birth as a result of hematogenous dissemination, which seeds the placenta; as a result of infected amniotic fluid in utero; or at the time of delivery as a result of fetal aspiration of tubercle bacilli in women with tuberculosis endometritis. On the rare occasions in which congenital tuberculosis is suspected, diagnostic evaluations and treatment of the neonate and mother should be initiated promptly.

Management of a newborn whose mother (or other household contact) is suspected of having tuberculosis is based on individual considerations. If possible, separation of the mother (or contact) and baby should be minimized. Differing circumstances and resulting recommendations are as follows:

- *Mother (or household contact) has a negative roentgenogram*—If the mother is asymptomatic, no separation of mother and infant is required. The mother is usually a candidate for treatment of tuberculosis infection. The newborn needs no special evaluation or therapy. Because the positive tuberculin test could be a marker of an unrecognized case of contagious tuberculosis within the household, other household members should have Mantoux skin tests with PPD and further evaluation.

- *Mother (or household contact) has an abnormal chest roentgenogram*—If the roentgenogram is abnormal, the mother and infant should be separated until the mother has been evaluated and, if active tuberculosis disease is found, until she is receiving antituberculosis therapy. Other household members should have Mantoux skin test with PPD and further evaluation.

- *Mother (or household contact) has an abnormal chest roentgenogram but no evidence of active disease*—If the mother's chest roentgenogram is abnormal but the history, physical examination, sputum smear, and roentgenogram indicate no evidence of active disease, the infant can be assumed to be at low risk of *M. tuberculosis* infection. The radiographic abnormality in this circumstance is probably due to another cause or to a quiescent focus of tuberculosis. In the latter case, the mother may develop contagious, active tuberculosis, if untreated, and should receive appropriate therapy, if not previously treated. She and her infant should receive follow-up care. Other household members should have a Mantoux skin test with PPD and further evaluation.

- *Mother (or household contact) has clinical or radiographic evidence of active, possibly contagious tuberculosis*—The mother (or household contact) should be reported immediately to the public health department so that investigation of all household members can be performed within several days. All contacts should have a tuberculin skin test, chest roentgenogram, and physical examination. The infant should be evaluated for congenital tuberculosis and should be tested for HIV infection. The mother and infant should be separated until both are receiving appropriate therapy and the mother is deemed to be noncontagious. Other household members should have skin testing and further evaluation.

If congenital tuberculosis is excluded, isoniazid is given until the infant is 3–4 months of age, at which time the Mantoux skin test with

PPD should be repeated. If the skin test is positive, the child should be reassessed for tuberculosis. If disease is not present, isoniazid should be continued for a total of at least 6 months; HIV-infected children should be treated for 12 months. If the skin test is negative and the mother and other family members with tuberculosis have good adherence and response to treatment and are no longer infectious, isoniazid may be discontinued. The infant should be evaluated at monthly intervals during treatment.

If the mother (or household contact) has disease due to multiple-drug-resistant *M. tuberculosis* or has poor adherence to treatment and directly observed therapy is not possible, the infant should be separated from the ill family member and bacillus Calmette–Guérin vaccination may be considered for the infant. Because the response to the vaccine in infants may be delayed and inadequate for prevention of tuberculosis, directly observed therapy is preferred.

Untoward effects of isoniazid therapy in newborns are rare. The incidence of hepatitis during isoniazid therapy is so low in otherwise healthy babies that routine determination of serum aminotransferase concentrations is not recommended. The maternal use of isoniazid is considered to be compatible with breastfeeding. Breastfeeding is considered safe during maternal antituberculosis therapy as long as the infant is not concurrently taking oral antituberculosis therapy. (If both mother and infant are taking antituberculosis therapy, excessive drug concentrations may occur in the neonate.) Breastfed infants of women taking isoniazid therapy should receive a multivitamin supplement, including pyridoxine. Drugs in breast milk should not be considered effective treatment or prophylaxis of the baby.

Bacillus Calmette–Guérin vaccine should be considered only for uninfected infants and children who are at high risk of intimate and prolonged exposure to patients with persistently infectious pulmonary tuberculosis, who cannot be removed from the source of exposure, and who cannot be placed on long-term preventive therapy. The vaccine also should be considered for infants who are continuously exposed to patients infected with *M. tuberculosis* that is resistant to isoniazid and rifampin and who cannot be removed from the source of exposure.

Spirochetal Infections

Syphilis

The incidence of syphilis in the United States continues to increase. All pregnant women should be serologically screened for syphilis as early as possible in pregnancy and again at delivery (as well as after exposure to an infected partner). Because false-negative serologic tests may occur in early primary infection and infection after the first prenatal visit is possible, patients who are considered to be at high risk for syphilis or who are from areas of high prevalence should be retested at the beginning of the third trimester.

The specificity of serologic testing is high if both a nontreponemal screening test (Venereal Disease Research Laboratory [VDRL] or Rapid Plasma Reagin [RPR] testing) and a subsequent treponemal serologic test are reactive. Microscopic dark-field and histologic examinations for spirochetes are most reliable when lesions are present.

Congenital syphilis is most often acquired through hematogenous transplacental infection of the fetus, although direct contact of the neonate with infectious lesions during or after birth can also result in infection. Transplacental infection can occur throughout pregnancy and at any stage of maternal infection.

Treatment for Pregnant Women

Pregnant women with syphilis should be treated with a penicillin regimen appropriate to the stage of infection. Women who are allergic to penicillin should be desensitized and then treated with the drug (Table 9–3). Tetracycline and doxycycline are contraindicated during pregnancy. Erythromycin is suboptimal because poor transplacental passage or poor patient compliance may result in failure to cure infection in the fetus.

All pregnant women, including those with syphilis, should receive HIV counseling, and education and testing should be recommended as a part of their regular prenatal care. Women with syphilis should be queried about substance use, especially cocaine. Results of the maternal serologic tests and treatment, if given, should be recorded in the neonate's medical record or be made available to the neonate's physician.

Table 9–3. Oral Desensitization Protocol for Penicillin V*

Suspension (U/ml)	Amount (ml)	Amount (U)	Cumulative Dose (U)†
1,000	0.1	100	100
1,000	0.2	200	300
1,000	0 4	400	700
1,000	0.8	800	1,500
1,000	1.6	1,600	3,100
1,000	3.2	3,200	6,300
1,000	6.4	6,400	12,700
10,000	1.2	12,000	24,700
10,000	2.4	24,000	48,700
10,000	4.8	48,000	96,700
80,000	1.0	80,000	176,700
80,000	2.0	160,000	336,700
80,000	4.0	320,000	656,700
80,000	8.0	640,000	1,296,700

* Observation period: 30 minutes before parenteral administration of penicillin.

† Dosing interval = 15 minutes; elapsed time = 3 hours 45 minutes; cumulative dose = 1.3 million U. The specific amount of drug was diluted in approximately 30 ml of water and given orally.

Modified with permission from Wendel GD Jr, Stark BJ, Jamison RB, Molina RD, Sullivan TJ. Penicillin allergy and desensitization in serious infections during pregnancy. N Engl J Med 1985;312:1229–1232.

Evaluation of Newborn Infants for Congenital Infection

No newborn should leave any hospital without determination of the syphilis serologic status of his or her mother. A neonate should be evaluated for congenital syphilis if he or she is born to a mother with a positive treponemal test who has one or more of the following conditions:

- Syphilis and HIV infection
- Untreated or inadequately treated syphilis
- Syphilis during pregnancy treated with a nonpenicillin regimen and inadequate regimen, such as erythromycin

- Syphilis during pregnancy treated with an appropriate penicillin regimen that failed to produce the expected decrease in nontreponemal antibody titer after therapy
- Syphilis treated less than 1 month before delivery (because treatment failures occur and the efficacy of treatment cannot be assumed)
- Syphilis treatment not documented
- Syphilis treated before pregnancy but with insufficient serologic follow-up during pregnancy to assess the response to treatment and current infection status

Neonates born to women with any of the preceding conditions should be evaluated for syphilis. This evaluation should include the following:

- Physical examination
- Quantitative nontreponemal serologic test for syphilis
- Cerebrospinal fluid evaluation, including a VDRL
- Long-bone X-ray (unless the diagnosis has been otherwise established)
- If available, determination of antitreponemal IgM antibody by a testing method recognized by the CDC, either as a standard or provisional method
- Other clinically indicated tests (eg, chest X-ray)

The VDRL or RPR test is commonly used to evaluate newborn infants for congenital infection with *Treponema pallidum*. For testing, serum from the neonate is preferred to cord blood because the latter can produce false-positive and false-negative results.

A diagnosis of congenital syphilis is frequently difficult to establish because clinical evidence of infection may not be apparent at birth and serologic test results may be equivocal or difficult to interpret. A reactive serologic test for syphilis (eg, VDRL, RPR, or fluorescent treponemal antibody absorption test) on neonatal blood does not necessarily indicate that the neonate is infected. If the reaction is caused only by passively transferred maternal antibody, the neonate's VDRL titer is usually lower than the mother's and reverts to negative in 4–6 months. A positive fluorescent treponemal antibody absorption test caused by passively transferred antibody may take up to 1 year to become negative. A persistently reactive serologic test for syphilis suggests infection, and a rising titer is almost diagnostic.

Clinical symptoms of early congenital syphilis are frequently absent or nonspecific. Long-bone X-rays may be useful in establishing a diagnosis in babies with suspected or proven congenital syphilis.

Moist, open syphilitic lesions are infectious. Standard precautions are sufficient for neonates with suspected or proven congenital syphilis. Health care personnel and parents should wear long gloves when handling the neonate. Individuals in intimate contact with the neonate before isolation precautions and treatment were instituted should be examined for the presence of lesions 2–3 weeks later and tested serologically for infection.

Parenteral penicillin G remains the preferred therapy for syphilis at any stage. Treatment of neonates with congenital syphilis is summarized in Table 9–4.

Lyme Disease

Lyme disease is caused by a spirochete (*Borrelia burgdorferi*) transmitted by deer ticks. Early stages of the disease are characterized by a distinctive bull's-eye skin lesion (erythema migrans), which occurs in 60–80% of patients, and nonspecific, flulike symptoms. Untreated disease can result in neurologic or cardiac manifestations within 4–6 weeks after the onset of early signs and symptoms. A late manifestation of Lyme disease is arthritis, usually intermittent inflammatory arthritis of a large joint. Untreated patients can develop joint involvement ranging from mild to moderate arthralgia to chronic destructive joint disease. No definitive early diagnostic tests, including serology, are commercially available. Patients in the later stages of Lyme disease will usually be seropositive, but false-positive and false-negative tests are common.

Suspicion of early maternal infection is based on a history of exposure to tick bites, the presence of the distinctive skin lesion, and nonspecific, flulike symptoms. Adequately treated patients may never develop antibodies to spirochetes.

Table 9–4. Recommended Treatment of Neonates (≤4 Weeks Old) with Proven or Possible Congenital Syphilis

Clinical Status of Newborn	Antimicrobial Therapy
Proven or highly probable disease	Aqueous crystalline penicillin G for 10–14 days*
Asymptomatic, normal CSF and radiographic examination when maternal treatment is:	
—None, inadequate penicillin dose, undocumented, failed, or reinfected	Aqueous crystalline penicillin G, IV, for 10–14 days *or** Clinical, serologic follow-up and benzathine penicillin G, IM, single dose†
—Adequate but given <1 month before delivery, mother's response to treatment is not demonstrated by a fourfold decrease in titer of a non-treponemal serologic test, or erythromycin therapy	Clinical, serologic follow-up and benthazine penicillin G, IM, single dose†

* If more than 1 day of therapy is missed, the entire course should be restarted.

† Some experts recommend aqueous crystalline penicillin G, as for proven or highly probable disease. Other experts would follow the baby without giving antibiotic therapy if both clinical and serologic follow-up can be ensured.

Abbreviations: CSF = cerebrospinal fluid; IM = intramuscularly; IV = intravenously.

Modified from American Academy of Pediatrics. Peter G, ed. 1997 Red book: report of the Committee on Infectious Diseases. 24th ed. Elk Grove Village, Illinois: AAP, 1997.

Spirochetes can cross the placenta and, in rare cases, have been found in the tissues of stillborn fetuses. However, the frequency and significance of fetal infection is unknown. Although malformations, intrauterine fetal death, prematurity, and rash in the newborn have occurred in association with infection in the pregnant mother, a causal relationship has not been established. Current data do not support counseling for pregnancy termination. The infant's health care provider should be informed when maternal disease is suspected.

Recommended treatment of suspected early disease in pregnant women is the same as for nonpregnant persons—amoxicillin, 500 mg three times a day for 2–3 weeks. For women who are allergic to penicillin, cefuroxime axetil or erythromycin is recommended for 2–3 weeks. Cefuroxime axetil is not acceptable for patients with immediate and anaphylactic hypersensitivity to penicillin unless they have undergone penicillin desensitization, which is an alternative method in patients who are unable to tolerate erythromycin. The best preventive measure is to avoid heavily wooded areas. If entrance into such areas is necessary, long-sleeved shirts and long pants tucked in at the ankle are helpful. Prophylactic antibiotic therapy for deer tick bites is not routinely recommended.

Toxoplasmosis

Toxoplasmosis is a protozoan infection caused by *Toxoplasma gondii*. As many as one third of women in the United States have antibodies to this organism. Infection is acquired from eating infected raw or poorly cooked meat and from exposure to infected domestic cats. Infected women are generally asymptomatic.

Although congenital infection is more common after maternal infection in the third trimester, the sequelae from first-trimester fetal infection are more severe. Congenital infection may result in chorioretinitis, hydrocephaly, microcephaly, and intracranial calcifications. Infants born to HIV- and toxoplasmosis-positive women should be evaluated for congenital toxoplasmosis.

The diagnosis of maternal infection is based on serologic antibody testing. Routine screening of pregnant women is not indicated, except in the presence of HIV infection. Because the presence of antibodies before pregnancy indicates immunity, the appropriate time to test for immunity to toxoplasmosis in women at risk is before conception. Demonstration of seroconversion is the best method of confirming the diagnosis of acute infection. A significant rise in IgG titer in paired samples taken 2–4 weeks apart (tested simultaneously) or the presence of very high titers most often indicates recent or current infection.

Although the presence of antitoxoplasma IgM antibodies is suggestive of acute infection, such IgM antibodies may persist for several years. Because false-positive results may be obtained in patients with rheumatoid factor, reference laboratory testing for the confirmation of IgM is important. The detection of IgA antibodies to toxoplasma is also indicative of acute infection. Confirmation of fetal infection is possible in some centers by culture of fetal blood or amniotic fluid. Therapy of infected mothers with the investigational macrolide antibiotic spiramycin (available through the FDA) may reduce the incidence of fetal infection but will not prevent sequelae in the fetus if congenital infection does occur. The combination of pyrimethamine and sulfadiazine has also been used and may decrease the severity of infection, although the efficacy of such therapy has not been proven. Routine neonatal screening for toxoplasmosis with early treatment of infected neonates may decrease the frequency of long-term sequelae.

Bibliography

American Academy of Pediatrics. Peter G, ed. 1997 Red book: report of the Committee on Infectious Diseases. 24th ed. Elk Grove Village, Illinois: AAP, 1997

American Academy of Pediatrics, Committee on Infectious Diseases. Update on timing of hepatitis B vaccination for premature infants and for children with lapsed immunization. Pediatrics 1994;94:403–404

American Academy of Pediatrics, Committee on Infectious Diseases and Committee on Fetus and Newborn. Respiratory syncytial virus immune globulin intravenous: indications for use. Pediatrics 1997;99:645–650

American Academy of Pediatrics, Committee on Infectious Diseases and Committee on Fetus and Newborn. Revised guidelines for prevention of early-onset group B streptococcal (GBS) infection. Pediatrics 1997;99:489–496

American Academy of Pediatrics, Committee on Pediatric AIDS. Human milk, breastfeeding, and transmission of human immunodeficiency virus in the United States. Pediatrics 1995;96:977–979

American Academy of Pediatrics, Provisional Committee on Pediatric AIDS. Perinatal human immunodeficiency virus testing. Pediatrics 1995;95:303–307

American College of Obstetricians and Gynecologists. Antimicrobial therapy for obstetric patients. ACOG Technical Bulletin 117. Washington, DC: ACOG, 1988

American College of Obstetricians and Gynecologists. Genital human papillomavirus infections. ACOG Technical Bulletin 193. Washington, DC: ACOG, 1994

American College of Obstetricians and Gynecologists. Hepatitis in pregnancy. Technical Bulletin 174. Washington, DC: ACOG, 1992

American College of Obstetricians and Gynecologists. Human immunodeficiency virus infections in pregnancy. Educational Bulletin 232. Washington, DC: ACOG, 1997

American College of Obstetricians and Gynecologists. Immunization during pregnancy. ACOG Technical Bulletin 160. Washington, DC: ACOG, 1991

American College of Obstetricians and Gynecologists. Perinatal viral and parasitic infections. ACOG Technical Bulletin 177. Washington, DC: ACOG, 1993

American College of Obstetricians and Gynecologists. Prevention of early-onset group B streptococcal disease in newborns. Committee Opinion 173. Washington, DC: ACOG, 1996

American College of Obstetricians and Gynecologists. Pulmonary disease in pregnancy. Technical Bulletin 224. Washington, DC: ACOG, 1996

American College of Obstetricians and Gynecologists. Rubella and pregnancy. ACOG Technical Bulletin 171. Washington, DC: ACOG, 1992

Centers for Disease Control and Prevention. Prevention of perinatal group B streptococcal disease: a public health perspective. MMWR Morb Mortal Wkly Rep 1996;45(RR-7):1–24

Centers for Disease Control and Prevention. Recommendations of the U.S. Public Health Service Task Force on the use of zidovudine to reduce perinatal transmission of human immunodeficiency virus. MMWR Morb Mortal Wkly Rep 1994;43(RR-11):1–20

Centers for Disease Control and Prevention. 1993 Sexually transmitted diseases treatment guidelines. MMWR Morb Mortal Wkly Rep 1993;42(RR-14):27–47

Chapter 10

Infection Control

Preventing infection in the healthy newborn nursery, the intensive care nursery, and other peripartum areas where newborns receive care may involve tasks that are easy to describe but functionally difficult to implement. The mother–newborn dyad is usually free from any significant infectious processes. When exposed to certain organisms, however, the outcome may be devastating for neonate or mother. Most infections of neonates in intensive care units are caused by pathogens acquired from the hospital environment. Prevention of these infections requires a multifaceted approach, including meticulous patient care techniques, elimination of inappropriate antibiotic use to avoid further alteration of the balance of colonizing flora, and careful attention to all aspects of infection control.

Today, health care providers must be aware of the consequences of their exposure, through the mother and fetus, to potentially life-threatening diseases. The importance of standard precautions for the prevention of occupationally acquired diseases in the health care environment has never been greater. Health care personnel should safeguard themselves against pathogens that may be contracted from patients.

Colonization in Neonates

Most neonates emerge from a sterile intrauterine environment. During and after birth, they are exposed to numerous microorganisms that colonize their skin, nasopharynx, and gastrointestinal tract. Ill neonates who are subjected to multiple invasive procedures frequently have colonization at multiple sites with a variety of organisms.

The skin of the newborn is a major initial site of bacterial colonization, particularly with *Staphylococcus aureus*. Colonizing strains of this organism are most commonly transmitted within the nursery rather than from the mother. Any break in the integrity of the protective skin affords an opportunity for infection to develop. Postpartum mastitis may indicate the presence of *S. aureus* in the nursery.

Nursery Admission Policies

An institution does not need restrictive nursery admission policies. Newborns transferred from a nursery at another hospital are usually admitted. Precautions should be taken to prevent the transmission of colonizing or infecting organisms from one neonate to another. Similarly, neonates may be moved safely from one nursery area to another under normal circumstances. Each neonate should be approached as though he or she harbored colonies of unique flora that should not be transmitted to any other neonate. To promote appropriate continuity of care, some neonates may need to be readmitted to the nursery after being discharged during the first 3 days of life. Newborns with suspected infectious diseases should not be readmitted to the normal newborn nursery. Newborns may be allowed to room in with mothers who are readmitted for management of complications.

Neonatal Intensive Care

Neonates who require intensive care are highly susceptible to infections from colonizing organisms. Because neonates colonized with pathogenic organisms may have no overt signs of illness, caregivers might not recognize the need to take special precautions to prevent spreading organisms capable of causing disease. Thus, caregivers may inadvertently carry these pathogenic organisms from neonates who have been colonized to neonates not previously colonized. As a result, a high proportion of the neonates in a single nursery may be colonized or infected with the same strains of bacteria. Respiratory tract and intestinal organisms are easily transmissible in such situations.

To minimize the transmission of infectious organisms, each individual working with these neonates and with the equipment used directly in their care should be meticulous when providing patient care. Personnel should wash their hands both before and after taking care of a neonate. Disposal of contaminated equipment or materials should always be accomplished using standard precautions and careful hand-washing.

Surveillance for Nosocomial Infection

The infection control committee of each hospital should work with perinatal care personnel to establish workable definitions of nosocomial infection for surveillance purposes. For obstetric patients, a nosocomial infection can be defined broadly as one that is neither present nor incubating at the time the patient is admitted to the hospital. Therefore, most cases of endometritis or urinary tract infection that occur postpartum are nosocomial, even though the causative organisms may be endogenous.

Nosocomial infection in newborns is more difficult to define. The broadest definition includes all infections that have an onset after birth, excluding only those known to have been transmitted transplacentally. Narrower definitions exclude infections that develop within 24–72 hours of birth, because these too may have been caused by organisms acquired from the mother rather than from the hospital environment. Definitions should include infections that become apparent within a certain period after a neonate's discharge. The definition selected should be applied consistently to allow uniform reporting and analysis of nosocomial infections.

Obstetric and nursery personnel should cooperate with hospital infection control personnel in conducting and reviewing the results of surveillance programs for nosocomial infections. This type of monitoring provides information about any unusual problems or clusters of infection, the risks associated with certain procedures or techniques, and the success of specific preventive measures. It can also provide temporal trends, allow comparison with other nurseries using standard definitions, and provide feedback to responsible personnel in the nursery.

Routine culturing of neonates' respiratory or gastrointestinal tract or skin for surveillance purposes is not recommended, but cultures of specimens from lesions or sites of infection can be helpful in identifying clusters of infection caused by a single strain of bacteria. This practice is especially important for pediatricians and others who care for the newborns to report confirmed or suspected postdischarge infections to nursery and hospital infection control personnel.

Although usually only clinically apparent infections should be recorded in the surveillance data, at times, especially during an outbreak of infection, it may be important to document organisms responsible for colonization of all neonates at certain sites. Clusters of infection that do not fit a standard definition may need to be investigated individually.

Both obstetric and nursery personnel are involved in providing perinatal care; therefore, precise communication between these groups about infectious diseases is essential. Nursery personnel should be notified in advance about the birth of a neonate who may have a congenital or perinatal infection or about a mother who is known to be infected with, or a chronic carrier of, an organism (eg, *Salmonella* species, hepatitis B virus [HBV], hepatitis C virus, hepatitis D virus, or herpes simplex virus). *Hand-washing before and after each patient contact remains the single most important routine practice in the control of nosocomial infections.*

Prevention and Control of Infections

Health Standards for Personnel

Obstetric and nursery personnel, as well as others who have significant contact with newborns, should be free of transmissible infectious diseases. Routine culturing of specimens such as nasal swabs obtained from personnel is not useful, although selective culturing may be of value when a pattern of infection is suspected. Each hospital should establish written policies and procedures for assessing the health of personnel assigned to perinatal care services, restricting their contact with patients when necessary, maintaining their health records, and reporting any illness that they may have. These policies and procedures should address screening for immunity to rubella, varicella–zoster virus, and HBV. Personnel should receive the Mantoux skin test with purified protein derivative for tuberculosis, and adequate treatment and noninfective status should be documented. Pregnancy should not exclude a female health care worker from being skin tested as part of a contact investigation or as part of a regular skin testing program. All susceptible, nonpregnant hospital personnel should be offered immunization against rubella, varicella–zoster virus, and HBV. Offering annual immunization of nursery personnel against prevalent strains of influenza virus is strongly encouraged.

Ideally, individuals with a respiratory, cutaneous, mucocutaneous, or gastrointestinal infection should not have direct contact with neonates. Personnel with exudative skin lesions or weeping dermatitis should refrain from all direct patient care and should not handle patient care equipment until the condition resolves. Personnel in contact with neonates should report personal infections, inability to wash hands (eg, because of casts or braces), and other conditions to their immediate supervisors and should be medically examined before working directly with neonates. Decisions regarding the exclusion of staff members from obstetric and nursery areas should be made on an individual basis. Employee health policies should be worded and applied in a way to ensure that personnel feel free to report infectious problems without fear of income loss.

Transmission of herpes simplex virus from infected personnel to neonates in newborn nurseries is rare. Personnel with cold sores who have direct contact with infants should cover and avoid touching their lesions and carefully observe hand-washing policies. Transmission of herpes simplex virus infection from personnel with genital lesions is not likely, provided that hand-washing policies are carefully observed. Personnel with herpetic hand infections (herpetic whitlow) should not participate directly in the care of patients until the lesions have healed.

Personnel in neonatal units are likely to be exposed to patients excreting cytomegalovirus. No evidence exists that transfer to another area of the hospital or to a different group of patients decreases the risk, because many hospitalized patients asymptomatically excrete cytomegalovirus. Acquisition of infection should be prevented by compliance with standard precautions. Women of childbearing age who work in neonatal units should be counseled about the relatively low risk of exposure should they become pregnant. A routine program of serologic testing for obstetric and nursery hospital employees is not recommended. Standard precautions should be used routinely by pregnant health care workers.

When possible, personnel assigned to obstetric or newborn areas should not be moved between or from other assigned areas of the hospital. If such movement cannot be avoided, the chance of spreading nosocomial infections should be minimized by strict adherence to standard precautions. Employee education regarding isolation precautions and other proper infection control techniques should be established and reviewed regularly. All personnel should be required to follow established infection control procedures strictly.

Hand-Washing

Medical and hospital personnel must follow careful hand-washing techniques to minimize transmission of disease. Personnel should remove rings, watches, and bracelets before washing their hands and entering the obstetric or nursery areas. Fingernails should be trimmed short, and no false fingernails or nail polish should be permitted. Antiseptic preparations should be used for scrubbing before entering the nursery, before providing care for neonates highly susceptible to infection, before performing invasive procedures, and after providing care for infected neonates. For routine hand-washing within the nursery, bactericidal soap and water may be sufficient.

The antiseptics most useful for hand-washing in the nursery are chlorhexidine gluconate (4%) and iodophor preparations; both are broad-spectrum bactericidal soaps. Iodophor preparations are often more drying to the skin. Hexachlorophene-based preparations may be especially useful during nursery outbreaks of *S. aureus* infection, but they are not recommended for routine hand-washing.

All antiseptic compounds are sensitizing or irritating to some people, and some individuals may need to use plain soap or mild detergents. Liquid soap dispensers and many hand-washing agents may become contaminated; disposable brushes or pads that contain an antiseptic hand-washing agent avoid this problem. Alcohol-containing foams kill bacteria satisfactorily when applied to clean hands and with sufficient contact (usually 2–3 minutes, in accordance with manufacturers' recommendations), but they are not sufficient for cleaning physically soiled hands, because transient organisms are not removed.

Before handling neonates for the first time on a work shift, personnel should scrub their hands and arms to a point above the elbow with an antiseptic soap. After 3 minutes of washing, the hands should be rinsed thoroughly and dried with paper towels.

A 10-second wash without a brush, but with soap and vigorous rubbing, is required before and after handling each neonate and after touching objects or surfaces likely to be contaminated with virulent microorganisms or hospital pathogens. Hand-washing facilities and materials must be easily accessible. Hand-washing is necessary even when gloves have been worn in direct contact with the infant. Hand-washing should immediately follow removal of gloves, before touching another infant.

Occupational Exposure to Bloodborne Pathogens

In 1991, the federal Occupational Safety and Health Administration (OSHA) issued regulations designed to minimize the transmission of human immunodeficiency virus (HIV), HBV, and other potentially infectious materials in the workplace (Appendix F). The regulations cover all employees in physicians' offices, hospitals, medical laboratories, and other health care facilities where workers could be reasonably anticipated to come into contact with blood and other potentially infectious material. The OSHA regulations require employers to implement an exposure control plan to minimize employees' exposure to bloodborne pathogens. The plan must contain the following components:

- Personal protective equipment for employees exposed to blood and other body fluids
- Adoption of certain work practice controls (eg, hand-washing facilities, disposal of contaminated needles, handling and storage of specimens)
- Housekeeping requirements

- Provision of HBV vaccination to employees
- Postexposure evaluation and follow-up procedures
- Employee training
- Use of warning labels
- Record-keeping requirements

These requirements are enforced by OSHA or, in the case of states with OSHA-approved comparable job safety and health plans, by state agencies. Violations are punishable by fines.

Exposure of Health Care Professionals to Human Immunodeficiency Virus

Health care workers who have had percutaneous or mucous membrane exposure to blood or bloody secretions from an HIV-infected mother or HIV-exposed or -infected newborn must be given medical evaluation and follow-up as prescribed in the OSHA regulations on occupational exposure to bloodborne pathogens. It is recommended that these steps be followed:

- Confirmation that the mother is HIV infected. It is recommended that all pregnant women be offered HIV counseling and testing. If this has not occurred routinely in the antepartum period, HIV counseling and testing with consent is recommended for all women whose status is unknown at the time of delivery. Voluntary testing requires consent in most states. If testing is refused, this should be documented.

- Evaluation of the exposed person, clinically and serologically, for evidence of HIV infection as soon as possible after the exposure. If the results are seronegative, retesting should be done at 6-week, 3-month, and 6-month intervals to determine whether transmission has occurred. Most exposed individuals who have been infected will undergo seroconversion within 12 weeks after exposure.

- Counseling for medical chemoprophylaxis should be offered to every exposed worker. U.S. Public Health Service guidelines should be followed, and antiretroviral treatment is recommended promptly for specific types of exposures.

Standard Precautions

The Centers for Disease Control and Prevention (CDC) recommends that blood and body fluid standard precautions should be used consistently for all patients. These new recommendations incorporate the prior concept of universal precautions to prevent transmission of bloodborne pathogens and recognizes the importance of all body fluids, secretions, and excretions in the transmission of nosocomial pathogens. These precautions apply to (1) blood; (2) all body fluids, secretions, and excretions except sweat, regardless of whether they contain visible blood; (3) nonintact skin; and (4) mucous membranes.

Recommended Isolation Precautions

The Hospital Infection Control Practices Advisory Committee of the CDC in 1996 issued new isolation guidelines for the care of hospitalized patients. These new guidelines are simpler than previous CDC recommendations and rely on very consistent strategies to prevent the spread of infection between infected and uninfected hospitalized patients. These recommendations state that "no guideline can address all the needs of the more than 6,000 US hospitals, which range in size from five beds to more than 1,500 beds and serve very different patient populations. Hospitals are encouraged to review the recommendations and to modify them according to what is possible, practical, and prudent." Therefore, with the new recommendations as a guide, each institution must create its own specific isolation policies. These isolation policies, supplemented by hospital policies and procedures for other aspects of infection and environmental control and occupational health, should result in policies that are "possible, practical, and prudent" for each hospital.

   These new guidelines rely on the routine and optimal performance of an expanded set of universal practices, designated standard precautions, designed for the care of all patients regardless of their diagnosis or presumed infection status; and pathogen- and syndrome-based precautions, designated transmission-based precautions, to be utilized in caring for patients who are infected or colonized with pathogens spread by the airborne, droplet, and/or contact routes.

   Since medical history and examination cannot reliably identify all patients infected with HIV or other bloodborne pathogens, the CDC recommends standard precautions for all patients to protect health care workers from infectious body fluids. These new, expanded precautions apply to blood, all body fluids, secretions, and excretions (regardless of whether they contain visible blood), nonintact skin, and mucous membranes. These general methods of infection prevention are designed to reduce the risk of transmission of microorganisms from both recognized and unrecognized sources of infection in hospitals. Standard precautions include some of the following techniques:

• Hand-washing is necessary after touching blood, body fluids, secretions, excretions, and contaminated items, whether or not gloves are worn. Hands should be washed immediately after removing gloves, between patient contacts, and when otherwise indicated to avoid transfer of microorganisms to other patients or environments.

• Gloves should be worn when touching blood, body fluids, secretions, excretions, and items contaminated with these fluids. Clean gloves should be used before touching mucous membranes and nonintact skin. Gloves should be promptly removed after use, before touching noncontaminated items and environmental surfaces, and before going to another patient.

• Masks, eye protection, and face shields should be worn to protect mucous membranes of the eyes, nose, and mouth during procedures and patient care activities likely to generate splashes or sprays of blood, body fluids, secretions, or excretions.

• Nonsterile gowns will protect skin and prevent the soiling of clothing during procedures and patient care activities likely to generate splashes or sprays of blood, body fluids, secretions, or excretions. Soiled gowns should be promptly removed.

• Patient care equipment that has been used should be handled in a manner that prevents skin and mucous membrane exposures and contamination of clothing.

• Linen soiled with blood and body fluids, secretions, and excretions should be handled, transported, and processed in a manner that prevents skin and mucous membrane exposure and contamination of clothing.

- Bloodborne pathogen exposure should be avoided by taking all precautions to prevent injuries when using, cleaning, and disposing of needles, scalpels, and other sharp instruments and devices.
- Mouthpieces, resuscitation bags, and other ventilation devices should be readily available in all patient care areas and used instead of mouth-to-mouth resuscitation.

Personnel caring for patients are frequently exposed to large amounts of bloody body fluids; standard precautions should be emphasized continually in patient care areas. In addition, soiled linen and contaminated disposable materials should be handled with gloves and disposed of according to federal and state statutes and regulations governing the disposal of infectious waste.

Dress Codes

Each hospital should establish dress codes for regular and part-time personnel who enter the labor, delivery, and nursery areas. Sterile, long-sleeved gowns should be worn by all personnel who have direct contact with the sterile field during vaginal deliveries, surgical obstetric procedures, and surgical procedures in the nursery. When personnel leave the operative room and while they are in the hospital, surgical scrub suits should be covered.

Some hospitals have approved more flexible dress codes for personnel who work in birthing rooms; however, CDC recommends that all health care workers who perform or assist in deliveries wear gloves, gowns, surgical masks, caps, and eye protection during the procedure. Wearing aprons or gowns made of impervious material during cesarean delivery may provide additional protection. Gloves should be worn when handling the placenta or the neonate until blood and amniotic fluid have been removed from the neonate's skin. Hands should be washed immediately after gloves are removed or when skin surfaces are contaminated with blood.

Recent studies have demonstrated that cover gowns are not necessary for regular personnel in the nursery or neonatal intensive care unit, as long as hand-washing standards are strictly enforced. When a neonate is held outside the bassinet by nursing or other neonatal intensive care unit personnel, a long-sleeved gown should be worn over the clothing and either discarded after use or maintained for use exclusively in the care of that neonate. If one gown is used for each neonate, the gowns should be changed regularly.

Caps, beard bags, and masks may be beneficial during certain surgical procedures, including umbilical vessel catheterization. Long hair should be restrained so that it does not touch the neonate or equipment during patient examinations or treatments. High-efficiency, disposable masks should be used, but even these masks remain effective for only a few hours. Masks should be worn so that they cover both the nose and the mouth and should be discarded as soon as they are removed from the nose and mouth.

Sterile gloves should be used during deliveries and all invasive procedures performed in either the obstetric or the nursery area. Disposable, nonsterile gloves may be useful in the care of patients in isolation or in the performance of procedures that may result in contamination of the hands.

Equipment

To avoid the need for unprotected emergency mouth-to-mouth resuscitation of patients, mouthpieces, endotracheal tubes, resuscitation bags and other ventilation devices, and suction equipment should be available for use in all areas where the need for resuscitation may arise. Personnel assisting in suctioning of the newborn should use mechanical devices. Equipment has been developed to allow wall suction to be used with valves that limit the amount of negative pressure generated and allow the individual to control when suctioning will occur. The use of mouth-controlled suctioning should be avoided. If mouth-controlled suctioning of the airway cannot be avoided, a trap should be placed in the line. Standard precautions should be used when any type of suctioning is performed.

Obstetric Considerations

The area where cesarean deliveries and tubal ligations are performed should be treated the same as the main operating room. Therefore, all persons present should wear appropriate operating room attire. For those close to the sterile surgical field, this attire includes clean scrub clothing, sterile operating room gowns, caps, masks, gloves, and shoe covers. For those not involved with the surgical field, a sterile operating room gown is not required. The surgical field should be prepared and draped according to standard recommendations. Shaving, if needed, should be done within 2 hours of the procedure. Clipping hair very close to the skin is preferred to shaving because it does not activate the bacteria that normally colonize the skin surface.

Intrauterine pressure catheters (for monitoring contractions or for amnioinfusion) or internal fetal electrodes (for fetal heart rate monitoring) should be inserted and maintained in accordance with standard sterile techniques. All devices and fluids used should be sterile. To minimize chances of contamination, the packing of the devices should be opened only at the time of their use and proper sterile techniques should be followed during their handling and insertion. Whenever possible, disposable items are preferable.

Neonatal Considerations

Invasive Procedures

Percutaneous placement of peripheral arterial or venous cannulas is associated with a lower risk of infection in neonates than is surgical placement. The cannulas should be removed promptly if signs of device-associated infection occur. A safe maximal duration of cannulation for intravascular catheters has not been established; the risks and benefits should be assessed daily for each neonate. Intravascular catheters should not be used or left in place unless they are clearly indicated for medical management. Each unit should have a written policy on the procedures governing the use of these catheters.

Arterial cannulas are an ideal pressure-monitoring device in a closed system, but often they are also used for obtaining blood samples. These samples should be obtained aseptically with precautions to avoid contamination of the system.

Total parenteral nutrition generally is safe but has been associated with infection, including bacteremia and fungemia. A cooperative team approach that involves pharmacists, nurses, and physicians is strongly recommended to reduce the incidence of infections and other complications. Meticulous attention should be given to aseptic insertion and maintenance of the cannula and to aseptic techniques of fluid administration. All parenteral nutrition fluids should be mixed in a central pharmacy, under a laminar flow hood. Because lipid emulsions are especially susceptible to contamination with a wide variety of bacteria and fungi that can proliferate to high concentrations within hours, particular caution must be taken in the storage and administration of these emulsions. Unit-dose amounts may be delivered from the pharmacy; if bottles of emulsion are kept in the nursery refrigerator, care should be taken to prevent contamination. Opened bottles must be discarded no later than 24 hours after the seal has been broken. Intravenous tubing, stopcocks, and flush syringes should be changed (using sterile technique) on a regular basis and no less frequently than every 72 hours. If an increased incidence of infection is noted, tubing should be changed more frequently.

Intravascular Flush Solutions

The hospital pharmacy should establish a system to ensure a satisfactory and safe means of providing sterile, unpreserved fluids to the nursery areas. Solutions with benzyl alcohol are contraindicated in neonates because their use may lead to severe metabolic acidosis, encephalopathy, or death. When the fluid administered is to contain heparin, it should be added to the fluid in the hospital pharmacy whenever possible. Flush solutions should be kept at room temperature no longer than 8 hours before being used or discarded. They should be labeled clearly with the time of opening or preparation.

Antibiotics

The efficacy of antibiotics used for prophylaxis in newborns has not been documented, and such use should be strongly discouraged. The relative frequencies of documented infection with different bacteria in neonates, along with patterns of antimicrobial susceptibility, should be monitored by the infection control committee. The most innocuous and specific antibiotic regimens should be selected after analysis of these data. The indiscriminate and inappropriate use of either systemic or topical antibiotics may alter the established flora of the neonate and result in the emergence of resistant strains of bacteria, making subsequent therapy for clinical infections more difficult and dangerous.

Isolation

The different categories of transmission-based isolation are listed in Table 10–1. Further details are outlined in the CDC "Guidelines for Isolation Precautions in Hospitals." These guidelines can be adapted whenever necessary to accommodate the special needs of pregnant mothers and neonates. These precautions are indicated for patients who are infected or colonized with certain transmissible pathogens; they are in addition to standard precautions that apply to all hospitalized patients.

Infected Postpartum Mothers

Most postpartum infections are caused by ascending endogenous organisms in the mother. The risk of infecting the neonate after birth with the same organisms is negligible. Therefore, the neonate need not be separated from a mother with a postpartum infection.

Mothers with communicable diseases (eg, group A streptococci) that are likely to be transmitted to the newborn should be separated from the newborn until the infection is no longer communicable, based on the natural history of the infection and the effectiveness of therapy in eliminating contagion. A mother with postpartum fever that is not due to a specific communicable cause can be allowed to feed and care for her newborn. With the exception of specific infections (see Chapter 9), breastfeeding is rarely contraindicated in maternal infection. Criteria for allowing mothers to handle neonates are as follows:

- Mother feels well enough to handle the baby.
- She washes her hands thoroughly under supervision.
- She wears a clean gown.
- She avoids contact of the baby with contaminated clothes, linen, dressings, or pads.

A mother with a respiratory tract infection should be made aware that the infection can be transmitted not only by droplets but also by hands and fomites. Therefore, she should practice strict hand-washing

Table 10–1. Transmission-Based Precautions for Hospitalized Patients*

Category of Precautions	Single Room	Masks	Gowns	Gloves
Airborne	Yes, with negative air pressure ventilation	Yes	No	No
Droplet	Yes†	Yes, for those close to patient	No	No
Contact	Yes†	No	Yes	Yes

* These recommendations are in addition to those for standard precautions for all patients.

† Preferred but not required. Grouping of children infected with the same pathogen into cohorts is acceptable.

Modified from American Academy of Pediatrics. Peter G, ed. 1997 Red book: report of the Committee on Infectious Diseases. 24th ed. Elk Grove Village, Illinois: AAP, 1997.

techniques and appropriately handle or dispose of contaminated tissues and any other items that may have come in contact with infectious secretions. If needed, she can wear a surgical mask to reduce the chance of droplet spread to her baby.

Postpartum mothers who are infected with nonobstetric-related communicable diseases should be treated according to the precautions and isolation techniques required by the specific disease. If the required guidelines cannot be followed safely on the obstetric unit, the patient should be transferred to the appropriate unit where such care can be provided.

Patients with abscesses or infected or draining wounds should have appropriate cover dressings. If it is not possible to cover the infected or draining wound completely, the patient should be placed in a separate room. Gloves and, if necessary, gowns should be worn during all contact with infected patients.

Cohorts

During an epidemic, neonates with overt infection and those who are colonized should be identified rapidly and placed in cohorts—separate areas where infants with similar exposures or symptoms receive care. If rapid identification of these neonates is not possible, separate cohorts should be established for neonates with disease, those who have been exposed, those who have not been exposed, and those who are newly admitted. The success of cohort programs depends largely on the willingness and ability of nursery and ancillary personnel to adhere strictly to the cohort system and to follow established practices.

Neonates with Infections

The housing of an infected neonate or one suspected of being infected depends on the overall condition of the neonate and the type of care required, the available space and facilities, the nurse-to-patient ratio, and the size and type of the neonatal care service. Other factors to be considered include the type of infection, the clinical manifestations, the source and possible modes of its transmission, and the number of colonized or infected neonates.

In many instances (a notable exception is neonatal varicella–zoster virus infection), it is unnecessary to isolate infected neonates if certain criteria are met:

1. Sufficient nursing and medical staff are on duty to provide comprehensive care.

2. Sufficient space is provided for a 4–6-foot aisle between neonatal stations.

3. Two or more sinks for hand-washing are available in each nursery room or area.

4. Continuing instruction is provided about the ways in which infections spread.

If these criteria are not met, an isolation room with separate scrub facilities is necessary. Physical separation with assignment of separate health care personnel for each area is best.

It has often been assumed that forced-air incubators provide adequate isolation for infected neonates. Although these incubators filter incoming air, they do not filter the air that is discharged into the nursery. They are therefore satisfactory for limited protective isolation of neonates but should not be relied on to prevent transmission of microorganisms from infected neonates to others.

When an isolation room is deemed necessary, blinds, windows, and other structural items must allow for ease of regular cleaning of this room. An intercom should be provided. Air from this room should be exhausted to the outside and not to the rest of the nursery.

Gastroenteritis/Abscess

Contact precautions should be observed when treating patients with gastroenteritis or draining lesions of abscesses that cannot be contained adequately by a dressing. All personnel should use gowns and disposable gloves when providing direct patient care. Contaminated items should be properly discarded. The environment may be heavily contaminated with the infecting microorganism, and these organisms are often transmitted on the hands of personnel to other neonates. If more than one neonate is infected, a cohort approach should be taken.

Congenital Infections

For neonates with congenital infections, the CDC recommends the following isolation precautions:

- Rubella: contact precautions (mask, gown, gloves, private room)
- Syphilis: standard precautions
- Cytomegalovirus: standard precautions
- Toxoplasmosis: standard precautions
- Herpes simplex virus: contact precautions for those neonates who may be clinically infected or those who were delivered either vaginally or by cesarean birth to women with active genital herpes infections

Viral Infections

Many viruses, such as respiratory syncytial virus, coxsackieviruses, or echoviruses, spread rapidly among neonates and personnel in a nursery. Such viral infections can be serious in neonates, sometimes resulting in death. Because neonates may shed selected viruses after their clinical illness has been resolved, they become reservoirs of infection. It is believed that the viruses, enteroviruses, and respiratory syncytial virus are transmitted predominantly by direct or indirect contact with the hands of personnel contaminated with virus-containing secretions or with contaminated environmental surfaces or fomites. Contact isolation may be required to prevent this type of spread, but specific requirements vary with the infecting virus. For example, respiratory syncytial virus is shed primarily from the respiratory tract, whereas coxsackieviruses and echoviruses can be shed from the throat or in the stool.

Neonates are usually ineffective disseminators of infectious bacterial or viral aerosols. Neonates with confirmed or possible infections caused by a viral agent that could be transmitted by the airborne route should be separated from other neonates by (1) transfer from the nursery area, (2) rooming-in with the mother, or (3) enclosure of all other neonates in the area in incubators.

Management of Nursery Outbreaks of Disease

Procedures for control of nursery epidemics depend on the microorganism responsible for the outbreak, the reservoir of infection, and the mode of transmission. An epidemiologic investigation should be undertaken to identify these factors. The hospital infection control practitioner and the proper health authorities should be notified promptly about all suspected or confirmed epidemics.

During epidemics, a comprehensive program of infection control is required. Even if an intensive investigation is not indicated, the results of the control measures should be evaluated to ensure that they have been effective and the problem has been resolved. Because many infections become apparent only after neonates leave the hospital, each hospital should establish a procedure to be used during a suspected or confirmed epidemic for disease surveillance of recently discharged neonates.

Environmental Control

The physician in charge and the nursing supervisor of the obstetric and nursery areas should work with the infection control officer and other appropriate groups (eg, representatives of the respiratory therapy service, central supply, and housekeeping) to establish an environmental control program for the labor, delivery, and nursery areas. This program should include specific procedures in a written policy manual for cleaning and disinfection or sterilization of patient care areas, equipment, and supplies. Consultation for specific details and problems is essential. Nursing supervisors should ensure that these procedures are carried out correctly.

Methods of Sterilization and Disinfection

All medical and hospital personnel should understand the difference between sterilization and disinfection. Sterilization is the destruction of all microorganisms, including spores; disinfection is simply a reduction in the number of contaminating microorganisms. High-level disinfection is the elimination or destruction of all microorganisms except spores. Cleaning is the physical removal of organic material or soil, including microorganisms, from objects.

Devices that enter tissue or the vascular system should be sterile. For neonates, devices that come into contact with mucous membranes or that have prolonged or intimate contact with skin should also be sterile. Much of the equipment required in perinatal care areas, however, can be used safely if it is satisfactorily cleaned and disinfected; clean, dry surfaces do not support the growth of microorganisms.

It is sometimes necessary to decontaminate equipment before it is cleaned and sterilized or disinfected in order to allow processing without exposing personnel to hazardous microbes. The equipment must be cleaned thoroughly to remove all blood, tissue, secretions, food, and other residue. Without thorough cleaning, no method of sterilization or disinfection can be effective. Furthermore, some chemical disinfectants are inactivated by organic materials.

Sterilization

Methods of sterilization include steam autoclaving, dry heat, and gaseous (ethylene oxide) or liquid chemical (eg, 2% glutaraldehyde) techniques. The preferred method of sterilization is steam autoclaving, because this is the least expensive method and provides the greatest margin of safety. Some equipment may be damaged by steam, however, and must be sterilized by another method.

Equipment made of material that absorbs ethylene oxide usually requires 8–12 hours of aeration after sterilization with ethylene oxide before it can be used again. Ethylene oxide sterilization of supplies or equipment should be preceded by a comprehensive review of data on the aeration time required for each material to be processed and the extent to which toxicity standards have been established. An ethylene oxide sterilization plan requires the presence of sufficient backup equipment to allow time for aeration.

Equipment that cannot be sterilized with steam or ethylene oxide may be satisfactorily sterilized after cleaning by immersion for 10 hours in acetic acid liquid sterilant or 2% glutaraldehyde or other acceptable liquid sporicide. This immersion should be followed by three rinses with sterile water (or tap water with at least 10 mg of hypochlorite per liter), thorough drying, and packaging in sterile wrappers.

High-Level Disinfection

Equipment that does not need to be sterilized may be subjected to high-level disinfection. Both hot-water pasteurization and chemical disinfection are satisfactory. Pasteurization of equipment requires immersing it in water at 80–85°C (176–185°F) for 15 minutes or 75°C (167°F) for 30 minutes. After air drying (preferably in a cabinet with heated, filtered air), disinfected items should be aseptically wrapped and stored until needed. Although spores are not eradicated by this method, bacterial and viral decontamination is adequate. The original reports of the equipment manufacturer should be consulted for a list of any parts or materials that may be warped or damaged at these temperatures.

The choice of liquid chemicals for high-level disinfection depends on the type of equipment to be disinfected. In many instances, immersion of the equipment for 20 minutes in 2% glutaraldehyde, followed by three rinses with sterile water (or tap water with at least 10 mg of hypochlorite per liter) and thorough drying, is satisfactory.

Cleaning and Disinfecting Noncritical Surfaces

Selection of Disinfectants

Although numerous disinfectants are available, no single agent or preparation is ideal for all purposes. Consideration should be given to the agent and its special use, as well as to the types of organisms likely to be contaminating the object that is to be disinfected. Special attention should be given to the recommended concentration of each disinfectant and to its time of exposure. Unnecessary exposure of neonates to disinfectants should be avoided, and strict adherence to manufacturers' recommendations is essential.

Quaternary ammonias, chlorine compounds, and phenolic compounds are satisfactory disinfectants. Use should be limited to disinfectant–detergent products registered by the U.S. Environmental Protection Agency and recommended by the manufacturer for nursery surfaces with which neonates have contact. Information about specific label claims of commercial germicides can be obtained from this agency.

General Housekeeping

The following order of cleaning is recommended:

1. Patient areas
2. Accessory areas
3. Adjacent halls

It is not known whether floor bacteria are a source of nosocomial infection, but regular cleaning prevents the accumulation of pathogenic bacteria. Disinfectant–detergents have been shown to be more effective than soap and water alone in cleaning floors, although hospital floors are rapidly recontaminated after disinfection. Available disinfectant–detergents may differ in effectiveness.

In the cleaning procedure, dust should not be dispersed into the air. Removal of dust by a dry vacuum machine, followed by wet vacuuming, is effective in cleaning and disinfecting hospital floors. Once dust has been removed, scrubbing with a mop and a disinfectant–detergent solution should be sufficient. Mop heads should be machine laundered and thoroughly dried daily.

Standard types of portable vacuum cleaners should not be used in nurseries or delivery areas because particulate matter and microbial contamination in the room may be disturbed and distributed by the exhaust jet. Vacuum cleaners that discharge outside the patient care area (ie, central vacuum cleaning systems or portable vacuums) should be used so that only the cleaning wand, floor tool, and high-efficiency, particulate air-filtered vacuum hose are brought into the patient care area.

Cabinet counters, work surfaces, and similar horizontal areas may be subject to heavy contamination during routine use. These areas should be cleaned once a day and between patient use with a disinfectant–detergent and clean cloths; friction cleaning is important to ensure physical removal of dirt and contaminating microorganisms. Surfaces that are contaminated by patient specimens or accidental spills should be carefully cleaned and disinfected.

Walls, windows, and storage shelves may be reservoirs of pathogenic microorganisms if grossly soiled or if dust and dirt are allowed to accumulate. These areas and similar noncritical surfaces should be scrubbed periodically with a disinfectant–detergent solution as part of the general housekeeping program.

Faucet aerators may be useful to reduce water splashing in sinks, but they are notoriously susceptible to contamination with a variety of hydrophilic bacteria. For this reason, removing aerators permanently may be preferred to periodic cleaning and disinfection. Sinks should have backsplashes to prevent the retention of pooling of water, a source of bacterial growth. Sinks should be scrubbed clean daily with a disinfectant–detergent; drain traps should not need routine cleaning or disinfection.

Written policies should be established for the removal and disposal of solid wastes. Sturdy plastic liners should be used in trash receptacles; these liners should be sealed before they are removed from the trash receptacles. In patient care areas, trash receptacles should be cleaned and disinfected regularly. Infectious material requires special handling and disposal.

Special housekeeping personnel should be assigned to clean the nursery. If the nursery is small, they may also be assigned to work in the obstetric areas or other clean areas of the hospital. The nursery should be cleaned daily when most neonates are not present. Intensive care nurseries should ideally be cleaned when traffic is minimal.

Cleaning and Disinfecting Patient Care Equipment

Incubators, Open Care Units, and Bassinets

After a neonate has been discharged, the care unit used by that neonate should be thoroughly cleaned and disinfected. A disinfectant–detergent registered by the U.S. Environmental Protection Agency is recommended for this purpose. Manufacturers' directions for use of a disinfectant–detergent should be followed carefully. A bassinet or incubator should never be cleaned when occupied. Infants who remain in the nursery for an extended period should be transferred periodically to a different, disinfected unit.

When a care unit is being cleaned and disinfected, all detachable parts should be removed and scrubbed meticulously. If the incubator has a fan, it should be cleaned and disinfected; the manufacturer's instructions should be followed to avoid equipment damage. The air filter should be maintained as recommended by the manufacturer. Mattresses should be replaced when the surface covering is broken, because such a break precludes effective disinfection or sterilization. Mattresses may be sterilized by heat or gas. Portholes and porthole cuffs and sleeves are easily contaminated, often heavily; cuffs should be replaced on a regular schedule or cleaned and disinfected frequently with freshly prepared mild soap or quaternary ammonium disinfectant–detergent solutions. Incubators not in use should be thoroughly dried by running the incubator hot without water in the reservoir for 24 hours after disinfection.

Evaporative humidifiers in incubators usually do not produce contaminated aerosols, but contaminated water reservoirs may be responsible for direct rather than airborne transmission of infection. Reservoirs should be filled with sterile water only; they should be drained and refilled with sterile water every 24 hours. In many areas of the United States and in hospitals with a central ventilation system, environmental humidity levels may be sufficiently high to eliminate the need for additional humidification in most cases, and water reservoirs may be left dry. If humidification is necessary, a source of humidity external to the incubator may be preferable to incubator humidifiers. An external humidifier can be changed daily and the equipment sent for cleaning and sterilization or disinfection.

Nebulizers, Water Traps, and Respiratory Support Equipment

Nebulizers and attached tubing should be replaced by clean, sterile equipment (or equipment that has been subjected to high-level disinfection) in accordance with established hospital policy. Failure to replace tubing may result in contamination of freshly cleaned equipment. Water traps should also be replaced regularly by autoclaved or disinfected equipment. Only sterile water should be used for nebulizers or water traps; residual water should be discarded when these containers are refilled. Water condensed in tubing loops should be removed and discarded and should not be allowed to reflux into the container.

Other Equipment

Cleaning and disinfection or sterilization of equipment should be performed between patients. Equipment that is used for only one patient should be replaced, cleaned, and disinfected or sterilized according to an established schedule. Disposable equipment should be replaced with approximately the same frequency as reusable equipment is recycled. Disposable equipment should never be reused.

Resuscitators, face masks, and other items used in direct contact with neonates should be dismantled, thoroughly cleaned, and sterilized, if possible. Alternately, the equipment may be subjected to high-level disinfection with liquid chemicals or by pasteurization. Equipment such as tubing for respiratory or oxygen therapy should be either sterilized or discarded after use. Stethoscopes and similar types of diagnostic instruments should be wiped with iodophor or alcohol before use, unless they are used for individual patients or the instruments become contaminated between usages.

Cultures of Environmental Surfaces and Equipment

Cultures of environmental surfaces and equipment may be useful as part of epidemiologic investigations, and an occasional, selective bacteriologic survey of particular patient care areas or equipment may help determine the effectiveness of existing procedures. These studies should be coordinated with the infection control committee and the microbiology laboratory.

Neonatal Linen

Procedures for laundering, making up packs, and delivering linen to the nursery should be established by the medical, nursing, laundry, and administrative staffs of the hospital. Each delivery of clean linen should contain sufficient linen for at least one 8-hour shift. Linen should be cleaned and transported in covered carts to the nursery areas. Autoclaving linen has not been shown to be effective in preventing infections in normal newborn nurseries or intensive care areas. No new garments or linen should be used for neonates without prior laundering.

It is acceptable to use disposable diapers rather than cloth diapers in a nursery. The use of nonsterile diapers has not been established as having a significant role in the epidemiology of neonatal disease.

Care of Soiled Linen

An established procedure for the disposal of soiled linen should be strictly followed. Chutes for the transfer of soiled linen from patient care areas to the laundry are not acceptable unless they are under negative air pressure. Soiled linen should be discarded into impervious plastic bags placed in hampers that are easy to clean and disinfect. Soiled diapers should be placed in special diaper receptacles immediately after removal from the neonate; they should never be rinsed in the nursery. All personnel should be aware that handling dirty diapers with bare hands can result in heavy contamination and transient colonization of the hands with microorganisms that cannot be easily eliminated with hand-washing and can be readily transmitted to the next neonate for whom they provide care.

Plastic bags of soiled diapers (reusable or disposable) and other linen should be sealed and removed from the nursery at least every 8 hours. Individuals who collect the bags of soiled diapers or linen need not enter the nursery if all bags are placed outside the nursery. Sealed bags of reusable, soiled nursery linens should be taken to the laundry at least twice each day; sealed bags of disposable diapers should also be taken away at least twice a day.

Laundering

Diapers and other nursery linens should be washed separately from other hospital linen and with products used to retain softness. Acidification neutralizes the alkalis used in the washing process and is responsible for the greatest bacterial destruction. Standard precautions should be taken in handling linen soiled with blood. Use of chlorine bleach should be considered for any items that are contaminated with blood.

The chemicals trichlorocarbanilide or the sodium salt of pentachlorophenol should not be used in hospital laundering because they may be harmful. To avoid the hazards associated with the use of such chemicals or enzymes in the hospital laundry, the physician in charge should be aware of all agents in use and should be informed before any changes are made in laundry chemicals or procedures. Therefore, caution should be exercised when new laundry or cleaning agents are introduced into the nursery or when procedures are changed.

Bibliography

American Academy of Pediatrics. Peter G, ed. 1997 Red book: report of the Committee on Infectious Diseases. 24th ed. Elk Grove Village, Illinois: AAP, 1997

Centers for Disease Control and Prevention. Update: provisional public health service recommendations for chemoprophylaxis after occupational exposure to HIV. MMWR Morb Mortal Wkly Rep 1996;45:468-472

Garner JS. Hospital Infectious Control Practices Advisory Committee. Guideline for isolation precautions in hospitals. Infect Control Hosp Epidemiol 1996;17:53–80

Chapter 11

Maternal and Newborn Nutrition

Maternal nutrition can contribute positively to maintaining or improving the mother's health as well as to the delivery of a healthy term newborn of an appropriate weight. Nutrition counseling is an integral part of perinatal care for all patients. It should focus on a well-balanced, varied nutritional food plan that is consistent with the patient's access to food and food preferences. Patient educational materials on nutrition are available from the American College of Obstetricians and Gynecologists, the U.S. Public Health Service, and the March of Dimes Birth Defects Foundation.

Dietary counseling and intervention based on special or individual needs are usually most effectively accomplished by referral to a nutritionist or registered dietitian. Each tertiary perinatal care center should have counseling programs available for the wide range of nutritional disorders that can be encountered clinically.

Preconception Care

Consumption of a balanced diet with appropriate distribution of the basic food pyramid groups is especially important during pregnancy. Diet can be affected by food preferences, cultural beliefs, and eating patterns.

A woman who is a complete vegan or food faddist or who has special dietary restrictions secondary to medical illnesses, such as phenylketonuria, diabetes mellitus, or renal disease, may need vitamin and mineral supplements. Women who fast, skip meals, or have eating disorders or unusual eating habits need to be identified. The patient's access to food and the ability to purchase food can be pertinent. One way to evaluate nutritional status is to calculate the woman's body mass index at the preconception visit (Table 11–1). Women who are underweight should be encouraged to gain weight. Overweight and obese women, however, should not be encouraged to lose weight.

Neural tube defects (NTDs), such as anencephaly and spina bifida, have multifactorial origins. The first occurrence of an NTD may be reduced if all women of reproductive age take 0.4 mg of folic acid daily both before conception and during the first trimester. In women with a history of NTD or a previous conception with an NTD, the recurrence rate (2–3%) with NTDs can be reduced more than 50% if the woman supplements her daily diet with 4 mg of folic acid for the month prior to conception and for the first trimester. This dose should be consumed singly, not as a multivitamin preparation, to avoid excess intake of other vitamins or minerals. The U.S. Food and Drug Administration has established new rules under which specified grain products are required to be fortified with folic acid at levels ranging from 0.43–1.4 mg per pound of product. These amounts are designed to enable women to more easily consume 0.4 mg of folic acid daily. However, these amounts of fortified folic acid are intended to keep the

Table 11–1. Recommended Ranges of Total Weight Gain for Pregnant Women, by Prepregnancy Body Mass Index for Singleton Gestation*

Weight-for-Height Category		Recommended Total Weight Gain	
Category	BMI†	kg	lb
Low	<19.8	12.5–18	28–40
Normal	19.8–26.0	11.5–16	25–35
High	26.0–29.0	7.0–11.5	15–25
Obese	≥29.0	<7.0	<15

* Young adolescents (<2 years after menarche) should strive for gains at the upper end of the range.

† BMI = body mass index [weight/(height²)].

Reprinted with permission from *Nutrition During Pregnancy* c.1990 by the National Academy of Sciences. Published by National Academy Press, Washington, DC.

daily intake of folic acid below 1 mg. Because the amount of folic acid added to fortified grain products may be less than the recommended amount of folic acid to prevent NTDs, supplementation is still recommended.

Nutrition in Pregnancy

Following the weight gain guidelines for singleton gestations (identified by the Institute of Medicine) improves the likelihood of delivering a normal-weight newborn (Table 11–1). Assessment of weight gain during pregnancy is important and should be documented appropriately, preferably on a form specifically designed for that purpose.

Goals for Weight Gain

Goals for weight gain during pregnancy should be based on individual needs. In general, caloric intake is calculated at 25–35 kcal/kg of optimal body weight. An additional 100–300 kcal per day is recommended during pregnancy. Because optimal outcome can occur over a relatively wide range of weight gain, the provider can be flexible. These recommendations can be adjusted to specific subgroups of patients such as teenagers and women who are obese, of lower socioeconomic status, or short.

The recommended daily dietary allowances (RDAs) and energy intake for adolescent and adult pregnant and lactating women are listed in Table 11–2. These recommendations can be considered a general guide to a balanced, nutritious diet for most healthy persons. If a patient is economically unable to meet nutritional needs, she should be referred to federal food and nutrition programs such as the Special Supplemental Food Program for Women, Infants, and Children.

Vitamin and Mineral Supplementation and Toxicity

Almost all pregnant women should be able to obtain the RDA for minerals and vitamins through their dietary intake. There is no requirement for routine supplementation, with the possible exception

Table 11–2. Recommended Daily Dietary Allowances for Adolescent and Adult Pregnant and Lactating Women

Nutrient (unit)	Status Pregnant	Lactating— First 6 Months
Energy (kcal)	+300	+500
Protein (g)	60	65
Fat-soluble vitamins		
Vitamin A (μg retinol equivalents)	800	1,300
Vitamin D (μg as cholecalciferol)	10	10
Vitamin E (mg alpha-tocopherol equivalents)	10	12
Vitamin K (μg)	65	65
Water-soluble vitamins		
Vitamin C (mg)	70	95
Thiamin (mg)	1.5	1.6
Riboflavin (mg)	1.6	1.8
Niacin (mg niacin equivalent)	17	20
Vitamin B_6 (mg)	2.2	2.1
Folate (μg)	400	280
Vitamin B_{12} (μg)	2.2	2.6
Minerals		
Calcium (mg)	1,200	1,200
Phosphorus (mg)	1,200	1,200
Magnesium (mg)	300	355
Iron (mg)	30	15
Zinc (mg)	15	19
Iodine (μg)	175	200
Selenium (μg)	65	75

Adapted and reprinted with permission from *Recommended Dietary Allowances, 10th Edition,* c. 1989 by the National Academy of Sciences. Published by National Academy Press, Washington, DC.

of iron. However, daily supplements should be given if the adequacy of a patient's diet is questionable or if she is at high nutritional risk. The latter category includes women with multiple gestations, substance users, complete vegans, women taking antiepileptic medications, and women with hemoglobinopathies.

Although vitamin A is essential, excessive vitamin A (>10,000 IU per day) may be associated with fetal malformations. The amount of vitamin A in standard prenatal vitamins (4,000–5,000 IU) is well below this toxic level. The use of beta carotene, the precursor of vitamin A found in fruits and vegetables, has not been shown to produce vitamin A toxicity. Excessive vitamin and mineral intake (ie, more than twice the RDA) should be avoided during pregnancy. For example, excess iodine is associated with congenital goiter, and excess vitamin A is associated with anomalies of bones, the urinary tract, and the central nervous system. There also may be toxicity of other fat-soluble vitamins (D, E, and K).

A daily supplement of ferrous iron (30 mg) is recommended as prophylaxis for iron deficiency. Ingestion between meals or at bedtime on an empty stomach will facilitate iron absorption. The treatment of iron-deficiency anemia requires doses of 60–120 mg of elemental iron each day.

Postpartum Guidelines

Postnatal dietary guidelines are similar to those established during pregnancy (Table 11–2). The minimal caloric requirement for adequate milk production in a woman of average size is 1,800 kcal per day. A balanced, nutritious diet will ensure both the quality and the quantity of the milk produced without depletion of maternal stores. Fluid intake by the mother is governed by thirst.

A vitamin–mineral supplement is not needed routinely. Mothers at nutritional risk should be given a multivitamin supplement with particular emphasis on calcium and vitamins B_{12} and D. Iron should be administered only if the mother herself needs it.

Maternal postpartum weight loss can occur at a rate of 2 pounds a month without affecting lactation. On average, a woman will retain 2 pounds above prepregnancy weight at 1 year postpartum. There is no relationship between body mass index or total weight gain and weight retention. Aging, rather than parity, is the major determinant of increases in a woman's weight over time.

Residual postpartum retention of weight gained during pregnancy that results in obesity is a concern. Special attention to lifestyle, including exercise and eating habits, will help these women return to a normal body mass index.

Neonatal Nutrition

Breastfeeding

At birth, the neonate's intestinal-tract host defense mechanism against bacterial and viral agents is incompletely developed. Colostrum and human milk contain a number of factors that promote immunologic development of the gastrointestinal tract and help to protect the infant from infection. In families with a strong history of allergy, breastfeeding is likely to be especially beneficial, and the ingestion of solid foods should be delayed until the infant is 6 months old.

Because human milk is the ideal food for neonates, mothers should be encouraged to breastfeed. In addition to promoting maternal–neonatal interaction, breastfeeding alone can satisfy the infant's nutritional needs for the first 4–6 months of life.

Prenatal counseling and education regarding methods of infant feeding may allow correction of misperceptions about feeding methods. Mothers who are hesitant to breastfeed can do so successfully with appropriate encouragement and education. If the mother chooses not to breastfeed, however, she should be supported in her decision.

Initiation of Breastfeeding

The successful management of breastfeeding begins during pregnancy. Prenatal care should include discussion of feeding plans and breast care. The breasts should be examined to determine whether the nipples are inverted or flat; a shield in the patient's brassiere may help to facilitate eversion. The areolar glands provide adequate lubrication during pregnancy and breastfeeding, and the use of special soaps or ointments should be discouraged. During prenatal visits to the pediatrician, the decision to breastfeed should be reinforced. The integration of breastfeeding into the total care of the infant in the first months of life should be discussed.

The mother should be offered the opportunity to breastfeed her newborn as soon as possible after delivery. Breastfeeding may be initiated in the first hour of life, unless medically contraindicated. The mother should be guided so that she can help the newborn latch on to the breast properly. Enough of the areola (at least $1/2$ inch) should be in the baby's mouth to permit the tongue to stroke the areola over the collecting ductals against the hard palate in the act of sucking.

After the mother and newborn have been transferred to the postpartum unit, they should be together as much as possible. When awake, the newborn should be encouraged to feed frequently (8–12 times per day or even more frequently) to stimulate milk production. Usually, it is wise to alternate the breast used to initiate the feeding and to equalize the time spent at each breast over the day. The duration of feeding at each breast should be guided by the infant's behavior. When satisfied, the infant will fall asleep or unlatch.

Intermittent bottle-feeding of a breastfed infant may lessen the success of breastfeeding. If the infant's appetite is partially satisfied by water or formula supplements, the infant will take less from the breast, and milk production will be diminished. Therefore, bottle-feeding a breastfed neonate should be discouraged. It is extremely unusual for breastfeeding infants to need any supplementation during the first week of life. Routine water and milk supplementation is contraindicated for healthy, full-term infants and most larger premature infants. If excessive weight loss or dehydration is evident during the first week of life in a breastfed infant, breastfeeding can be preserved and enhanced through the administration of formula by means of a nursing supplementer. Observation of breastfeeding by a trained expert and advice to ensure effective nursing is needed in such situations.

Many mothers wish to breastfeed their sick or preterm neonates and should be encouraged to do so. Feeding human milk to a small or ill baby provides a variety of hormonal, enzymatic, immunologic, and cellular benefits. Although breastfed preterm babies may gain weight at a slower rate than formula-fed babies, the unique advantages of human milk balance concerns about the difficulties in achieving intrauterine accretion rates with human milk.

Monitoring the Breastfed Newborn

An adequately nourished newborn is usually considered to be one who takes at least eight feedings per day and sleeps well between feedings. It is also important to ensure that the neonate urinates at least six times each day, stools at least three times a day in the first week of life, and gains weight over time. The healthy neonate may actually feed 12–14 times each day and produce a small, moist stool with many of the feedings. A physician or nurse should examine the neonate during the first 2 weeks of life, regardless of the infant's age upon discharge. If discharge occurs at less than 24 hours of age, the neonate should be reexamined within 48 hours of discharge. Failure to regain birth weight by 2 weeks of age in the term neonate requires a careful evaluation of the feeding techniques being used and the adequacy of breastfeeding.

Contraindications to Breastfeeding

Contraindications to breastfeeding include certain maternal infectious diseases and maternal medications. Endometritis or mastitis being treated with antibiotics is not a contraindication to breastfeeding. Mothers with active herpes simplex virus infection may breastfeed their neonates if they have no vesicular lesions in the breast area, as long as the mother observes careful hand-washing techniques (see the section "Hand-Washing" under "Prevention and Control of Infections" in Chapter 10). Otherwise, the infections discussed in the following paragraphs are contraindications to breastfeeding.

Mothers with active tuberculosis may breastfeed their babies only after they have received adequate therapy and are considered noninfectious. The neonate should be examined for infection and provided with appropriate treatment, if necessary. Cytomegalovirus is excreted in human milk. Mothers with identified primary cytomegalovirus infection should not breastfeed during the acute phase of illness. Mothers who test positive for hepatitis B virus surface antigen (HBsAg) may breastfeed, but their infants must receive hepatitis B virus immune globulin and vaccine.

Human immunodeficiency virus (HIV) has been found in the milk of a small number of HIV-infected women whose milk was cultured. The relative risk of infection of newborns from this source is unknown. In the United States and other developed countries where formula is safe and readily available, women infected with HIV should be counseled to neither breastfeed their neonates nor serve as milk donors. The effects on the infant of medications taken by a nursing mother have been closely studied. The American Academy of Pediatrics Committee on Drugs reviewed the current data on the transfer of drugs and other chemicals into human milk. There are only a few drugs that, taken by the mother, are absolute contraindications to breastfeeding (Table 11–3). The mother should discuss the use of these medications

Table 11–3. Drugs That Are Contraindicated During Breastfeeding

Drug	Reason for Concern, Reported Sign or Symptom in Infant, or Effect on Lactation
Bromocriptine	Suppresses lactation; may be hazardous to the mother
Cocaine	Cocaine intoxication
Cyclophosphamide	Possible immune suppression; unknown effect on growth or association with carcinogenesis; neutropenia
Cyclosporine	Possible immune suppression; unknown effect on growth or association with carcinogenesis
Doxorubicin*	Possible immune suppression; unknown effect on growth or association with carcinogenesis
Ergotamine	Vomiting, diarrhea, convulsions (at doses used in migraine medications)
Lithium	One third to one half of therapeutic blood concentration in infants
Methotrexate	Possible immune suppression; unknown effect on growth or association with carcinogenesis; neutropenia
Phencyclidine	Potent hallucinogen
Phenindione	Anticoagulant; increased prothrombin and partial thromboplastin time in one infant; not used in United States
Radioactive iodine and other radiolabeled elements	Contraindications to breastfeeding for various periods

* Drug is concentrated in human milk.
American Academy of Pediatrics, Committee on Drugs. The transfer of drugs and other chemicals into human milk. Pediatrics 1994;93:137–150.

with her obstetrician and pediatrician if she wishes to continue breast-feeding. They must determine whether the drug therapy is really necessary, whether safer drugs are available, and whether the baby's drug exposure may be minimized by having the mother take the medication after feedings. If the drug presents a risk to the baby, the baby should be carefully monitored to detect any adverse effects, and consideration should be given to measuring blood concentrations. Oral contraceptives may be used by breastfeeding women once lactation has been established.

Human Milk Collection and Storage

There is general agreement that the use of pooled donor human milk is the least satisfactory regimen for routine feeding of small or ill infants. Concern over transmission of infectious diseases has led to heat treatment of most banked human milk, reducing its beneficial aspects. In addition, the composition of donor human milk depends on the donor's diet, environmental exposure, and lifestyle and may pose unknown risks to the infant. Consequently, human milk banks have declined in number in the United States and have avoided use of pooled milk. Careful monitoring of donors and laboratory evaluation of donated milk is required by the Human Milk Banking Association of North America.

Mothers who have tested positive for HIV antibody or HBsAg should not provide stored milk for their babies because of the risk to other infants. Although mothers who are HBsAg positive may breast-feed their babies after the babies have received hepatitis B immune globulin and vaccine, it is preferable not to store milk that is potentially contaminated with hepatitis B virus in the nursery.

Women who donate milk for other infants should be interviewed carefully regarding past and current infectious diseases, use of drugs and medicines, and other factors that may impair the quality or safety of the milk that they provide. Before they are accepted as milk donors, they should be tested for HIV, HBsAg, and tuberculosis. Because seroconversion may occur, ideally the milk should be stored and the donor retested at 4–6 months for HIV before the milk is consumed. Women whose test results are positive should not be accepted as donors. These tests should be repeated periodically for donors who continue to provide milk or who seek reinstatement as a donor. The potential risks should be explained to mothers whose infants are to receive donated milk.

All women who provide milk for infants should be instructed in the proper techniques of milk collection in order to prevent bacterial contamination. Careful hand-washing is critical, and the nipples should be wiped with cotton and plain water before the milk is expressed. The first 5–10 ml of milk contains a large number of bacteria; discarding this portion greatly decreases the contamination of the expressed samples. Although manual expression, when performed correctly, yields relatively clean milk, many women prefer to use a breast pump. All parts of the pump that are in contact with milk should be washed carefully with hot, soapy water after each use.

Expressed milk can be refrigerated in sterile glass or plastic containers for 48 hours without an increase in bacterial contamination. If it must be stored for longer periods, it can be frozen in the freezing compartments of refrigerators for 2–3 weeks, or in a deep freeze at $-20°C \pm 2°C$ ($-4°F \pm 3.6°F$) for several months.

Frozen expressed milk should be thawed quickly under running water, using precautions to avoid contamination from the water, or thawed gradually in the refrigerator at 4°C (39.2°F). It should not be left at room temperatures for long periods, nor should it be subjected to extremely hot water or to microwave ovens. The very high temperatures that may be reached with the latter methods can destroy valuable components of the milk. Once this milk has been thawed, it may be refrigerated for up to 24 hours.

There is no consensus on standards of the microbiologic quality of expressed milk. In general, each milliliter of expressed human milk contains 10^3–10^4 colony-forming units of normal skin bacteria, such as *Staphylococcus epidermidis* and diphtheroids; this milk can be fed to infants with no ill effects. The presence of gram-negative rods in the milk indicates a problem in the collection technique. Feeding intolerance has been reported with milk containing more than 10^2 colony-forming units of gram-negative bacteria per milliliter, and higher levels have been associated with suspected sepsis. Bacteria levels in milk can be controlled by heat treatment, which entails heating the milk to 56°C (132.8°F) for 30 minutes, which will also inactivate HIV. Heat treatment leads to a 15% loss of secretory immunoglobulin A, a 25% loss of lactoferrin and folate, a 75% loss of phosphatase, and total elimination of beneficial cellular elements. Expressed milk samples are seldom routinely screened for bacterial count. Such screening should be carried out, however, when there are concerns about the expression techniques being used and when intestinal intolerance of the milk by the infant is suspected. When the milk is to be given by continuous infusion at room temperature, thus creating a risk of bacterial proliferation in the container and tubing, the syringe and tubing should be changed every 12 hours.

Formula Preparation

Formula selection and control should be directed by the physician. New formulas should be reviewed by the appropriate hospital committees and the director of the nursery before use. For mothers who intend to breastfeed their infants, distribution of formula packages upon discharge should be discouraged. For mothers who intend to feed their infants with formula, the distribution of formula packages upon discharge should be consistent with the physician's written orders. The physician should write orders for the formula to be used and the amount to be given at each feeding.

Most hospitals now use prepared formula units with separate nipples that are readily attached to the bottles just before use. These units need not be refrigerated and may be stored in a convenient, clean, cool area. The sterile cap should be kept on the nipple until the neonate is ready to be fed.

If there is a special area where nipples are uncapped and placed on the bottle, it should be kept very clean and should be used only for formula preparation. Alternatively, nipples may be uncapped and attached to bottles at the mother's bedside just before feeding. The formula and nipple unit should be used as soon as possible, certainly within 4 hours after the bottle is uncapped, and then discarded.

Aseptic technique should be used for preparing infant formulas from concentrated liquids or powders. Aseptic technique involves mixing concentrated liquid or powder with clean water in clean containers using clean utensils. Containers and utensils are considered clean after they have been boiled for 5 minutes and allowed to cool for 1 hour. Information regarding the risk of using unboiled municipal tap water is not available.

Vitamin and Mineral Supplementation

Infants who are breastfed may show evidence of vitamin D deficiency if their mothers have a low intake of vitamin D or little exposure to sunlight, either antepartum or postpartum. If it is suspected that the mother's vitamin D status is not optimal, the infant should receive a supplement of 400 IU of vitamin D per day. This is particularly important if the infant is dark-skinned or if there is little possibility of significant exposure to sunlight.

Recent recommendations by the American Dental Association and the American Academy of Pediatrics indicate that fluoride supplementation for both breast- and bottle-fed infants can begin at 6 months of age.

Although the iron content of human milk is low, the bioavailability is high: 50% of the iron is absorbed by infants who are exclusively breastfed. Breastfed infants should be given supplemental elemental iron (2–3 mg/kg per day) when they reach 6 months of age. Iron-containing formulas with up to 12 mg of elemental iron per liter of formula should be used for all formula-fed infants. Further iron supplementation is not necessary. Infants consuming commercial infant formulas do not need vitamin and mineral supplementation for the first 6 months of life.

Feedings for Preterm Infants

Preterm infants who weigh more than 1,500 g at birth grow adequately if they are fed their mother's milk or a regular 67-kcal/dl infant formula designed for term infants, although preterm babies retain calcium and phosphorus at rates slower than the fetal accretion rates. Very low-birth-weight babies are better nourished if they are fed either a 67–80-kcal/dl formula especially designed for preterm neonates or their own mother's milk fortified by a commercial mixture. Special formulas for small preterm babies contain easily digested and absorbed lipids (15–50% medium-chain triglycerides), additional protein, easily absorbed carbohydrates (glucose polymers and lactose), and enough added calcium and phosphorus to achieve a bone mineralization rate faster than that achieved by means of regular infant formulas or unfortified human milk. Sufficient sodium is added to ensure positive sodium balance for growth, whereas additional trace metals and vitamins are included to meet, at least in part, the special needs of the preterm infant.

Human milk has a number of special features that make its use desirable in feeding preterm babies. It contains antiinfection factors and has a triglyceride structure that results in excellent fat absorption. The lipase in human milk facilitates fat digestion and supplements the deficient quantity of pancreatic lipase of the preterm baby. However, human milk does not provide adequate protein, calcium, or phosphorus to meet the needs of rapidly growing small preterm babies. This deficiency can be corrected by adding nutritionally well-balanced and commercially available dry or liquid human milk fortifiers.

Bibliography

American Academy of Pediatrics. Peter G, ed. 1997 Red book: report of the Committee on Infectious Diseases. 24th ed. Elk Grove Village, Illinois: AAP, 1997

American Academy of Pediatrics, Committee on Drugs. The transfer of drugs and other chemicals into human breast milk. Pediatrics 1994;93:137–150

American Academy of Pediatrics, Committee on Nutrition. Pediatric nutrition handbook. 4th ed. Elk Grove Village, Illinois: AAP, in press

American College of Obstetricians and Gynecologists. Vitamin A supplementation during pregnancy. Committee Opinion 157. Washington, DC: ACOG, 1995

Briggs GG, Freeman RK, Yaffe SJ. Drugs in pregnancy and lactation: a reference guide to fetal and neonatal risk. 4th ed. Baltimore, Maryland: Williams & Wilkins, 1994

Institute of Medicine, Subcommittee on Nutritional Status and Weight Gain During Pregnancy. Nutrition during pregnancy, part I: weight gain. Washington, DC: National Academy Press, 1990

Institute of Medicine, Subcommittee on Nutritional Status and Weight Gain During Pregnancy. Nutrition during pregnancy, part II: nutrient supplement. Washington, DC: National Academy Press, 1990

Institute of Medicine, Subcommittee on Nutrition During Lactation. Nutrition during lactation. Washington, DC: National Academy Press, 1991

National Research Council, Subcommittee on the Tenth Edition on RDAs. Recommended dietary allowances. 10th ed. Washington, DC: National Academy Press, 1989

Appendix A

ACOG Antepartum Record

DATE _____

NAME _____
     LAST   FIRST   MIDDLE

ID # _____ HOSPITAL OF DELIVERY _____

NEWBORN'S PHYSICIAN _____ REFERRED BY _____

FINAL EDD _____ PRIMARY PROVIDER/GROUP _____

BIRTH DATE	AGE	RACE	MARITAL STATUS	ADDRESS:
MONTH DAY YEAR			S M W D SEP	
OCCUPATION			EDUCATION	ZIP: PHONE: (H) (O)
☐ HOMEMAKER			(LAST GRADE COMPLETED)	INSURANCE CARRIER / MEDICAID #
☐ OUTSIDE WORK				
☐ STUDENT Type of Work				
HUSBAND/FATHER OF BABY:			PHONE:	EMERGENCY CONTACT: PHONE:

TOTAL PREG	FULL TERM	PREMATURE	AB. INDUCED	AB. SPONTANEOUS	ECTOPICS	MULTIPLE BIRTHS	LIVING

MENSTRUAL HISTORY

LMP: ☐ DEFINITE ☐ APPROXIMATE (MONTH KNOWN)   MENSES MONTHLY ☐ YES ☐ NO   FREQUENCY: Q _____ DAYS   MENARCHE _____ (AGE ONSET)
     ☐ UNKNOWN ☐ NORMAL AMOUNT/DURATION   PRIOR MENSES _____ DATE   ON BCP AT CONCEPT. ☐ YES ☐ NO   hCG + ____ / ____ /
     ☐ FINAL _____

PAST PREGNANCIES (LAST SIX)

DATE MONTH / YEAR	GA WEEKS	LENGTH OF LABOR	BIRTH WEIGHT	SEX M/F	TYPE DELIVERY	ANES.	PLACE OF DELIVERY	PRETERM LABOR YES / NO	COMMENTS / COMPLICATIONS

PAST MEDICAL HISTORY

	O Neg + Pos	DETAIL POSITIVE REMARKS INCLUDE DATE & TREATMENT		O Neg + Pos	DETAIL POSITIVE REMARKS INCLUDE DATE & TREATMENT
1. DIABETES			16. D (Rh) SENSITIZED		
2. HYPERTENSION			17. PULMONARY (TB, ASTHMA)		
3. HEART DISEASE			18. ALLERGIES (DRUGS)		
4. AUTOIMMUNE DISORDER			19. BREAST		
5. KIDNEY DISEASE / UTI			20. GYN SURGERY		
6. NEUROLOGIC/EPILEPSY					
7. PSYCHIATRIC			21. OPERATIONS / HOSPITALIZATIONS (YEAR & REASON)		
8. HEPATITIS / LIVER DISEASE					
9. VARICOSITIES / PHLEBITIS					
10. THYROID DYSFUNCTION			22. ANESTHETIC COMPLICATIONS		
11. TRAUMA/DOMESTIC VIOLENCE			23. HISTORY OF ABNORMAL PAP		
12. HISTORY OF BLOOD TRANSFUS.			24. UTERINE ANOMALY/DES		

	AMT/DAY PREPREG	AMT/DAY PREG	#YEARS USE			
				25. INFERTILITY		
13. TOBACCO				26. RELEVANT FAMILY HISTORY		
14. ALCOHOL						
15. STREET DRUGS				27. OTHER		

COMMENTS: _____

ACOG ANTEPARTUM RECORD (FORM A)

296   Guidelines for Perinatal Care

Patient Addressograph

SYMPTOMS SINCE LMP

GENETIC SCREENING/TERATOLOGY COUNSELING
INCLUDES PATIENT, BABY'S FATHER, OR ANYONE IN EITHER FAMILY WITH:

	YES	NO			YES	NO
1. PATIENT'S AGE ≥ 35 YEARS				12. MENTAL RETARDATION/AUTISM		
2. THALASSEMIA (ITALIAN, GREEK, MEDITERRANEAN, OR ASIAN BACKGROUND) MCV < 80				IF YES, WAS PERSON TESTED FOR FRAGILE X?		
3. NEURAL TUBE DEFECT (MENINGOMYELOCELE, SPINA BIFIDA, OR ANENCEPHALY)				13. OTHER INHERITED GENETIC OR CHROMOSOMAL DISORDER		
4. CONGENITAL HEART DEFECT				14. MATERNAL METABOLIC DISORDER (EG, INSULIN-DEPENDENT DIABETES, PKU)		
5. DOWN SYNDROME				15. PATIENT OR BABY'S FATHER HAD A CHILD WITH. BIRTH DEFECTS NOT LISTED ABOVE		
6. TAY-SACHS (EG, JEWISH, CAJUN, FRENCH CANADIAN)						
7. SICKLE CELL DISEASE OR TRAIT (AFRICAN)				16. RECURRENT PREGNANCY LOSS, OR A STILLBIRTH		
8. HEMOPHILIA				17. MEDICATIONS/STREET DRUGS/ALCOHOL SINCE LAST MENSTRUAL PERIOD		
9. MUSCULAR DYSTROPHY						
10. CYSTIC FIBROSIS				IF YES, AGENT(S)		
11. HUNTINGTON CHOREA				18. ANY OTHER		

COMMENTS/COUNSELING: _____

INFECTION HISTORY	YES	NO			YES	NO
1. HIGH RISK HEPATITIS B/IMMUNIZED?				4. RASH OR VIRAL ILLNESS SINCE LAST MENSTRUAL PERIOD		
2. LIVE WITH SOMEONE WITH TB OR EXPOSED TO TB				5. HISTORY OF STD, GC, CHLAMYDIA, HPV, SYPHILIS		
3. PATIENT OR PARTNER HAS HISTORY OF GENITAL HERPES				6. OTHER (SEE COMMENTS)		

COMMENTS: _____

INTERVIEWER'S SIGNATURE _____

INITIAL PHYSICAL EXAMINATION

DATE ___ / ___ / ___   PREPREGNANCY WEIGHT ___   HEIGHT ___   BP ___

1. HEENT	☐ NORMAL	☐ ABNORMAL	12. VULVA	☐ NORMAL	☐ CONDYLOMA	☐ LESIONS	
2. FUNDI	☐ NORMAL	☐ ABNORMAL	13. VAGINA	☐ NORMAL	☐ INFLAMMATION	☐ DISCHARGE	
3. TEETH	☐ NORMAL	☐ ABNORMAL	14. CERVIX	☐ NORMAL	☐ INFLAMMATION	☐ LESIONS	
4. THYROID	☐ NORMAL	☐ ABNORMAL	15. UTERUS SIZE	___ WEEKS		☐ FIBROIDS	
5. BREASTS	☐ NORMAL	☐ ABNORMAL	16. ADNEXA	☐ NORMAL	☐ MASS		
6. LUNGS	☐ NORMAL	☐ ABNORMAL	17. RECTUM	☐ NORMAL	☐ ABNORMAL		
7. HEART	☐ NORMAL	☐ ABNORMAL	18. DIAGONAL CONJUGATE	☐ REACHED	☐ NO	___ CM	
8. ABDOMEN	☐ NORMAL	☐ ABNORMAL	19. SPINES	☐ AVERAGE	☐ PROMINENT	☐ BLUNT	
9. EXTREMITIES	☐ NORMAL	☐ ABNORMAL	20. SACRUM	☐ CONCAVE	☐ STRAIGHT	☐ ANTERIOR	
10. SKIN	☐ NORMAL	☐ ABNORMAL	21. SUBPUBIC ARCH	☐ NORMAL	☐ WIDE	☐ NARROW	
11. LYMPH NODES	☐ NORMAL	☐ ABNORMAL	22. GYNECOID PELVIC TYPE	☐ YES	☐ NO		

COMMENTS (Number and explain abnormals): _____

EXAM BY _____

ACOG ANTEPARTUM RECORD (FORM B)

Patient Addressograph

NAME _____
   LAST   FIRST   MIDDLE

DRUG ALLERGY:

RELIGIOUS/CULTURAL CONSIDERATIONS _____   ANESTHESIA CONSULT PLANNED   ☐ YES   ☐ NO

PROBLEMS/PLANS	MEDICATION LIST:	Start date	Stop date
1.	1.		
2.	2.		
3.	3.		
4.	4.		
5.	5.		
6.	6.		

EDD CONFIRMATION

INITIAL EDD:

LMP ____ / ____ / ____   = EDD ____ / ____ /

INITIAL EXAM ____ / ____ / ____ = ____ WKS = EDD ____ / ____ /

ULTRASOUND ____ / ____ / ____ = ____ WKS = EDD ____ / ____ /

INITIAL EDD ____ / ____ / ____   INITIALED BY _____

18–20-WEEK EDD UPDATE:

QUICKENING ____ / ____ / ____ +22 WKS = ____ / ____ /

FUNDAL HT. AT UMBIL. ____ / ____ / ____ +20 WKS = ____ / ____ /

FHT W/ FETOSCOPE ____ / ____ / ____ +20 WKS = ____ / ____ /

ULTRASOUND ____ / ____ / ____ = ____WKS = ____ / ____ /

FINAL EDD ____ / ____ / ____   INITIALED BY _____

VISIT DATE ____ (YEAR)	WEEKS GEST. (BEST EST.)	FUNDAL HEIGHT (CM)	PRESENTATION	FHR	FETAL MOVEMENT	PRETERM LABOR SIGNS/SYMPTOMS: + =PRESENT O=ABSENT	CERVIX EXAM. (DIL/EFF/STA.)	BLOOD PRESSURE	EDEMA	WEIGHT	URINE (GLUCOSE/ALBUMIN)	NEXT APPOINTMENT	PROVIDER (INITIALS)	COMMENTS:

PROBLEMS: _____

COMMENTS: _____

ACOG ANTEPARTUM RECORD (FORM C)

LABORATORY AND EDUCATION

INITIAL LABS	DATE	RESULT	REVIEWED
BLOOD TYPE	/ /	A B AB O	
D (Rh) TYPE	/ /		
ANTIBODY SCREEN	/ /		
HCT/HGB	/ /	_____ % _____ g/dL	
PAP TEST	/ /	NORMAL / ABNORMAL / _____	
RUBELLA	/ /		
VDRL	/ /		
URINE CULTURE/SCREEN	/ /		
HBsAg	/ /		
HIV COUNSELING/TESTING	/ /	☐ POS ☐ NEG ☐ DECLINED	

OPTIONAL LABS	DATE	RESULT	
HGB ELECTROPHORESIS	/ /	AA AS SS AC SC AF ↑A₂	
PPD	/ /		
CHLAMYDIA	/ /		
GC	/ /		
TAY-SACHS	/ /		
OTHER			

COMMENTS/ADDITIONAL LABS

8–18-WEEK LABS (WHEN INDICATED/ELECTED)	DATE	RESULT	
ULTRASOUND	/ /		
MSAFP/MULTIPLE MARKERS	/ /		
AMNIO/CVS	/ /		
KARYOTYPE	/ /	46, XX OR 46, XY / OTHER____	
AMNIOTIC FLUID (AFP)	/ /	NORMAL____ ABNORMAL____	

24–28-WEEK LABS (WHEN INDICATED)	DATE	RESULT	
HCT/HGB	/ /	_____ % _____ g/dL	
DIABETES SCREEN	/ /	1 HOUR_____	
GTT (IF SCREEN ABNORMAL)	/ /	____FBS ____1 HOUR	
		____2 HOUR ____3 HOUR	
D (Rh) ANTIBODY SCREEN	/ /		
D IMMUNE GLOBULIN (RHIG) GIVEN (28 WKS)	/ /	SIGNATURE _____	

32–36-WEEK LABS (WHEN INDICATED)	DATE	RESULT	
HCT/HGB (RECOMMENDED)	/ /	_____ % _____ g/dL	
ULTRASOUND	/ /		
VDRL	/ /		
GC	/ /		
CHLAMYDIA	/ /		
GROUP B STREP (35-37 WKS)	/ /		

PLANS/EDUCATION (COUNSELED ☐)

☐ ANESTHESIA PLANS _____
☐ TOXOPLASMOSIS PRECAUTIONS (CATS/RAW MEAT) _____
☐ CHILDBIRTH CLASSES _____
☐ PHYSICAL/SEXUAL ACTIVITY _____
☐ LABOR SIGNS _____
☐ NUTRITION COUNSELING _____
☐ BREAST OR BOTTLE FEEDING _____
☐ NEWBORN CAR SEAT _____
☐ POSTPARTUM BIRTH CONTROL _____
☐ ENVIRONMENTAL/WORK HAZARDS _____

☐ TUBAL STERILIZATION _____
☐ VBAC COUNSELING _____
☐ CIRCUMCISION _____
☐ TRAVEL _____
☐ LIFESTYLE, TOBACCO, ALCOHOL _____
REQUESTS _____

TUBAL STERILIZATION   DATE   INITIALS
CONSENT SIGNED ____/____/____   _____

AA201 AA128   12345/10987

PROVIDER SIGNATURE (AS REQUIRED) _____

Appendix B

Early Pregnancy Risk Identification for Consultation

Risk Factor	Recommended Consultation*
Medical history/conditions	
Asthma	
Symptomatic on medication	Obstetrician–gynecologist
Severe (multiple hospitalizations)	MFM subspecialist
Cardiac disease	
Cyanotic, prior MI, aortic stenosis, primary pulmonary hypertension, Marfan syndrome, prosthetic valve, AHA Class II or greater	MFM subspecialist
Other	Obstetrician–gynecologist
Diabetes mellitus	
Class A–C	Obstetrician–gynecologist
Class D or greater	MFM subspecialist
Drug/alcohol use	Obstetrician–gynecologist
Epilepsy (on medication)	Obstetrician–gynecologist
Family history of genetic problems (Down syndrome, Tay–Sachs disease)	MFM subspecialist
Hemoglobinopathy (SS, SC, S-thal)	MFM subspecialist
Hypertension	
Chronic, with renal or heart disease	MFM subspecialist
Chronic, without renal or heart disease	Obstetrician–gynecologist
Prior pulmonary embolus/deep vein thrombosis	Obstetrician–gynecologist
Psychiatric illness	Obstetrician–gynecologist
Pulmonary disease	
Severe obstructive or restrictive	MFM subspecialist
Moderate	Obstetrician–gynecologist
Renal disease	
Chronic, creatinine ≥3 with or without hypertension	MFM subspecialist
Chronic, other	Obstetrician–gynecologist

Continued

Early Pregnancy Risk Identification for Consultation *(continued)*

Risk Factor	Recommended Consultation*
Medical history/conditions *(continued)*	
Requirement for prolonged anticoagulation	MFM subspecialist
Severe systemic disease	MFM subspecialist
Obstetric history/conditions	
Age ≥35 at delivery	Obstetrician–gynecologist
Cesarean delivery, prior classical or vertical incision	Obstetrician–gynecologist
Incompetent cervix	Obstetrician–gynecologist
Prior fetal structural or chromosomal abnormality	MFM subspecialist
Prior neonatal death	Obstetrician–gynecologist
Prior fetal death	Obstetrician–gynecologist
Prior preterm delivery or preterm PROM	Obstetrician–gynecologist
Prior low birth weight (<2,500 g)	Obstetrician–gynecologist
Second-trimester pregnancy loss	Obstetrician–gynecologist
Uterine leiomyomata or malformation	Obstetrician–gynecologist
Initial laboratory tests	
HIV	
Symptomatic or low CD4 count	MFM subspecialist
Other	Obstetrician–gynecologist
CDE (Rh) or other blood group isoimmunization (excluding ABO, Lewis)	MFM subspecialist
Initial examination: condylomata (extensive, covering vulva/vaginal opening)	Obstetrician–gynecologist

* At the time of consultation, continued patient care should be determined to be by collaboration with the referring care provider or by transfer of care.

Abbreviations: MFM = maternal–fetal medicine; MI = myocardial infarction; AHA = American Heart Association; PROM = premature rupture of membranes; HIV = human immunodeficiency virus.

Modified from March of Dimes Birth Defects Foundation, Committee on Perinatal Health. Toward improving the outcome of pregnancy: the 90s and beyond. White Plains, New York: March of Dimes Birth Defects Foundation, 1993.

Appendix C

Ongoing Pregnancy Risk Identification for Consultation

Risk Factor	Recommended Consultation*
Medical history/conditions	
Drug/alcohol use	Obstetrician–gynecologist
Proteinuria (≥2+ by catheter sample, unexplained by urinary tract infection)	Obstetrician–gynecologist
Pyelonephritis	Obstetrician–gynecologist
Severe systemic disease that adversely affects pregnancy	MFM subspecialist
Obstetric history/conditions	
Blood pressure elevation (diastolic ≥90 mm Hg), no proteinuria	Obstetrician–gynecologist
Fetal growth restriction suspected	Obstetrician–gynecologist
Fetal abnormality suspected by ultrasound	
Anencephaly	Obstetrician–gynecologist
Other	MFM subspecialist
Fetal demise	Obstetrician–gynecologist
Gestational age 41 weeks (to be seen by 42 weeks)	Obstetrician–gynecologist
Gestational diabetes mellitus	Obstetrician–gynecologist
Herpes, active lesions 36 weeks	Obstetrician–gynecologist
Hydramnios by ultrasound	Obstetrician–gynecologist
Hyperemesis, persisting beyond first trimester	Obstetrician–gynecologist
Multiple gestation	Obstetrician–gynecologist
Oligohydramnios by ultrasound	Obstetrician–gynecologist
Preterm labor, threatened, <37 weeks	Obstetrician–gynecologist
Premature rupture of membranes	Obstetrician–gynecologist
Vaginal bleeding ≥14 weeks	Obstetrician–gynecologist

Continued

Ongoing Pregnancy Risk Identification for Consultation *(continued)*

Risk Factor	Recommended Consultation*
Examination/laboratory findings	
Abnormal MSAFP (low or high)	Obstetrician–gynecologist
Abnormal Pap test	Obstetrician–gynecologist
Anemia (Hct <28%, unresponsive to iron therapy)	Obstetrician–gynecologist
Condylomata (extensive, covering labia/vaginal opening)	Obstetrician–gynecologist
HIV	
Symptomatic or low CD4 count	MFM subspecialist
Other	Obstetrician–gynecologist
CDE (Rh) or other blood group isoimmunization (excluding ABO, Lewis)	MFM subspecialist

* At the time of consultation, continued patient care should be determined to be by collaboration with the referring care provider or by transfer of care.

Abbreviations: MFM = maternal–fetal medicine; MSAFP = maternal serum alpha-fetoprotein; Hct = hematocrit; HIV = human immunodeficiency virus.

Modified from March of Dimes Birth Defects Foundation, Committee on Perinatal Health. Toward improving the outcome of pregnancy: the 90s and beyond. White Plains, New York: March of Dimes Birth Defects Foundation, 1993.

Appendix D

Federal Requirements for Patient Screening and Transfer

In 1986 the United States Congress first enacted legal requirements specifying how Medicare-participating hospitals with emergency services must handle individuals with emergency medical conditions or women who are in labor. Since then, the patient screening and transfer law has undergone numerous refinements and revisions. The most recent regulations, promulgated by the Health Care Financing Administration, became effective on July 22, 1994. Physicians should expect that this law will continue to evolve and that there will be additional modifications to it in the future.

Requirements for an Appropriate Medical Screening Examination

Federal law requires that all Medicare-participating hospitals with emergency services must provide an "appropriate medical screening examination" for any individual who comes to the emergency department for medical treatment or examination to determine whether the patient has an emergency medical condition. This examination must be made within the capability of the hospital's emergency department, including ancillary services routinely available to the emergency department. For example, "[i]f a hospital has a department of obstetrics and gynecology, the hospital is responsible for adopting procedures under which the staff and resources of that department are available to treat a woman in labor who comes to its emergency department."

Medical screening examinations must also ". . . be conducted by individuals determined qualified by hospital by-laws or rules and regulations." Thus, it is up to a hospital to designate who is a "qualified medical person" to provide an appropriate medical screening examination. The law does not require that physicians perform all screening examinations. Therefore, a hospital can determine under what circumstances a physician is required to provide medical screening and when screening can be done by a nonphysician.

Determining Whether a Patient Has an Emergency Medical Condition

The legal definition of "emergency medical condition" is not the same as the medical one. Under the law, it is defined as follows:

A medical condition manifesting itself by acute symptoms of sufficient severity (including severe pain, psychiatric disturbances and/or symptoms of substance abuse) such that the absence of immediate attention could reasonably be expected to result in—

(A) Placing the health of the individual (or, with respect to a pregnant woman, the health of the woman or her unborn child) in serious jeopardy;

(B) Serious impairment to bodily functions; or

(C) Serious dysfunction of any bodily organ or part.

It is important to note that, in the case of a pregnant woman who presents to a hospital emergency room, the health of the fetus must also be considered in determining whether an "emergency medical condition" exists.

Special Determination of Emergency Medical Conditions for Pregnant Women

The definition of an emergency medical condition also makes specific reference to a pregnant woman who is having contractions. It provides that an emergency medical condition exists if a pregnant woman is having contractions and ". . . there is inadequate time to effect a safe transfer to another hospital before delivery; or that transfer may pose a threat to the health or safety of the woman or the unborn child." An emergency medical condition does not exist, even when a woman is having contractions, as long as there is adequate time to effect a safe transfer before delivery and the transfer will not pose a threat to the health or safety of the mother or fetus.

The latest regulations also define labor to mean:

> . . . the process of childbirth beginning with the latent phase of labor or early phase of labor and continuing through delivery of the placenta. A woman experiencing contractions is in true labor unless a physician certifies that after a reasonable time of observation the woman is in false labor.

Unless the definition is revised, it creates a new requirement that only a physician may certify that a woman is in false labor.

Patients with Emergency Medical Conditions

Once a patient comes to an emergency room, is appropriately screened, and is determined to have an emergency medical condition, the physician has two choices as to how to proceed. The physician may:

1. Treat the patient and stabilize her condition.
2. Transfer the patient to another medical facility in accordance with specific procedures outlined below.

In situations in which a woman is experiencing contractions and meets the other criteria outlined above for an emergency medical condition, the only way to stabilize the patient is to deliver the child and the placenta.

Patients Can Refuse to Consent to Treatment

If a patient refuses to consent to treatment, the hospital has fulfilled its obligations under the law. If a patient refuses to consent to treatment, however, the following steps must be taken:

1. The patient must be informed of the risks and benefits of the examination or treatment or both.

2. The medical record must contain a description of the examination and treatment that was refused by the patient.

3. The hospital must take all reasonable steps to secure the patient's written informed refusal. The written document must indicate that the person has been informed of the risks and benefits of the examination or treatment or both.

Procedures for Transferring a Patient to Another Medical Facility

In general, a patient who meets the criteria of an emergency medical condition may not be transferred until he or she is stabilized. There are, however, some exceptions to this prohibition.

The patient may request a transfer, in writing, after being informed of the hospital's obligations under the law and the risks of transfer. The unstabilized patient's written request for transfer must indicate the reasons for the request and that the patient is aware of the risks and benefits of transfer.

An unstabilized patient may also be transferred if a physician signs a written certification that:

> based upon the information available at the time of transfer, the medical benefits reasonably expected from the provision of appropriate medical treatment at another medical facility outweigh the increased risks to the individual or, in the case of a woman in labor, to the woman or the unborn child, from being transferred.

The certification must contain a summary of the risks and benefits of transfer.

If a physician is not physically present in the emergency department at the time of the transfer of a patient, a qualified medical person can sign the certification described above after consulting with a physician who authorizes the transfer. The physician must countersign the certification later.

Patients Can Refuse to Consent to Transfer

If the hospital offers to transfer a patient, in accordance with the appropriate procedures, and the patient refuses to consent to transfer, the hospital has also fulfilled its obligations under the law. When a patient refuses to consent to the transfer, the hospital must take the following steps:

1. The patient must be informed of the risks and benefits of the transfer.

2. The medical record must contain a description of the proposed transfer that was refused by the patient.

3. The hospital must take all reasonable steps to secure the patient's written informed refusal. The written document must indicate that the person has been informed of the risks and benefits of the transfer and the reasons for the patient's refusal.

Additional Requirements of the Transferring and Receiving Hospitals

The transferring hospital must comply with the following requirements in order to ensure that the transfer was appropriate:

1. The receiving hospital must have space and qualified personnel to treat the patient and must have agreed to accept the transfer. A hospital with specialized capabilities, such as a neonatal intensive care unit, may not refuse to accept patients if space is available.

2. The transferring hospital must minimize the risks to the patient's health, and the transfer must be executed through the use of qualified personnel and transportation equipment.

3. The transferring hospital must send to the receiving hospital all medical records related to the emergency condition that are available at the time of transfer. These records include available history, records related to the emergency medical condition, observations of signs or symptoms, preliminary diagnosis, results

of diagnostic studies or telephone reports of the studies, treatment provided, results of any tests and informed written consent or certification, and the name of any on-call physician who has refused or failed to appear within a reasonable time to provide necessary stabilizing treatment. Other records not yet available must be sent as soon as practicable.

General Requirements

1. Medical records related to transfers must be retained by both the transferring and receiving hospitals for 5 years from the date of the transfer.

2. Hospitals are required to report to the Health Care Financing Administration or the state survey agency within 72 hours from the time of the transfer any time it has reason to believe it may have received a patient who was transferred in an unstable medical condition.

3. Hospitals are required to post signs in areas such as entrances, admitting areas, waiting rooms, and emergency departments with respect to their obligations under the patient screening and transfer law.

4. Hospitals are also required to post signs stating whether the hospital participates in the Medicaid program under a state-approved plan. This requirement applies to all hospitals, not only those that participate in Medicare.

5. Hospitals must keep a list of physicians who are on call after the initial examination to provide treatment to stabilize a patient with an emergency medical condition.

6. Hospitals must keep a central log of all individuals who come to the emergency department seeking assistance and the result of each individual's visit.

7. A hospital may not delay providing appropriate medical screening to inquire about payment method or insurance status.

Enforcement and Penalties

Physicians and hospitals violating these federal requirements for patient screening and transfer are subject to civil monetary penalties of up to $50,000 for each violation and to termination from the Medicare program. Hospitals are prohibited from penalizing physicians who report violations of the law or who refuse to transfer an individual with an unstabilized emergency medical condition.

Appendix E

Standard Terminology for Reporting of Reproductive Health Statistics in the United States*

The adoption of standard definitions and reporting requirements for reproductive health statistics will provide an improved basis for standardization and uniformity in the design, implementation, and evaluation of intervention strategies. The reduction of maternal and infant mortality and the improvement of the health of our nation's mothers and infants are the ultimate goals. The collection and analysis of reliable statistical data are an essential part of in-depth investigations and incorporate case finding, individual review, and analysis of risk factors. These studies could then yield valuable clinical information for practitioners, aiding them in improved case management for high-risk patients, which would result in decreased morbidity and mortality.

Both the collection and the use of statistics have been hampered by lack of understanding of differences in definitions, statistical tabulations, and reporting requirements among state, national, and international bodies. Misapplication and misinterpretation of data may lead to erroneous comparisons and conclusions. For example, specific requirements for reporting of fetal deaths have often been misinterpreted as implying a weight or gestational age for viability. Distinctions can and should be made among (1) the definition of an event, (2) the reporting requirements for the event, and (3) the statistical tabulation and interpretation of the data. The definition indicates the meaning of a term (for example, *live birth*, *fetal death*, or *maternal death*). A re-

---

* This document has been modified. Different states use different birth weight and gestational age criteria to define fetal death. The Committee on Obstetric Practice of the American College of Obstetricians and Gynecologists recommends that perinatal mortality statistics be based on a gestational weight of 500 g.

porting requirement is that part of the defined event for which reporting is mandatory or desired. Statistical tabulations connote the presentation of data for the purpose of analysis and interpretation of existing and future conditions. The data should be collected in a manner that will allow them to be presented in different ways for different users. Adjustments should be made for variations in reporting before comparisons among data are attempted.

If information is collected and presented in a standardized manner, comparisons between the new data and the data obtained by previous reporting requirements can be delineated clearly and can contribute to improved public understanding of reproductive health statistics. For ease in assimilating this information, it is divided into three sections: (1) definitions, (2) statistical tabulations, and (3) reporting requirements/recommendations. Some of the definitions and recommendations are a departure from those currently or historically accepted; however, these recommendations were agreed upon by the interorganizational group that was brought together to review terminology related to reproductive health issues.

Definitions

Live birth: The complete expulsion or extraction from the mother of a product of human conception, irrespective of the duration of pregnancy, which, after such expulsion or extraction, breathes or shows any other evidence of life, such as beating of the heart, pulsation of the umbilical cord, or definite movement of voluntary muscles, whether or not the umbilical cord has been cut or the placenta is attached. Heartbeats are to be distinguished from transient cardiac contractions; respirations are to be distinguished from fleeting respiratory efforts or gasps.

Birth weight: The weight of a neonate determined immediately after delivery or as soon thereafter as feasible. It should be expressed to the nearest gram.

Gestational age: The number of weeks that have elapsed between the first day of the last normal menstrual period (not the presumed time of conception) and the date of delivery, irrespective of whether the gestation results in a live birth or a fetal death.

Neonate:

> *Low birth weight*—Any neonate, regardless of gestational age, whose weight at birth is less than 2,500 g.
>
> *Preterm**—Any neonate whose birth occurs through the end of the last day of the 37th week (259th day) following the onset of the last menstrual period.
>
> *Term**—Any neonate whose birth occurs from the beginning of the first day (260th day) of the 38th week through the end of the last day of the 42nd week (294th day) following the onset of the last menstrual period.
>
> *Postterm*—Any neonate whose birth occurs from the beginning of the first day (295th day) of the 43rd week following the onset of the last menstrual period.

Fetal death: Death prior to the complete expulsion or extraction from the mother of a product of human conception, fetus and placenta, irrespective of the duration of pregnancy; the death is indicated by the fact that, after such expulsion or extraction, the fetus does not breathe or show any other evidence of life, such as beating of the heart, pulsation of the umbilical cord, or definite movement of voluntary muscles. Heartbeats are to be distinguished from transient cardiac contractions; respirations are to be distinguished from fleeting respiratory efforts or gasps. This definition excludes induced termination of pregnancy.

---

* These definitions are for statistical purposes and are not intended to affect clinical management. Appropriate assessment of fetal maturity for purposes of clinical management is delineated in Chapter 4.

Statisticians making a determination of the status of a neonate, namely preterm or term, should define preterm as less than 259 days and term as 259 days to less than 294 days in order to ensure comparable calculations with the medical community. Statisticians, by formula, subtract the date of the first day of the last menstrual period from the date of birth, whereas physicians include the first day, thus accounting for the difference.

Neonatal death: Death of a liveborn neonate before the neonate becomes 28 days old (up to and including 27 days, 23 hours, and 59 minutes from the moment of birth).

Infant death: Any death at any time from birth up to, but not including, 1 year of age (364 days, 23 hours, and 59 minutes from the moment of birth).

Maternal death:* The death of a woman from any cause related to or aggravated by pregnancy or its management (regardless of the duration or site of pregnancy), but not from accidental or incidental causes.

Direct obstetric death—The death of a woman resulting from obstetric complications of pregnancy, labor, or the puerperium; from interventions, omissions, or treatment; or from a chain of events resulting from any of these.

Indirect obstetric death—The death of a woman resulting from a previously existing disease or a disease that developed during pregnancy, labor, or the puerperium that was not due to direct obstetric causes, although the physiologic effects of pregnancy were partially responsible for the death.

In 1987, the Centers for Disease Control and Prevention (CDC) collaborated with the Maternal Mortality Special Interest Group of the American College of Obstetricians and Gynecologists (ACOG), the Association of Vital Records and Health Statistics, and state and local health departments to initiate the National Pregnancy Mortality Surveillance System. The CDC/ACOG Maternal Mortality Study Group introduced two new terms, which are being used by the CDC and increasingly by some states and researchers. The study group differentiates between pregnancy-associated and pregnancy-related deaths.

---

* Death occurring to a woman during pregnancy or after its termination from causes not related to the pregnancy or to its complications or management is not considered a maternal death. Nonmaternal deaths may result from accidental causes (eg, auto accident or gunshot wound) or incidental causes (eg, concurrent malignancy).

Pregnancy-associated death: The death of any woman, from any cause, while pregnant or within 1 calendar year of termination of pregnancy, regardless of the duration and the site of pregnancy.

Pregnancy-related death: A pregnancy-associated death resulting from (1) complications of the pregnancy itself, (2) the chain of events initiated by the pregnancy that led to death, or (3) aggravation of an unrelated condition by the physiologic or pharmacologic effects of the pregnancy that subsequently caused death.

Induced termination of pregnancy: The purposeful interruption of an intrauterine pregnancy with the intention other than to produce a liveborn infant, and which does not result in a live birth. This definition excludes management of prolonged retention of products of conception following fetal death.

Statistical Tabulations

Statistical tabulations for vital events related to pregnancy provide the medical and statistical community with valuable information on reproductive health and generate data on trends apparent in this country and worldwide. This information often is disaggregated and used to examine specific events over time or within selected geographic locations. In informing the public about health issues, media sources often report various statistical measures. Heightened public interest in health-related issues makes it essential that the medical community understand and have the capacity to interpret these statistics.

The following explanations of statistical tabulations are intended to provide the reader with a better understanding of the measures used for events related to reproduction.

Rate: A measure of the frequency of some event in relation to a unit of population during a specified time period, such as a year; events in the numerator of the rate occur to individuals in the denominator. Rates express the risk of the event in the specified population during a particular time. Rates are generally expressed as units of population in the denominator (per 1,000, per

100,000, etc). For example, the 1982 teenage birth rate was 52.9 live births per 1,000 women 15–19 years of age.

Ratios: A term that expresses a relationship of one element to a different element (where the numerator is not necessarily a subset of the denominator). A ratio is generally expressed per 1,000 of the denominator element. For example, the sex ratio of live births for 1982 was 1,051 males per 1,000 females.

In the formulae that follow, *period* refers to a calendar year.

Live Birth Measures

These measures are designed to show the rate at which childbearing is occurring in the population. The *crude birth rate*, which relates the total number of births to the total population, indicates the impact of fertility on population growth. The *general fertility rate* is a more specific measure of fertility because it relates the number of births to the population at risk, namely, women of childbearing age (assumed to be ages 15–44 years). An even more specific set of rates, the *age-specific birth rate*, relates the number of births to women of specific ages directly to the total number of women in that age group. Formulae for these measures follow:

$$\text{Crude birth rate} = \frac{\text{Number of live births to women of all ages during a calendar year} \times 1{,}000}{\text{Total estimated mid-year population}}$$

$$\text{General fertility rate} = \frac{\text{Number of live births to women of all ages during a calendar year} \times 1{,}000}{\text{Estimated mid-year population of women 15–44 years of age}}$$

$$\text{General pregnancy rate} = \frac{\text{Number of live births + number of fetal deaths + number of induced terminations of pregnancy during a calendar year} \times 1{,}000}{\text{Estimated mid-year population of women 15–44 years of age}}$$

$$\text{Age-specific birth rate} = \frac{\text{Number of live births to women in a specific age group during a calendar year} \times 1{,}000}{\text{Estimated mid-year population of women in same age group}}$$

$$\text{Total fertility rate} = \text{The sum of age-specific birth rates of women at each age group 10--14 through 45--49.}$$

Five-year age groups are used; therefore, the sum is multiplied by 5. This rate can also be computed by using single years of age.

Because the birth weight of the infant is included on the birth certificate, it is possible to tabulate and focus an analysis on selected groups of live births, for example, those weighing 500 g or more.

Births can be tabulated by where they occur. Thus, they can be shown by place of occurrence, by place of residence, and by kind of setting of delivery, such as at a hospital or home. Most tabulations of vital statistics are routinely calculated by place of residence of the mother, but they could be tabulated on another basis as well. What is essential, however, is that the classification be the same for all events under consideration for a specific measure.

Fetal Mortality Measures

The population at risk for fetal mortality is the number of live births plus the number of fetal deaths in a year. Fetal death indices indicate the magnitude of late pregnancy losses.

It is recognized that most states report fetal deaths on the basis of gestational age. However, birth weight can be more accurately measured than can gestational age. Therefore, it is recommended that states adopt minimum reporting requirements of fetal deaths based on and labeled as specific birth weight rather than gestational age (see "Fetal Death" under "Reporting Requirements/Recommendations," below). In addition, statistical tabulations of fetal deaths should include, at a minimum, fetal deaths of 500 g or more.

Fetal death rate =

$$\frac{\text{Number of fetal deaths } (x \text{ weight or more}) \text{ during a period} \times 1,000}{\text{Number of fetal deaths } (x \text{ weight or more}) + \text{number of live births during the same period}}$$

Fetal death ratio =

$$\frac{\text{Number of fetal deaths } (x \text{ weight or more}) \text{ during a period} \times 1,000}{\text{Number of live births during the same period}}$$

It is recognized that states will not be able to immediately translate data from gestational age to weight, and, for comparative purposes, it may be desirable to know fetal death rates for various gestational periods. Therefore, the collection of both weight and gestational age is recommended to allow for these comparisons. When calculating fetal death rates based on gestational age, the number of weeks or more of stated or presumed gestation can be substituted for weight in the above formulae.

Perinatal Mortality Measures

Indices of perinatal mortality combine fetal deaths and live births with only brief survival (up to a few days or weeks) on the assumption that similar factors are associated with these losses. The population at risk is the total number of live births plus fetal deaths, or alternatively, the number of live births. Perinatal mortality indices can vary as to age of the fetus and the infant who is included in the particular tabulation. However, the concept itself cuts across all the calculations.

It is recommended that perinatal mortality measures be based on and labeled with specific weight rather than gestational age (see "Reporting Requirements/Recommendations," below).

Perinatal mortality rate =

$$\frac{\begin{array}{c}\text{Number of infant deaths of less than} \\ x \text{ days} + \text{number of fetal deaths} \\ \text{(with stated or presumed weight} \\ \text{of } y \text{ or more}) \text{ during the same period} \times 1,000\end{array}}{\text{Number of live births during the same period}}$$

It is recognized that states will not be able to immediately translate data from gestational age to weight, and for purposes of comparability, knowledge of gestational age (based on last menstrual period) may be required and should be collected. When perinatal death rates based on gestational age are calculated, the number of weeks of a stated or presumed gestational age can be substituted for weight in the above formulae. When comparisons based on gestational age are desired, the generally accepted breakdown is as follows:

- Perinatal period I includes infant deaths occurring at less than 7 days and fetal deaths with a stated or presumed period of gestation of 28 weeks or more.

- Perinatal period II includes infant deaths occurring at less than 28 days and fetal deaths with a stated or presumed period of gestation of 20 weeks or more.

- Perinatal period III includes infant deaths occurring at less than 7 days and fetal deaths with a stated or presumed gestation of 20 weeks or more.

Perinatal measures can be specific for race and other characteristics. Perinatal events can be tabulated by where they occur. Thus, they can be shown by place of occurrence, by place of residence, and by place of delivery, such as at a hospital or home. Most tabulations of vital statistics are routinely calculated by place of residence of the mother, but they could be tabulated by place of occurrence. What is essential, however, is that the classification be the same for all events under consideration for a specific measure.

Indices of infant mortality are designed to show the likelihood that live births with certain characteristics will survive the first year of life or, conversely, will die during the first year of life. For infant mortality, the "population at risk" is approximated by live births that occur in a calendar year. One can compare the infant mortality rate of different population groups, such as that between white and black infants. Interest sometimes focuses on two different periods in the first year of an infant's life, such as the very early period before the infant becomes 28 days old (up through 27 days, 23 hours, and 59 minutes from the moment of birth), called the *neonatal period*; and the later period starting at the end of the 28th day up to, but not including, 1 year of age

(364 days, 23 hours, and 59 minutes), called the *postneonatal period.* Accordingly, two indices reflect these differences, namely, the neonatal mortality rate and the postneonatal mortality rate. The neonatal period can be divided further for statistical tabulations as follows:

- Neonatal period I is from the moment of birth through 23 hours and 59 minutes.
- Neonatal period II starts at the end of the 24th hour of life through 6 days, 23 hours, and 59 minutes.
- Neonatal period III starts at the end of the 7th day of life through 27 days, 23 hours, and 59 minutes.

$$\text{Infant mortality rate} = \frac{\text{Number of infant deaths (neonatal and postneonatal) during a period} \times 1,000}{\text{Number of live births during the same period}}$$

$$\text{Neonatal mortality rate} = \frac{\text{Number of neonatal deaths during a period} \times 1,000}{\text{Number of live births during the same period}}$$

$$\text{Postneonatal mortality rate} = \frac{\text{Number of postneonatal deaths during a period} \times 1,000}{\text{Number of live births during the same period}}$$

The denominator for the postneonatal mortality rate can also be calculated by subtracting the number of neonatal deaths from the number of live births. This denominator more accurately defines the population at risk of death in the postneonatal period. In addition, it should be noted that infant deaths can be broken down into birth weight categories, if desired, for comparative purposes when birth and death records are linked (see "Reporting Requirements/Recommendations," below).

Maternal Mortality Measures

Measures of maternal mortality are designed to indicate the likelihood that a pregnant woman will die from complications of pregnancy, childbirth, or the puerperium. Accordingly, the population at risk is an approximation of the population of pregnant women in a year; the approximation is usually taken to be the number of live births. Maternal mortality can be examined in terms of characteristics of the woman, such as age, race, and cause of death. The maternal mortality rate measures the risk of death from deliveries and complications of pregnancy, childbirth, and the puerperium.

The group exposed to risk consists of all women who have been pregnant at some time during the period. Thus, the population at risk should theoretically include all fetal deaths (reported and unreported), all induced terminations of pregnancy, and all live births. Because most states do not require the reporting of all fetal deaths and a large number of states still do not require reporting of induced terminations of pregnancy, the entire population at risk cannot be included in the denominator. Therefore, the total number of live births has become the generally accepted denominator. It is recommended that when complete ascertainment of the denominator (that is, the number of pregnant women) is achieved, a modified maternal mortality rate should be defined, in addition to the traditional rate. The rate is most frequently expressed per 100,000 live births, as follows:

$$\text{Maternal mortality rate} = \frac{\text{Number of deaths attributed to maternal conditions during a period} \times 100,000}{\text{Number of live births during the same period}}$$

Death rates for specified maternal causes are computed by restricting the numerator to the specified cause. The maternal mortality rates specific for race and age groups are computed by appropriately restricting both the numerator and the denominator to the specified group. Caution should be used in interpreting rates in small geographic areas; it may not be possible to generate race- and age-specific rates.

For statistical comparisons with the World Health Organization (WHO), it is recommended that two tabulations of statistics be prepared: (1) maternal deaths within 42 days of the end of pregnancy (WHO) and (2) maternal deaths with no time limitation for comparison within the United States.

The CDC uses the following statistical measures of pregnancy-related mortality:

$$\text{Pregnancy mortality ratio} = \frac{\text{Number of pregnancy-related deaths during a period} \times 100,000}{\text{Number of live births during the same period}}$$

$$\text{Pregnancy mortality rate} = \frac{\text{Number of pregnancy-related deaths during a period} \times 100,000}{\text{Number of pregnancies (live births, fetal deaths, induced and spontaneous abortions, ectopic pregnancies, and molar pregnancies)}}$$

Measures of Induced Termination of Pregnancy

Measures of induced pregnancy termination parallel those of fetal deaths but refer to "induced" events. The population at risk for induced termination of pregnancy is taken to be live births in a year, which is used as a surrogate measure of pregnancies. Because this is not actually the total population at risk, this measure is generally considered a ratio.

$$\text{Induced termination of pregnancy ratio I} = \frac{\text{Number of induced terminations occurring during a period} \times 1,000}{\text{Number of live births occurring during the same period}}$$

Another measure is one that, by also including an estimate of pregnancies that do not result in live births, more closely approximates the population at risk:

$$\text{Induced termination of pregnancy ratio II} = \frac{\text{Number of induced terminations occurring during a period} \times 1{,}000}{\text{Number of induced terminations of pregnancies + live births + reported fetal deaths during the same period}}$$

Still a third measure is a rate that provides information on the probability that a woman of a certain age or race will have an induced termination of pregnancy:

$$\text{Induced termination of pregnancy rate} = \frac{\text{Number of induced terminations occurring during a period} \times 1{,}000}{\text{Female population aged 15–44 years}}$$

Sometimes indices for induced termination are specific for certain characteristics of the woman; that is, they can refer to women of particular age or race groups.

Reporting Requirements/Recommendations

Reporting requirements for vital events related to reproductive health enable the collection of data that are essential to the calculation of statistical tabulations in order to examine trends and changes at the local, state, and national levels. The data used in statistical tabulations may be only a portion of those collected, due to the need for consistency in a tabulation and to the variations in reporting requirements from state to state. For instance, although a few states require that all fetal deaths, regardless of length of gestation, be reported, statistical tabulations of fetal death rates by the National Center for Health Statistics utilize only those fetal deaths occurring at 20 weeks or more gestation.

Live Birth

It is generally recognized that all states report all live births, as defined in the definitions section of this document. It is recommended that all live births be reported, regardless of birth weight, length of gestation, or survival time.

Fetal Death

Reporting requirements for fetal deaths now vary from state to state. At present, most states require reporting of fetal deaths by gestational age. It is generally recognized that birth weight can be measured more accurately than can gestational age. The 1977 revision of the *Model State Vital Statistics Act and Regulations* recommends reporting of all spontaneous losses occurring at 20 weeks or more of gestation or weighing 350 g or more.

It must be emphasized that a specific birth weight criterion for reporting of fetal deaths does not imply a point of viability and should be chosen instead for its feasibility in collecting useful data.

Current statistical tabulations of fetal deaths include, at a minimum, fetal deaths of 500 g or more. Furthermore, 27 states have adopted the requirement of reporting deaths of more than 20 weeks of gestation. Therefore, it is recommended that all state fetal death report forms include birth weight and gestational age.

Perinatal Mortality

Perinatal mortality indices generally combine fetal deaths and live births that survive only briefly (up to a few days or weeks). Because reporting requirements of fetal deaths vary from state to state, perinatal mortality reporting will also vary (see definitions of perinatal periods under "Perinatal Mortality Measures").

As with fetal deaths, it is recommended that perinatal mortality be weight specific. However, for purposes of comparability, knowledge of gestational age (based on last menstrual period) should be collected.

Infant Mortality

All states require that all infant deaths (neonatal plus postneonatal), as defined in the section "Definitions" in this document, be reported.

Infant deaths by birth weight are not routinely available for the United States as a whole because birth weight information is not collected on the death certificate. However, because birth weight is reported on the birth certificate, it is possible to obtain information on infant deaths by birth weight by linking together the birth certificate and the death certificate for the same infant. At present, most states link birth and death certificates. A national linked birth certificate and infant death certificate file is now available.

In addition, it is recommended that infant death reports include the exact interval from birth rather than categories such as "neonatal" or "postneonatal." This, too, will allow for more specific age-related death analyses.

Maternal Mortality

Every state is required to report all maternal deaths. Because annual deaths attributed to maternal mortality approximate only 300, emphasis must be placed on in-depth investigations. Case finding, together with individual review and analysis of risk factors contributing to maternal deaths, is of the highest importance. Collection of data regarding these rare events is critical, when combined, as it should be, with educational review by those closest to the case, usually the obstetrician–gynecologists in the hospital and the surrounding region. Such analysis can yield clinical information about risk factors associated with, for example, detection and treatment of ectopic pregnancies or with anesthesia. This clinical information can then be gathered and exchanged to help practitioners identify risk factors that contribute to maternal death and associated conditions.

The CDC/ACOG Maternal Mortality Study Group has also designed a new system of classifying pregnancy-related deaths after review of the case. This system differentiates between the immediate and underlying causes of death as stated on the death certificate, associated obstetric and medical conditions or complications, and the outcome of pregnancy. For example, if a woman died of a hemorrhage that resulted from a ruptured ectopic pregnancy, the immediate cause of death would be classified as "hemorrhage," the associated obstetric condition would be classified as "ruptured fallopian tube," and the outcome of pregnancy would be "ectopic pregnancy." This classification scheme allows analysis of the chain of events that led to the death.

Induced Termination of Pregnancy

The United States has no national system for reporting induced termination of pregnancy. State health departments vary greatly in their approaches to the compilation of these data, from compiling no data to (1) periodically requesting hospitals, clinics, and/or physicians performing the procedures to voluntarily report total number of procedures performed; (2) requiring (by legislative or regulatory authority) hospitals, clinics, and/or physicians to periodically report aggregate level data on number or number and characteristics of procedures; or (3) requiring (by legal or regulatory authority) hospitals, clinics, and/or physicians to periodically report individual data on each procedure performed.

Since 1969, the CDC Division of Reproductive Health has published an annual Abortion Surveillance Report based on data provided from state health departments, when available, and from data voluntarily provided to the CDC from hospitals and clinics in states with no data available from health departments. In addition to information on the number and characteristics of induced terminations of pregnancy, the Abortion Surveillance Report contains information from the CDC abortion mortality surveillance, which was begun with the cooperation of state health departments in 1972. Investigation and review of each related death by epidemiologists in the Division of Reproductive Health result in improved detailed nosological identification of abortion mortality by type of risk.*

Since 1977, the National Center for Health Statistics has analyzed the induced terminations of pregnancy occurring in up to 13 states in which individual reports of induced termination are submitted to state vital registration offices. In addition, the Alan Guttmacher Institute, a private organization, publishes information on induced termination

---

* The CDC Abortion Surveillance Report includes information on events categorized by the CDC as abortions (legal, illegal, and spontaneous). Although this terminology predates the recommendations in this document and is at variance with the definition herein, it has been commonly used and understood to include induced termination of pregnancy.

that it obtains from a nationwide survey of providers of induced termination.

Collecting information on the number of induced terminations of pregnancy, the characteristics of women having such procedures, and the number and characteristics of all deaths related to induced termination of pregnancy would be extremely valuable in identifying and evaluating risk factors for specific population groups and for the public in general. By gathering these data, studies could be instituted with practitioners. Knowing the outcomes could further the body of knowledge and ultimately reduce the risks.

Therefore, we urge state health departments that compile statistics on induced termination of pregnancy to evaluate and improve the quality of their data. Furthermore, we urge state health departments that do not compile such statistics to explore mechanisms for initiating their collection.

Rates of Vaginal Births After Cesarean Delivery

About 24% of the births in the United States are cesarean births. One third of these cesarean births are repeat cesarean deliveries. The safety of vaginal birth after a previous low transverse cesarean delivery (VBAC) when established criteria are met has been demonstrated in many studies.

The literature evaluating VBAC generally focuses on the criteria for a trial of labor after cesarean delivery, the safety of a trial of labor, and the success rate of such trials. The latter rate has usually been quoted as 60–80%, depending on selection criteria and other variables. Given the current focus on cost-containment in health care, the VBAC rate is a often used as a measurement of obstetric practice by hospital quality-assurance committees, insurers, and government agencies.

To facilitate an accurate comparison of VBAC rates between providers and between institutions, standardized definitions based on readily available numbers should be used. Although there are some women in whom a trial of labor is absolutely contraindicated, it may be difficult to accurately identify this group. This applies to a small number of women, however, and will not have a substantial impact on the VBAC rate. For this reason, women who are not candidates for a trial of labor are included in the denominator used to calculate the VBAC rate. Two methods for defining VBAC rates are proposed:

$$1. \quad \text{VBAC rate} = \frac{\text{Total number of VBACs}}{\substack{\text{Total number of women with prior cesarean} \\ \text{deliveries (including women who were} \\ \text{candidates for a trial of labor but declined} \\ \text{and women who were not candidates}}} \times 100$$

$$2. \quad \substack{\text{Trial of labor} \\ \text{success rate}} = \frac{\text{VBAC}}{\substack{\text{Number of women who had a} \\ \text{trial of labor after cesarean delivery}}} \times 100$$

Clearly, these rates are interrelated. However, calculations based on the rates as defined allow a more accurate comparison of practice between providers and between institutions.

Current Reporting Requirements

The following general fetal death reporting requirements, as of March 1991, should be brought into conformity with the recommendations in this report:

≥20 weeks of gestation:

Alabama	Iowa	Oklahoma
Alaska	Maryland*	Oregon*
Arizona*	Minnesota	Texas
California	Montana	Utah
Connecticut	Nebraska	Vermont*
Delaware	Nevada	Washington
Florida	New Jersey	West Virginia
Guam	North Carolina	Wyoming
Illinois	North Dakota	
Indiana	Ohio	

* Modifiers apply.

≥20 *weeks of gestation or birth weight of* ≥500 *g:*

District of Columbia

≥20 *weeks of gestation or birth weight of* ≥350 *g:*

Idaho	Massachusetts	New Hampshire
Kentucky	Mississippi	South Carolina
Louisiana	Missouri	Wisconsin

Birth weight of >350 *g:*

Kansas

≥20 *weeks of gestation or birth weight of* ≥400 *g:*

Michigan

Birth weight of ≥500 *g:*

New Mexico
South Dakota
Tennessee*

≥5 *months of gestation:*

Puerto Rico

≥16 *weeks of gestation:*

Pennsylvania

All products of human conception:

American Samoa	Maine	Rhode Island
Arkansas	New York City	Virginia
Colorado	New York State	Virgin Islands
Georgia	Northern Mariana	
Hawaii	Islands	

* Modifiers apply.

Appendix F

Occupational Safety and Health Administration Regulations on Occupational Exposure to Bloodborne Pathogens*

In 1970, the U.S. Congress enacted the Occupational Safety and Health Act to protect workers from unsafe and unhealthy conditions in the workplace. To oversee this effort, the law also created the Occupational Safety and Health Administration (OSHA) within the U.S. Department of Labor. The Occupational Safety and Health Administration has the responsibility for developing and implementing job safety and health standards and regulations. Its standards and regulations apply to all employers and employees. To promote and ensure compliance with its standards, OSHA has the authority to conduct unannounced workplace inspections. It also maintains a reporting and record-keeping system to monitor job-related injuries and illnesses. Failure to comply with OSHA standards may result in the assessment of civil or criminal penalties.

In December 1991, OSHA issued new regulations on occupational exposure to bloodborne pathogens that are designed to minimize the transmission of human immunodeficiency virus (HIV), hepatitis B virus (HBV), and other potentially infectious materials in the workplace. The regulations cover all employees in physician offices, hospitals, medical laboratories, and other health care facilities where workers could be "reasonably anticipated" as a result of performing their job duties to come into contact with blood and other potentially infectious materials.

* Modified with permission from Kaminetzky HN, Rutledge P. OSHA regulations and medical practice. Prim Care Update Ob/Gyn 1995;2:143–149. Elsevier Science Inc.

Approved State Plans

Under the federal law that created OSHA, states are encouraged to develop and operate—under OSHA guidance—state job safety and health plans. Currently, 23 states and 2 territories have OSHA-approved plans, which require them to provide standards and enforcement programs that are at least as effective as the federal standards. They are:

Alaska	Michigan	Tennessee
Arizona	Minnesota	Utah
California	Nevada	Vermont
Connecticut*	New Mexico	Virgin Islands
Hawaii	New York*	Virginia
Indiana	North Carolina	Washington
Iowa	Oregon	Wyoming
Kentucky	Puerto Rico	
Maryland	South Carolina	

A list of these state OSHA offices is appended; call the number listed to receive a copy of the state's standards on occupational exposure to bloodborne pathogens. In Connecticut and New York, the state plans cover state and local government employees only; the private sector is covered by the federal OSHA standard. In addition, states with an OSHA-approved state plan must comply with the federal OSHA standard.

Complying with the Regulations

Exposure Control Plan

In order to comply with the regulations, health care employers are required to prepare a written "Exposure Control Plan" designed to eliminate or minimize employee exposure to bloodborne pathogens. This plan must list all job classifications in which employees are likely to be exposed to infectious materials and the relevant tasks and procedures performed by these employees. Infectious materials include blood, semen, vaginal secretions, peritoneal fluid, amniotic

* The state OSHA plan covers state and local government employees only.

fluid, any body fluid visibly contaminated with blood, all body fluids in which it is impossible to differentiate between the body fluids, any unfixed human tissue or organ (living or dead), as well as HIV-containing cell or tissue cultures, organ cultures, and HIV- or HBV-containing culture medium or other solutions.

Under the plan, employers are required to adopt universal precautions, engineering and work practice controls, and personal protective equipment requirements. Employers must also establish a schedule for implementing the following:

- Housekeeping requirements
- Employee training and record-keeping requirements
- HBV vaccination for employees and postexposure evaluation and follow-up procedures
- Communication of hazards

A detailed discussion of each of these requirements follows. The plan must be accessible to employees and made available to OSHA upon request. Employers must review and update the plan annually and as necessary to reflect workplace changes.

Mandatory Universal Precautions

The regulations require that universal precautions must be used to prevent contact with blood or other potentially infectious materials. It is OSHA's intention to follow the Centers for Disease Control and Prevention guidelines on universal precautions. As defined by the Centers for Disease Control and Prevention, the concept of universal precautions requires the employer and employee to assume that blood and other body fluids are infectious and must be handled accordingly.

Engineering and Work Practice Controls

Specific engineering and work practice controls for the workplace must be implemented and examined for effectiveness on a regular schedule. These controls include the following:

1. Employers are required to provide hand-washing facilities that are readily accessible to employees; when this is not feasible, employ-

ees must be provided with an antiseptic hand cleanser with clean cloth/paper towels or antiseptic towelettes. It is the employer's responsibility to ensure that employees wash their hands immediately after gloves and other protective garments are removed.

2. Contaminated needles and other contaminated sharp objects shall not be bent, recapped, or removed unless the employer can demonstrate that no alternative is feasible or that a specific medical procedure requires such action. Shearing or breaking of contaminated needles is prohibited. Recapping or needle removal must be accomplished by a mechanical device or a one-handed technique. Contaminated reusable sharp objects shall be placed in appropriate containers until properly reprocessed; these containers must be puncture resistant, leakproof, and labeled or color coded in accordance with the regulations for easy identification.

3. Eating, drinking, smoking, applying cosmetics or lip balm, and handling contact lenses are prohibited in work areas where there is a reasonable likelihood of exposure to potentially infectious materials.

4. Food and drink must not be kept in refrigerators, freezers, shelves, cabinets, or on countertops where blood or other potentially infectious materials are present.

5. All procedures involving blood or other infectious materials shall be performed in a manner to minimize splashing, spraying, spattering, and creating droplets; mouth pipetting/suctioning of blood or other potentially infectious materials is prohibited.

6. Specimens of blood or other potentially infectious materials must be placed in closed containers that prevent leakage during collection, handling, processing, storage, transport, or shipping; containers must be labeled or color coded in accordance with the regulations for easy identification. However, when a facility uses universal precautions in the handling of all specimens, the required labeling or color coding of specimens is not necessary as long as containers are recognizable as containing specimens; this exemption applies only while the specimens and containers remain in the facility. If outside contamination of the primary container occurs, it must be placed within a second container that

is leakproof, puncture resistant, and labeled or color coded accordingly.

7. Equipment that could be contaminated with blood or other infectious materials must be examined prior to servicing or shipping and shall be decontaminated as necessary, unless the employer can demonstrate that decontamination of the equipment or parts of the equipment is not feasible. A label must be attached to the equipment stating which parts remain contaminated. The employer must ensure that this information is conveyed to all affected employees, the servicing representative, and/or the manufacturer prior to handling, servicing, or shipping so that the necessary precautions will be taken.

Personal Protective Equipment

The regulations also stress the importance of appropriate personal protective equipment that employers are required to provide at no cost to employees whose job duties expose them to blood and other infectious materials. Appropriate personal protective equipment includes but is not limited to gloves, gowns, laboratory coats, face shields or masks, eye protection, mouthpieces, resuscitation bags, pocket masks, or other ventilation devices. As defined by OSHA, personal protective equipment is considered "appropriate" if it prevents blood or other potentially infectious materials from reaching an employee's work clothes and skin, eyes, mouth, or other mucous membranes under normal conditions of use.

Employers must ensure that the employee uses appropriate personal protective equipment unless the employer can demonstrate that the employee temporarily declined to use the equipment, when under rare and extraordinary circumstances, it was the employee's professional judgment that use of personal protective equipment would have prevented the delivery of health care services or would have posed an increased hazard to the safety of the worker or co-worker. When an employee makes this judgment, the circumstances shall be investigated and documented in order to determine whether changes can be made to prevent such situations in the future.

Personal protective equipment in the appropriate sizes must be accessible at the worksite or issued to employees. The employer shall provide for laundering and disposal of personal protective equipment, as well as repair and replace this equipment when necessary to maintain its effectiveness, at no cost to the employee. If a garment(s) is penetrated by blood or other infectious materials, it must be removed immediately or as soon as feasible. All personal protective equipment must be removed before leaving the work area, whereupon it shall be placed in a designated area or storage container for washing or disposal.

Gloves must be worn when it can reasonably be anticipated that the employee may have hand contact with blood, other potentially infectious materials, mucous membranes, and nonintact skin; when performing vascular access procedures; and when handling or touching contaminated surfaces. Disposable gloves shall be replaced as soon as practical when contaminated or when torn or punctured; they shall not be washed or decontaminated for reuse. Utility gloves may be decontaminated for reuse but must be discarded if a glove is cracked, peeling, torn, punctured, or shows other signs of deterioration.

Masks in combination with goggles or protective eye shields must be worn whenever splashes, spray, spatter, or droplets of blood may be created and eye, nose, or mouth contamination can reasonably be anticipated. Gowns and other protective body clothing such as, but not limited to, gowns, aprons, lab coats, clinic jackets, or similar outer garments, shall be worn in occupational exposure situations. The type and characteristics will depend upon the task and degree of exposure anticipated. Surgical caps or hoods and/or shoe covers must be worn in situations in which "gross contamination" can reasonably be anticipated (eg, autopsies, orthopedic surgery).

Housekeeping

Employers must ensure that the worksite is maintained in a clean and sanitary condition and shall develop and implement a written schedule for cleaning and method of decontamination based upon the location within the facility, type of surface to be cleaned, type of soil present, and tasks or procedures being performed in the area. All equipment and working surfaces shall be cleaned and decontaminated after contact with blood or other potentially infectious materials. Contaminated work surfaces shall be decontaminated with an appropriate disinfectant after tasks and procedures are completed; immediately or as soon as feasible when surfaces are contaminated or after any spill of blood or other potentially infectious materials; and at the end of the work shift if the surface may have become contaminated since the last cleaning. Protective covering (eg, plastic wrap, aluminum foil, or imperviously backed absorbent paper used to cover equipment and environmental surfaces) must be removed and replaced as soon as feasible upon contamination or at the end of the work shift if they may have become contaminated during the shift. All bins, pails, cans, and similar containers intended for reuse shall be inspected and decontaminated on a regularly scheduled basis and cleaned immediately or as soon as feasible upon visible contamination.

Broken glassware that may be contaminated must not be picked up directly with the hands; it must be cleaned up using a brush and dustpan, tongs, or forceps. Contaminated reusable sharp objects must not be stored or processed in a manner that requires employees to reach by hand into the containers in which these sharp objects have been placed. Containers for contaminated sharp objects must be closable, puncture resistant, leakproof on the sides and bottom, and labeled or color coded in accordance with the regulations. During use, containers for contaminated sharp objects shall be easily accessible to personnel and located as close as possible to the immediate area where sharp objects are used. Additionally, these containers must be maintained upright throughout use, replaced routinely, and not be allowed to be overfilled. Reusable containers shall not be opened, emptied, or cleaned manually or in any other manner that would expose employees to the risk of percutaneous injury. Containers of contaminated disposable sharp objects and personal protective equipment are defined as regulated waste; such containers must prevent the spillage or protrusion of contents during handling, storage, transport, or shipping.

Contaminated laundry shall be handled as little as possible and must be placed in bags or containers at the location where it was used;

it must not be sorted or rinsed in the location of use. Contaminated laundry shall be transported in clearly labeled or color-coded bags or containers in accordance with the regulations. Employers shall ensure that employees who have contact with contaminated laundry wear protective gloves and other appropriate personal protective equipment. When a facility ships contaminated laundry offsite to a second facility that does not use universal precautions in handling all laundry, the facility generating the contaminated laundry must clearly mark or color code the bags or containers with appropriate biohazard labels.

Hepatitis B Vaccination

Employers are required to provide the vaccination for HBV free of charge to all employees who are at risk for occupational exposure. The vaccine must be provided within 10 days of an employee's initial assignment, except in the following cases:

- The employee has previously received the complete HBV vaccination series.
- Antibody testing has revealed that the employee is immune.
- The vaccine is contraindicated for medical reasons.

The regulations prohibit employers from making employees participate in a prescreening program as a prerequisite for receiving the vaccination. Employees who refuse the vaccination must sign a "Hepatitis B Vaccine Declination" form stating that they have declined the vaccine. If the U.S. Public Health Service ever recommends booster doses of HBV vaccine, they must also be provided to employees free of charge. The employee, however, is allowed to change his or her mind and elect to receive the vaccine at any time at the employer's expense.

Postexposure Evaluation and Follow-Up

Following a report of an employee exposure incident, the employer must make immediately available to the exposed employee a confidential medical evaluation and follow-up, including at least the following:

1. Documentation of the route(s) of exposure and the circumstances under which the exposure occurred

2. Identification and documentation of the individual who is the source of the blood or potentially infectious material, unless the employer can establish that such identification is not feasible or is prohibited by state or local law. The source individual's blood shall be tested as soon as possible and after consent is obtained, in order to determine HBV or HIV infectivity. If consent is not obtained, the employer must document that legally required consent cannot be obtained. If the source individual's consent is not required by law, the source individual's blood if available shall be tested and the results documented. However, when the source individual is already known to be infected with HBV or HIV, blood testing for HBV or HIV is not required. Results of the source individual's blood test shall be made available to the exposed employee, and the employee shall be informed of all applicable laws concerning the disclosure of the source individual's identity and infectious status.

3. Collection and testing of the exposed employee's blood for HBV and HIV serologic status as soon as feasible after the employee gives consent. If the employee consents to baseline blood collection but does not give consent at that time for HIV serologic testing, the sample shall be preserved for 90 days. Testing of the blood shall take place within the 90 days if the employee decides to do so.

4. Postexposure prophylaxis when medically indicated, as recommended by the U.S. Public Health Service

5. Counseling

6. Evaluation of reported illnesses

The employer must ensure that the health professional responsible for the employee's HBV vaccination is provided a copy of the OSHA regulation on bloodborne pathogens. In the case of a health professional evaluating an exposed employee, the employer shall ensure that the health professional is provided the following information:

• A copy of the OSHA bloodborne pathogens regulations

• A description of the exposed employee's duties as they relate to the exposure incident

- Documentation of the routes of exposure and circumstances under which exposure occurred
- Results of the source individual's blood testing, if available
- All medical records relevant to the appropriate treatment of the exposed employee, including vaccination status, which is the employer's responsibility to maintain

The employer must obtain and provide the employee with a copy of the evaluating health professional's written opinion within 15 days of completion. The health professional's written opinion for HBV vaccination shall be limited to whether HBV vaccination is indicated for the employee and if the employee has received such vaccination. The health professional's written opinion for postexposure evaluation and follow-up shall be limited to the following:

- The employee has been informed of the results of the evaluation.
- The employee has been told about any medical conditions resulting from exposure to blood or other potentially infectious materials that require further evaluation or treatment.

All other findings or diagnoses must remain confidential and shall not be included in the written report.

Communications of Hazards to Employees

Warning Labels and Signs

The regulations require warning labels on containers of regulated waste and refrigerators and freezers containing blood or other potentially infectious materials. Warning labels must also be affixed to containers used to store, transport, or ship blood or other potentially infectious materials. The warnings must be fluorescent orange or orange-red; however, red bags or red containers may be substituted for labels.

Employee Training

Employers must ensure that all employees at risk for occupational exposure participate in a training program at no cost to employees and during working hours. Training shall take place at the time of an employee's initial assignment to tasks that risk exposure and at least annually thereafter. Annual training for employees shall be provided within 1 year of their previous training. Additional training must be provided when changes such as modifications of tasks or procedures or introduction of new tasks and procedures affect the worker's exposure risk. The training must be conducted by a person knowledgeable about the subject matter, and the material shall be presented at an educational level appropriate to the employees. The training program at a minimum must include the following:

1. A copy of the bloodborne pathogens regulations and an explanation of their contents

2. A general explanation of the epidemiology and symptoms of bloodborne diseases

3. An explanation of the modes of transmission of bloodborne diseases

4. An explanation of the employer's Exposure Control Plan and information on how the employee can obtain a copy of the plan

5. An explanation of the appropriate methods for identifying tasks and other activities that may involve exposure

6. An explanation of the methods that will prevent or reduce exposure (including appropriate engineering controls, work practices, and personal protective equipment)

7. Information on the types, proper use, location, removal, handling, decontamination, and disposal of personal protective equipment

8. An explanation of the basis for selection of personal protective equipment

9. Information on the HBV vaccine (efficacy, safety, method of administration, benefits of being vaccinated, and that the vaccine will be offered free of charge)

10. Information on the appropriate actions to take and persons to contact in an emergency involving blood or other infectious materials

11. An explanation of the procedure for follow-up if an exposure incident occurs (including the method for reporting incident and the medical follow-up that may be available)

12. Information on the postexposure evaluation and follow-up that the employer is required to provide for the employee

13. An explanation of the signs and labels and/or color-coding requirements

14. An opportunity for interactive questions and answers with the person conducting the training session.

Record-Keeping Requirements

The employer shall maintain an accurate record for each employee at risk for occupational exposure that includes the following:

• The name and social security number of employee

• The employee's HBV vaccination status (dates and any medical information relative to the employee's ability to receive the vaccination)

• The results of examinations, medical testing, and follow-up procedures

• The employer's copy of the health professional's written evaluation as required following an exposure incident

• A copy of the information provided to the health professional as required following an exposure incident

The employer shall ensure the confidentiality of employee records; information shall not be disclosed without the employee's written consent. The employer is required to maintain records for the duration of employment plus 30 years. The employer must also maintain records of the training sessions that include the dates, the names and qualifications of persons who conducted training sessions, and the names and job titles of employees who attended sessions. These records shall be maintained for 3 years from the date the training session occurred.

All records shall be made available to the assistant secretary of OSHA for examination and copying, including employee medical records, for which the employee's consent is not needed. In the event of an employer going out of business, these records must be transferred to the new owner or must be offered to the National Institute for Occupational Safety and Health.

The bloodborne pathogens regulations are just one of the OSHA standards that physician offices must follow to be in compliance. Other OSHA regulations include standards on the hazards of chemicals in the workplace, compressed gases, office equipment, and an action plan in case of fire. An emergency hotline number has been established by OSHA to report emergencies: 1-800-321-OSHA.

States with Approved Plans

States administering their own occupational safety and health programs through plans approved under section 18(b) of the Occupational Safety and Health Act of 1970 must adopt standards and enforce requirements that are at least as effective as the federal requirements.

There are currently 25 states with state plans: 23 cover the private and public (state and local government) sectors and 2 cover the public sector only.

Alaska
Alaska Department of Labor
1111 West Eighth Street, Room 306
Juneau, AK 99801
907-465-2700

Arizona
Industrial Commission of Arizona
800 West Washington
Phoenix, AZ 85007
602-542-5795

California
California Department of Industrial Relations
45 Fremont Street
San Francisco, CA 94105
415-972-8835

Connecticut*
Connecticut Department of Labor
200 Folly Brook Boulevard
Wethersfield, CT 06109
860-566-5123

Hawaii
Hawaii Department of Labor and Industrial Relations
830 Punchbowl Street
Honolulu, HI 96813
808-586-8844

Indiana
Indiana Department of Labor
State Office Building
402 West Washington Street
Room W195
Indianapolis, IN 46204
317-232-2378

Iowa
Iowa Division of Labor Services
1000 East Grand Avenue
Des Moines, IA 50319
515-281-3447

Kentucky
Kentucky Labor Cabinet
1047 U.S. Highway 127 South, Suite 2
Frankfort, KY 40601
502-564-3070

Maryland
Maryland Division of Labor and Industry
Department of Labor, Licensing and Regulation
501 St Paul Place, 2nd Floor
Baltimore, MD 21202-2272
410-333-4179

*State plan covers state and local government employees only.

Michigan
Michigan Department of Consumer and Industry Services
4th Floor, Law Building
PO Box 30004
Lansing, MI 48909
517-373-7230

Minnesota
Minnesota Department of Labor and Industry
443 Lafayette Road
St Paul, MN 55155
612-296-2342

Nevada
Nevada Division of Industrial Relations
400 West King Street
Carson City, NV 89710
702-687-3032

New Mexico
New Mexico Environment Department
PO Box 26110
1190 St Francis Drive
Santa Fe, NM 87502
505-827-2850

New York*
New York Department of Labor
W. Averell Harriman State Office Building—12
Room 500
Albany, NY 12240
518-457-2741

North Carolina
North Carolina Department of Labor
319 Chapanoke Road
Raleigh, NC 27603
919-662-4585

Oregon
Department of Consumer and Business Services
Oregon Occupational Safety and Health Division
Labor and Industries Building, Room 430
Salem, OR 97310
503-378-3272

Puerto Rico
Puerto Rico Department of Labor and Human Resources
Prudencio Rivera Martinez Building
505 Munoz Rivera Avenue
Hato Rey, PR 00918
809-754-2119

South Carolina
South Carolina Department of Labor, Licensing and
    Regulation
3600 Forest Drive
PO Box 11329
Columbia, SC 29211-1329
803-734-9594

Tennessee
Tennessee Department of Labor
710 James Robertson Parkway
Nashville, TN 37243-0659
615-741-2582

Utah
Industrial Commission of Utah
160 East 300 South, 3rd Floor
PO Box 146600
Salt Lake City, UT 84114
801-530-6898

Vermont
Vermont Department of Labor and Industry
National Life Building—Drawer 20
120 State Street
Montpelier, VT 05620
802-828-2288

Virgin Islands
Virgin Islands Department of Labor
2131 Hospital Street
Box 890, Christiansted
St Croix, VI 00820-4666
809-773-1994

Virginia
Virginia Department of Labor and Industry
Powers–Taylor Building
13 South 13th Street
Richmond, VA 23219
804-786-2377

Washington
Washington Department of Labor and Industries
General Administration Building
PO Box 44000
Olympia, WA 98504-4000
360-902-4200

Wyoming
Worker's Safety and Compensation Division
Wyoming Department of Employment
Herschler Building
2nd Floor East
122 West 25 Street
Cheyenne, WY 82002
307-777-7786

Appendix G

AAP Policy Statements and ACOG Committee Opinions and Educational Bulletins

American Academy of Pediatrics Policy Statements

Ad Hoc Task Force on Definition of the Medical Home

American Academy of Pediatrics. Ad Hoc Task Force on Definition of the Medical Home. The medical home. Pediatrics 1992;90:774

Committee on Adolescence

American Academy of Pediatrics, Committee on Adolescence. Adolescent pregnancy. Pediatrics 1989;83:132–134 (reaffirmed 1992)

American Academy of Pediatrics, Committee on Adolescence. Counseling the adolescent about pregnancy options. Pediatrics 1989;83: 135–137 (reaffirmed 1992)

Committee on Bioethics

American Academy of Pediatrics, Committee on Bioethics. Ethics and the care of critically ill infants and children. Pediatrics 1996;98: 149–152

American Academy of Pediatrics, Committee on Bioethics. Fetal therapy: ethical considerations. Pediatrics 1988;81:898–899 (reaffirmed 1992)

American Academy of Pediatrics, Committee on Bioethics. Guidelines on forgoing life-sustaining medical treatment. Pediatrics 1994; 93:532–536

Committee on Children with Disabilities

American Academy of Pediatrics, Committee on Children with Disabilities. Guidelines for home care of infants, children, and adolescents with chronic disease. Pediatrics 1995; 96:161–164

Committee on Drugs

American Academy of Pediatrics, Committee on Drugs. Guidelines for monitoring and management of pediatric patients during and after sedation for diagnostic and therapeutic procedures. Pediatrics 1992;89:1110–1115 (reaffirmed 1995)

American Academy of Pediatrics, Committee on Drugs. Neonatal drug withdrawal. Pediatrics 1983;72:895–902 (reaffirmed 1990)

American Academy of Pediatrics, Committee on Drugs. The transfer of drugs and other chemicals into human breast milk. Pediatrics 1994;93:137–150

Committee on Fetus and Newborn

American Academy of Pediatrics, Committee on Fetus and Newborn. Advanced practice in neonatal nursing (RE9257). AAP News 1992; 8:17 (reaffirmed 1995)

American Academy of Pediatrics, Committee on Fetus and Newborn. Hospital stay for healthy term newborns. Pediatrics 1995;96:788–790

American Academy of Pediatrics, Committee on Fetus and Newborn. The initiation or withdrawal of treatment for high-risk newborns. Pediatrics 1995;96:362–363

American Academy of Pediatrics, Committee on Fetus and Newborn, Committee on Drugs, Section on Anesthesiology, and Section on Surgery. Neonatal anesthesia. Pediatrics 1987;80:446

American Academy of Pediatrics, Committee on Fetus and Newborn. Perinatal care at the threshold of viability. Pediatrics 1995;96:974–976

American Academy of Pediatrics, Committee on Fetus and Newborn. Recommendations on extracorporeal membrane oxygenation. Pediatrics 1990;85:618–619 (reaffirmed 1996)

American Academy of Pediatrics, Committee on Fetus and Newborn. Surfactant replacement therapy for respiratory distress syndrome. Pediatrics 1991;87:946–947

American Academy of Pediatrics, Committee on Fetus and Newborn, and American College of Obstetricians and Gynecologists. Use and abuse of the Apgar score. Pediatrics 1996;98:141–142

Committee on Genetics

American Academy of Pediatrics, Committee on Genetics. Folic acid for the prevention of neural tube defects. Pediatrics 1993;92:493–494

American Academy of Pediatrics, Committee on Genetics. Issues in newborn screening. Pediatrics 1992;89:345–349 (reaffirmed 1995)

American Academy of Pediatrics, Committee on Genetics. Maternal phenylketonuria. Pediatrics 1991;88:1284–1285 (reaffirmed 1994)

American Academy of Pediatrics, Committee on Genetics. Maternal serum alpha-fetoprotein screening. Pediatrics 1991;88:1282–1283 (reaffirmed 1994)

American Academy of Pediatrics, Committee on Genetics. Newborn screening fact sheets. Pediatrics 1996;98:473–501

American Academy of Pediatrics, Committee on Genetics. Prenatal genetic diagnosis for pediatricians. Pediatrics 1994;93:1010–1015

Committee on Infectious Diseases

American Academy of Pediatrics. Peter G, ed. 1997 Red book: report of the Committee on Infectious Diseases. 24th ed. Elk Grove Village, Illinois: AAP, 1997

American Academy of Pediatrics, Committee on Infectious Diseases. Reassessment of the indications for ribavirin therapy in respiratory syncytial virus infections. Pediatrics 1996;97:137–140

American Academy of Pediatrics, Committee on Infectious Diseases and Committee on Fetus and Newborn. Respiratory syncytial virus immune globulin intravenous: indications for use. Pediatrics 1997;99:645–650

American Academy of Pediatrics, Committee on Infectious Diseases and Committee on Fetus and Newborn. Revised guidelines for prevention of early-onset group B streptococcal (GBS) infection. Pediatrics 1997;99:489-496

American Academy of Pediatrics, Committee on Infectious Diseases. Update on timing of hepatitis B vaccination for premature infants and for children with lapsed immunization. Pediatrics 1994;94:403–404

Committee on Injury and Poison Prevention

American Academy of Pediatrics, Committee on Injury and Poison Prevention. Safe transportation of newborns discharged from the hospital. Pediatrics 1990;86:486–487 (reaffirmed 1993)

American Academy of Pediatrics, Committee on Injury and Poison Prevention and Committee on Fetus and Newborn. Safe transportation of premature and low birth weight infants. Pediatrics 1996; 97:758–760

Committee on Nutrition

American Academy of Pediatrics, Committee on Nutrition. Aluminum toxicity in infants and children. Pediatrics 1996;97:413–416

American Academy of Pediatrics, Committee on Nutrition. Encouraging breast-feeding. Pediatrics 1980;65:657–658 (reaffirmed 1994)

American Academy of Pediatrics, Committee on Nutrition. Hypoallergenic infant formulas. Pediatrics 1989;83:1068–1069

American Academy of Pediatrics, Committee on Nutrition. Iron-fortified infant formulas. Pediatrics 1989;84:1114–1115 (reaffirmed 1993)

American Academy of Pediatrics, Committee on Nutrition. Pediatric nutrition handbook. 4th ed. Elk Grove Village, Illinois: AAP (expected publication date November 1997)

American Academy of Pediatrics, Committee on Nutrition. Soy-protein formulas: recommendations for use in infant feeding. Pediatrics 1983;72:359–363 (reaffirmed 1991)

Committee on Pediatric AIDS

American Academy of Pediatrics, Committee on Pediatric AIDS. Human milk, breastfeeding, and transmission of human immunodeficiency virus in the United States. Pediatrics 1995;96:977–979

Committee on Practice and Ambulatory Medicine

American Academy of Pediatrics, Committee on Practice and Ambulatory Medicine and Section on Ophthalmology. Eye examination and vision screening in infants, children, and young adults. Pediatrics 1996;98:153–157

American Academy of Pediatrics, Committee on Practice and Ambulatory Medicine. Recommendations for preventive pediatric health care. Pediatrics 1995;96:373–374

American Academy of Pediatrics, Committee on Practice and Ambulatory Medicine and Committee on Fetus and Newborn. The role of the primary care pediatrician in the management of high-risk newborn infants. Pediatrics 1996;98:786–788

Committee on Psychosocial Aspects of Child and Family Health

American Academy of Pediatrics, Committee on Psychosocial Aspects of Child and Family Health. Guidelines for Health Supervision III. Elk Grove Village, Illinois: AAP 1997

American Academy of Pediatrics, Committee on Psychosocial Aspects of Child and Family Health. The prenatal visit. Pediatrics 1996; 97:141–142

Committee on State Government Affairs

American Academy of Pediatrics. Post-delivery care for mothers and newborns act. In: Policy reference guide of the American Academy of Pediatrics. Elk Grove Village, Illinois: AAP, 1996

Committee on Substance Abuse

American Academy of Pediatrics, Committee on Substance Abuse. Alcohol use and abuse: a pediatric concern. Pediatrics 1995;95:439–442

American Academy of Pediatrics, Committee on Substance Abuse. Drug-exposed infants. Pediatrics 1995;96:364–367

American Academy of Pediatrics, Committee on Substance Abuse and Committee on Children with Disabilities. Fetal alcohol syndrome and fetal alcohol effects. Pediatrics 1993;91:1004–1006

Joint Committee on Infant Hearing

American Academy of Pediatrics, Joint Committee on Infant Hearing. Joint Committee on Infant Hearing 1994 position statement. Pediatrics 1995;95:152–156

Neonatal Resuscitation Steering Committee

Bloom RS, Cropley C, eds. Textbook of neonatal resuscitation. American Academy of Pediatrics/American Heart Association NRP Steering Committee. Dallas, TX: American Heart Association, 1994

Provisional Committee on Pediatric AIDS

American Academy of Pediatrics, Provisional Committee on Pediatric AIDS. Perinatal human immunodeficiency virus testing. Pediatrics 1995;95:303–307

Provisional Committee on Quality Improvement

American Academy of Pediatrics, Provisional Committee on Quality Improvement and Subcommittee on Hyperbilirubinemia. Practice Parameter. Management of hyperbilirubinemia in the healthy term newborn. Pediatrics 1994;94:558–565

Section on Endocrinology

American Academy of Pediatrics, AAP Section on Endocrinology and Committee on Genetics, and American Thyroid Association

Committee on Public Health. Newborn screening for congenital hypothyroidism: recommended guidelines. Pediatrics 1993; 91:1203–1209 (reaffirmed 1996)

Section on Ophthalmology

American Academy of Pediatrics, Section on Ophthalmology, American Association for Pediatric Ophthalmology and Strabismus, and American Academy of Ophthalmology. Screening examination of premature infants for retinopathy of prematurity. Pediatrics 1997;100:273

Task Force on Breast-Feeding

American Academy of Pediatrics, Task Force on Breast-Feeding. The promotion of breast-feeding. Pediatrics 1982;69:654–661

Task Force on Circumcision

American Academy of Pediatrics, Task Force on Circumcision. Report of the Task Force on Circumcision. Pediatrics 1989;84: 388–391. (Erratum in Pediatrics 1989;84:761)

Task Force on Infant Positioning and SIDS

American Academy of Pediatrics, AAP Task Force on Infant Positioning and SIDS. Positioning and SIDS. Pediatrics 1992;89:1120–1126 (reaffirmed 1994)

American Academy of Pediatrics, Task Force on Infant Positioning and SIDS. Positioning and sudden infant death syndrome (SIDS): update. Pediatrics 1996;98:1216–1218

Task Force on Interhospital Transport

American Academy of Pediatrics, Task Force on Interhospital Transport. Guidelines for air and ground transport of neonatal and pediatric patients. Elk Grove Village, Illinois: AAP, 1993:75–83

Task Force on Prolonged Infantile Apnea

American Academy of Pediatrics, Task Force on Prolonged Infantile Apnea. Prolonged infantile apnea: 1985. Pediatrics 1985;76:129–131 (reaffirmed 1995)

Vitamin K Ad Hoc Task Force

American Academy of Pediatrics, Vitamin K Ad Hoc Task Force. Controversies concerning vitamin K and the newborn. Pediatrics 1993;91:1001–1003

ACOG Committee Opinions

Committee on Ethics

Committee on Genetics

Committee on Obstetric Practice

145 Statement on Surgical Assistants (joint with Committee on Gynecologic Practice) (November 1994; reaffirmed 1996)

147 Antenatal Corticosteroid Therapy for Fetal Maturation (December 1994)

149 Financial Influences on Mode of Delivery (December 1994; reaffirmed 1996)

157 Vitamin A Supplementation During Pregnancy (September 1995)

158 Guidelines for Diagnostic Imaging During Pregnancy (September 1995; reaffirmed 1997)

163 Perinatal Care at the Threshold of Viability (joint with AAP Committee on Fetus and Newborn) (November 1995)

167 Perinatal and Infant Mortality Statistics (December 1995)

172 Home Uterine Activity Monitoring (May 1996)

173 Prevention of Early-Onset Group B Streptococcal Disease in Newborns (June 1996)

174 Use and Abuse of the Apgar Score (joint with AAP Committee on Fetus and Newborn) (July 1996)

175 Scope of Services for Uncomplicated Obstetric Care (September 1996)

179 Rate of Vaginal Births After Cesarean Delivery (November 1996)

180 New Ultrasound Output Display Standard (November 1996)

ACOG Educational Bulletins

General

Obstetrics

151 Automobile Passenger Restraints for Children and Pregnant Women (January 1991)

159 Fetal Macrosomia (September 1991)

160 Immunization During Pregnancy (October 1991)

161 Trauma During Pregnancy (November 1991)

163 Fetal and Neonatal Neurologic Injury (January 1992)

168 Cardiac Disease in Pregnancy (June 1992)

171 Rubella and Pregnancy (August 1992)

174 Hepatitis in Pregnancy (November 1992)

176 Diagnosis and Management of Fetal Death (January 1993)

177 Perinatal Viral and Parasitic Infections (February 1993)

179 Nutrition During Pregnancy (April 1993)

180 Smoking and Reproductive Health (May 1993)

181 Thyroid Disease in Pregnancy (June 1993)

187 Ultrasonography in Pregnancy (December 1993)

188 Antepartum Fetal Surveillance (January 1994)

189 Exercise During Pregnancy and the Postpartum Period (February 1994)

195 Substance Abuse in Pregnancy (July 1994)

196 Operative Vaginal Delivery (August 1994)

200 Diabetes and Pregnancy (December 1994)

205 Preconceptional Care (May 1995)

206 Preterm Labor (June 1995)

207 Fetal Heart Rate Patterns: Monitoring, Interpretation, and Management (July 1995)

208 Genetic Technologies (July 1995)

216 Umbilical Artery Blood Acid–Base Analysis (November 1995)

217 Induction of Labor (December 1995)

218 Dystocia and the Augmentation of Labor (December 1995)

219 Hypertension in Pregnancy (January 1996)

220 Hemoglobinopathies in Pregnancy (February 1996)

Reproductive Endocrinology and Fertility

Index

Milk, human *(continued)*
  cytomegalovirus transmission
    by, 208
  expressed
    bacteria levels in, 289, 290
    freezing of, 289
    heat treatment of, 289
    refrigerating of, 289
  human immunodeficiency
    virus DNA in, 220
  for preterm babies, 292
  production of
    caloric requirements for,
      283
    stimulation of, 285
  transmission of human im-
    munodeficiency virus by,
    218
Milk banks, 288
  cytomegalovirus transmission
    by, 208
Mineral supplementation
  for newborn, 291
  postpartum, 283
  preconception, 279
  during pregnancy, 281, 283
Mineral toxicity, 283
*Model State Vital Statistics Act
  and Regulations* 1977,
    revision of, 324
Monitoring equipment, for high-
  risk neonate, mother's
  familiarity with, 170
Mop heads, 272
Morphine, 198
Mortality
  fetal. *See* Fetal death
  maternal, *xvii*
    cesarean delivery after,
      neonatal survival and,
      140
    defined, 314
    direct obstetric, 314
    from hemorrhage, 140

Mortality, maternal *(continued)*
    indirect obstetric, 314
    measures of, 321–322
    pregnancy-associated, 315,
      322
    reporting requirements/
      recommendations, 325–
      326
  neonatal. *See* Neonatal
    mortality
  perinatal, 7
    measures, 318–320
    reporting requirements/
      recommendations, 324
Mortality rate
  calculation of, 320
  decline in, *xix*
  maternal, pregnancy, 322
  postneonatal, calculation of,
    320
Mother
  assessment of fetal movement
    by, 85
  evaluation of, for discharge
    from hospital, 172
  familiarity with newborn care,
    discharge from hospital
    and, 167–168
  for high-risk neonate, 170–
    171
  follow-up care for, 176–177
  hepatitis B virus infection in,
    209–211
    transmission to newborn,
      209
  herpex-simplex virus-infected,
    contact of newborn with,
    217
  human immunodeficiency
    virus infection in
    transmission to newborn,
      218
  written authorization for
    disclosing, 152, 219

Religion, blood products and,
143
Renal disease, risk assessment for
consultation, early
pregnancy, 299
Renal failure, 138
Report, reporting
follow-up, 56
for interhospital transport, 55
requirements and recommendations, 323–328
Reproductive health statistics,
standard terminology for
reporting, in the United
States, 311–312
definitions, 312–315
fetal mortality measures, 317–
318
live birth measures, 316–317
maternal mortality measures,
321–322
measures of induced termination of pregnancy, 322–
323
perinatal mortality measures,
318–320
statistical tabulations, 315–316
Reproductive risks, patient
awareness of, 9, 10t
Respiratory depression, narcotic-
induced, 121
Respiratory distress syndrome,
134, 194
postnatal corticosteroid
therapy for, 195
surfactant replacement therapy
in, 194–195
Respiratory support equipment,
cleaning and disinfection
of, 275
Respiratory syncytial virus, 223–
224
prevention, 223

Respiratory therapists, in specialty
and subspecialty care
facility, 24
Respiratory tract
infection, mother with, transmission to newborn, 265,
266
of newborn, culturing for
infection surveillance,
253
Resuscitation, of newborn, 115–
116, 171
Apgar score for, 116–117
in delivery room, 124–125
drugs and volume expansion,
120, 121, 124
acidosis, 121
bradycardia, 121
hypovolemia, 121
external cardiac massage, 119–
120, 120f
maintenance of body temperature, 117
narcotic-induced respiratory
depression, 121
personnel for, 14
during cesarean delivery,
113
qualifications for performing,
115–116
responsibility for, 115–116, 122
suctioning, 117–118
ventilation, 118–119
Resuscitation area, in neonatal
functional area, 35–36
Resuscitation equipment
for interhospital transport, 57
in neonatal continuing care
unit, 39
in neonatal intermediate care
unit, 40
Resuscitator, cleaning and
sterilization of, 275